Yearbook of Paediatric Endocrinology 2015

Yearbook of Paediatric Endocrinology 2015

Endorsed by the European Society for Paediatric Endocrinology

Editors

Ken Ong
Ze'ev Hochberg

Associate Editors

Carla Bizzarri
Evangelia Charmandari
Stefano Cianfarani
Nicolas De Roux
Khalid Hussain
Christopher J H Kelnar
Wieland Kiess
Outi Mäkitie
Orit Pinhas-Hamiel
Michel Polak
Olle Söder
Martin Wabitsch

haymarket®

Yearbook of Paediatric Endocrinology 2015

Sponsored by a grant from Pfizer

British Library Cataloguing in Publication Data.
A catalogue record for this book is available from the British Library.

ISBN 978-0-9566456-4-7

Published by Haymarket Medical, Teddington Studios, Broom Road, Teddington TW11 9BE.

Haymarket is certified by BSI to environmental standard ISO 14001

Printed by Stephens & George Print Group, Merthyr Tydfil, Wales.

PEFC Certified

This product is from sustainably managed forests and controlled sources

PEFC/16-33-254

www.pefc.org

Editors

Ken Ong

Medical Research Council Epidemiology Unit
Wellcome Trust-MRC Institute of Metabolic Science, University of Cambridge
Box 285, Cambridge Biomedical Campus
Cambridge CB2 0QQ, UK
Tel. +44 1223 769207, Fax +44 1223 330316
Email ken.ong@mrc-epid.cam.ac.uk

Ze'ev Hochberg

Technion-Israel Institute of Technology, POB 9602
IL-31096 Haifa, Israel
Email rprzeev@tx.technion.ac.il

Associate Editors

Carla Bizzarri

Division of Endocrinology, Metabolism and Diabetes
Unit of Endocrinology and Diabetes
'Bambino Gesù' Children's Hospital
IRCCS, Rome, Italy
Email carla.bizzarri@opbg.net

Evangelia Charmandari

Division of Endocrinology, Metabolism and Diabetes
First Department of Pediatrics, University of Athens Medical School
'Aghia Sophia' Children's Hospital
GR-11527 Athens, Greece
Tel. +30 210 7794023, Fax +30 210 7759167
Email evangelia.charmandari@googlemail.com

Stefano Cianfarani

DPUO 'Bambino Gesù' Children's Hospital –
'Tor Vergata' University, Rome, Italy
Department of Women's and Children's Health
Karolinska Institutet, Stockholm, Sweden
P.zza Sant'Onofrio, 4, IT-00165 Rome, Italy
Tel. +39 06 6859 3074, Fax +39 06 6859 2508
Email stefano.cianfarani@uniroma2.it

Nicolas de Roux
INSERM U 690, Laboratoire d'Hormonologie, AP-HP
Hôpital Robert Debré, 48 Boulevard Sérurier
FR-75019 Paris, France
Tel. +33 1 40 03 19 85, Fax +33 1 40 40 91 95
Email nicolas.deroux@inserm.fr

Khalid Hussain
Clinical and Molecular Genetics Unit
The Developmental Endocrinology Research Group
Institute of Child Health
University College London
30 Guilford Street, London WC1N 1EH, UK
Tel. +44 20 7 905 2128, Fax +44 20 7 404 6191
Email khalid.hussain@ucl.ac.uk

Christopher J H Kelnar
Honorary Professor of Paediatric Endocrinology
University of Edinburgh
9 Easter Belmont Road, Edinburgh EH12 6EX, UK
Tel. +44 131 337 3195
Email christopher.kelnar@gmail.com

Wieland Kiess
Hospital for Children and Adolescents
Centre for Pediatric Research, University of Leipzig
Leipzig, Germany
Email wieland.kiess@medizin.uni-leipzig.de

Outi Mäkitie
Pediatric Endocrinology and Metabolic Bone Diseases
Children's Hospital
Helsinki University Central Hospital and University of Helsinki
PO Box 281, FI-00029 Helsinki, Finland
Tel. +358 9 4711, Fax +358 9 471 75888
Email outi.makitie@helsinki.fi

Orit Pinhas-Hamiel
Pediatric Endocrinology and Diabetes Unit
Safra Children's Hospital
Sheba Medical Center Ramat-Gan
IL-52621 Ramat-Gan, Israel
Tel. +972 3 5305015, Fax +972 3 5305055
Email orit.hamiel@sheba.health.gov.il

Michel Polak
Paediatric Endocrinology, Gynecology and Diabetology, INSERM U1016, Institut IMAGINE
Université Paris Descartes, Hôpital Necker-Enfants Malades
149, rue de Sèvres, FR-75015 Paris, France
Tel. +33 1 44 49 48 03/02, Fax +33 1 44 38 16 48
Email michel.polak@nck.aphp.fr

Olle Söder
Pediatric Endocrinology Unit, Q2:08
Department of Women's and Children's Health
Karolinska Institutet and University Hospital, Solna
SE-171 76 Stockholm, Sweden
Tel. +46 8 517 75124, Fax +46 8 517 75128
Email olle.soder@ki.se

Martin Wabitsch
Division of Pediatric Endocrinology and Diabetes, and Endocrine Research Laboratory
Department of Pediatrics and Adolescent Medicine (www.ped-u.de)
Ulm University, Eythstrasse 24, DE-89075 Ulm, Germany
Tel. +49 731 5005 7400, Fax +49 731 5005 7407
Email martin.wabitsch@uniklinik-ulm.de

Table of Contents

Preface

The Yearbook 2015 summarises the highlights of publications from June 2014 to May 2015. Time and again we are amazed by the enormous advances in medical science over a single year, covering the diverse fields of clinical research, genetics and genomics, proteomics and metabolomics, molecular biology, systems biology, population genetics, immunology and evolutionary biology, as they apply to our work as paediatric endocrinologists. Although most of our readers are clinicians, we strongly believe that the basic understanding of physiology and disease mechanisms will inform advances in diagnosis and therapy.

Some highlights of this 2015 collection include major advances in clinical treatments for hypophosphataemic rickets and achondroplasia, physiological cortisol replacement, early use of sulfonylurea in neonatal diabetes, early growth hormone therapy in Prader-Willi syndrome, early low-dose estrogen replacement in Turner syndrome and timely reviews of drugs that cause weight gain and weight loss. Of the basic research discoveries, we draw your attention to GPR101 mutations in gigantism, developmental genes associated with hypospadias, insulin and insulin-like growth factor 1 receptors in the expression of imprinted genes, dynamic 4D imaging of the growth plate and rare bioinactive forms of leptin and parathyroid hormone.

On this page each year we cite some important science anniversaries. In 1915, Albert Einstein introduced his general theory of relativity, widely regarded as the most remarkable scientific contribution of the 20th century. A Google search reveals that the terms endocrinology and hormones were still unknown in 1915.

We are grateful to our 12 Associate Editors and their coauthors, who have completed an enormous task to discern this year's advances and provide their chapters in a timely fashion. These are obviously their personal choices, and we acknowledge that as such they cannot be a complete coverage of all this year's highlights. We thank Helmuth Dörr for his contribution over the last three years, and welcome Carla Bizzarri, who edits the chapter on 'Oncology and chronic disease'. We welcome also Wieland Kiess who replaces Francesco Chiarelli on 'Type 1 diabetes'.

This is the 12th edition of the Yearbook, which has been continuously supported by Pfizer Ltd. We thank our previous publisher Karger AG, and look forward to working with Haymarket on this and future volumes.

Ze'ev Hochberg (Haifa)
Ken Ong (Cambridge)

Pituitary and Neuroendocrinology

Carles Gaston-Massuet[a], Nicolas de Roux[b] and Evelien F Gevers[a,c]

[a]Department of Endocrinology, William Harvey Research Institute, Queen Mary University London, London, UK

[b]Inserm U1141, Biochemistry Laboratory, Robert Debré Hopsital, Paris Diderot University, Paris, France

[c]Department of Paediatric Endocrinology, The Royal London Hospital, Barts Health Trust, London, UK

As usual, the year in research in pituitary and neuroendocrinology has been very rich and the selection of the most interesting papers has not been easy. The number of papers reporting new mechanisms but also new physiological functions of old or new proteins increases every year. We have selected a few papers that reflect this evolution. The investigation of neuroendocrine mechanisms of endocrine disease requires mostly rodent models since there is little opportunity to investigate these mechanisms in humans. The in vivo strategy in rodents may be highly informative but it is a long, and often complex process that can be very disappointing after one or two years of intensive laboratory investigations. It was therefore necessary to implement complementary approaches such as in vitro investigation of hypothalamic neurons, which is now feasible. The possibility to differentiate hypothalamic neurons from human pluripotent stem cells is a real progress. This opens new perspectives to delineate novel mechanisms of endocrine diseases but also to develop new therapeutic approaches.

Novel genes

Dysfunctional *SEMA3E* signaling underlies gonadotropin-releasing hormone neuron deficiency in Kallmann syndrome

Cariboni A, Andre V, Chauvet S, Cassatella D, Davidson K, Caramello A, Fantin A, Bouloux P, Mann F, Ruhrberg C

UCL Institute of Ophthalmology, University College London, London, UK and University of Milan, Department of Pharmacological and Biomolecular Sciences, Milan, Italy

J Clin Invest 2015;125:2413–2428

Background: Individuals with an inherited deficiency in gonadotropin-releasing hormone (GnRH) have impaired reproduction function. Multiple genes have now been linked to GnRH deficiency. The exact molecular mechanisms of the GnRH deficiency have been elucidated for few of them. In this paper, Cariboni et al report an elegant study describing the role of the Sema3a signalling pathway in the neurodevelopment of GnRH neurons.
Methods: Exome analysis of patients with Kallmann syndrome. In vitro and in vivo analysis of Sema3E function in mice.
Results: A very rare missense mutation (R619C) of SEMA3E was found in two brothers who have Kallmann syndrome (KS). Recombinant wild-type SEMA3E protected maturing GnRH neurons from cell death by triggering a plexin D1-dependent (PLXND1-dependent) activation of PI3K-mediated survival signalling. In contrast, recombinant SEMA3E carrying the KS-associated mutation did not protect GnRH neurons from death. In murine models, lack of either SEMA3E or PLXND1 increased apoptosis of GnRH neurons in the developing brain, reducing innervation of the adult median eminence by GnRH-positive neurites. GnRH neuron deficiency in male mice was accompanied by impaired testes growth, a characteristic feature of KS. A genetic interaction between PLXND1 and CHD7, another gene linked to KS was then demonstrated.
Conclusion: SEMA3E loss-of-function mutation causes an enhanced death of GnRH neurons during development. This mechanism is a new cause of Kallmann syndrome.

The findings of this study are novel for several reasons. First, SEMA3E is a new gene linked to Kallmann syndrome. Although mutations in SEMA3A, another gene of the SEMA3 family, have already been described in KS, the molecular mechanism causing GnRH deficiency is different.

SEMA3A loss-of-function mutations cause an ectopic migration of GnRH neurons along mispatterned axons in the nose. Second, the R619C mutation impaired the neuroprotective effect of SEMA3E on GnRH neuron death. The effect of SEMA3E on GnRH neuron survival is related to the developmental stage of GnRH neurons. This demonstrates that GnRH neurons adapt their phenotypes in accordance with the territories in which they travel during their long migration from the nose to the hypothalamus. Third, the oligogenic inheritance pattern of KS has now been reported by several groups. Various combinations of mutations in different genes have been characterised. This oligogenicity may explain the heterogeneity of the phenotype. Here, Cariboni et al showed that Plxnd1 genetically interacts with Chd7 in the neurodevelopment of GnRH neurons. This result is original as it proposes functional interactions between two proteins belonging to different biochemical pathways.

Gigantism and acromegaly due to Xq26 microduplications and GPR101 mutation

Trivellin G, Daly AF, Faucz FR, Yuan B, Rostomyan L, Larco DO, Schernthaner-Reiter MH, Szarek E, Leal LF, Caberg JH, Castermans E, Villa C, Dimopoulos A, Chittiboina P, Xekouki P, Shah N, Metzger D, Lysy PA, Ferrante E, Strebkova N, Mazerkina N, Zatelli MC, Lodish M, Horvath A, de Alexandre RB, Manning AD, Levy I, Keil MF, Sierra Mde L, Palmeira L, Coppieters W, Georges M, Naves LA, Jamar M, Bours V, Wu TJ, Choong CS, Bertherat J, Chanson P, Kamenicky P, Farrell WE, Barlier A, Quezado M, Bjelobaba I, Stojilkovic SS, Wess J, Costanzi S, Liu P, Lupski JR, Beckers A, Stratakis CA
National Institutes of Health, Clinical Research Center, Bethesda, MD, USA and Department of Endocrinology, Centre Hospitalier Universitaire de Liège, Domaine Universitaire du Sart-Tilman, Liege, Belgium
albert.beckers@chu.ulg.ac.be; stratakc@mail.nih.gov
N Engl J Med 2014;371:2363–2374

Background: Hypersecretion of growth hormone can lead to gigantism in children or acromegaly in adults. Non-syndromic gigantism is mostly due to pituitary adenomas, either sporadic or familial isolated pituitary adenomas (FIPA). FIPA can be due to mutations in aryl hydrocarbon receptor-interacting protein (AIP) but other genetic causes remain to be identified.
Methods: Genetic analysis was performed in 13 patients with childhood onset gigantism without mutations in AIP. High-definition analysis, long range PCR and Sanger sequencing was performed to identify the breakpoint of the duplication found. qRT-PCR was used to measure levels of expression of the duplicated genes.
Results: A micro-duplication on chromosome Xq26.3 was identified in all 13 patients. Duplication of four genes in the region was shared by all patients: *CD40LG, ARHGEF6, RBMX* and *GPR101*. Sanger sequencing of these genes in the 13 patients and 43 other patients with gigantism revealed no nucleotide variance. Quantitative RT-PCR showed strong upregulation of *GPR101* but not the other duplicated genes *CD40LG, ARHGEF6* or *RBMX*. This result was confirmed by finding increased immune-reactivity of GPR101 in the adenoma tissue. The Xq26.3 duplication was not identified in 248 patients with sporadic acromegaly, however, another mutation in *GPR101* (c.924G>C) was identified in 11 patients with sporadic GH adenoma.
Conclusions: Microduplication of chromosome Xq26.3 was found in the rare paediatric form of gigantism, X-linked acrogigantism (X-LAG). The genomic duplication results in overexpression of the orphan G-protein-coupled receptor GPR101, suggesting duplication of *GPR101* as the likely cause of X-LAG.

The authors identify a genomic duplication of chromosome Xq26.3, resulting in increased GPR101 expression as the cause of early onset X-linked acrogigantism (X-LAG). Interestingly, the duplication was found in all children with onset of gigantism before the age of five years. It therefore allows us to categorise children with gigantism in two clinical phenotypes: an early childhood form with a typical onset in infancy and a form with a typical onset at over five years old. Interestingly, all affected patients had severe and treatment-resistant disease, requiring medical therapy, repeated neurosurgery combined with GH receptor antagonist treatment or radiotherapy. The function of GPR101 is still unknown and further work is needed to understand the mechanism resulting in pituitary adenoma formation and GH oversecretion.

Gonadotrope-specific deletion of Dicer results in severely suppressed gonadotropins and fertility defects

Wang H, Graham I, Hastings R, Gunewardena S, Brinkmeier ML, Conn PM, Camper SA, Kumar TR
Departments of Molecular and Integrative Physiology, Flow Cytometry Core Laboratory, University of Kansas Medical Center, Kansas City, KS, USA
tkumar@kumc.edu
J Biol Chem 2015;290:2699–2714

Background: LH and FSH are heterodimeric glycoproteins expressed in gonadotropes that act on gonads and promote their development and functions including steroidogenesis and gametogenesis. Post-transcriptional regulation of gonadotropin subunits is not well understood.
Methods: To test if microRNAs regulate the hormone-specific gonadotropin-beta subunits in vivo, Dicer was specifically deleted in gonadotropes by a Cre-lox genetic approach in mice.
Results: It was found that Dicer-dependent microRNAs, predicted in silico to bind gonadotropin-beta subunit mRNAs, were suppressed in purified gonadotropes of mutant mice. Loss of these microRNAs resulted in profound suppression of gonadotropin-beta subunit proteins. In addition to suppression of basal levels, interestingly, the post-gonadectomy-induced rise in pituitary gonadotropin synthesis and secretion were also both abolished, indicating a defective gonadal negative feedback control.
Conclusions: Dicer-dependent microRNAs are essential for gonadotropin homeostasis and fertility in mice. MicroRNAs are also required in gonadal feedback control of gonadotropin synthesis and secretion. Thus, Dicer-dependent microRNAs confer a new layer of transcriptional and post-transcriptional regulation in gonadotropes to orchestrate the hypothalamus-pituitary-gonadal axis physiology.

This robust paper uncovers another layer of regulation of hormone production in gonadotropes: post-transcriptional regulation of LH and FSH beta by non-coding microRNAs. Only 5% of the human genome is coding DNA, but ~75% of it is transcribed, giving rise to abundant non-coding RNA. MicroRNAs (miRNAs) are small non-coding RNA molecules, containing ~22 nucleotides which can lead to RNA silencing and post-transcriptional regulation of gene expression by binding to complementary RNA. miRNAs have recently emerged as critical regulators of tissue development and gene expression at multiple levels including mRNA expression, turnover, stability and translational control. For example, Lin28/Lin28b inhibits the maturation of miRNAs of the let7 family and both Lin28 and let7 are involved in the regulation of puberty. Clusters of miRNAs have been predicted to bind to 3′-UTRs of mouse *Lhb* and *Fshb* mRNAs, but their functional significance in vivo was unknown. Dicer is an evolutionarily conserved endoribonuclease that synthesises miRNAs and small interfering RNAs from double-stranded RNA.

The authors created a mouse model in which Dicer is deleted selectively in gonadotropes. The findings provide overwhelming evidence that suppression of Dicer-dependent miRNAs reduces LH and FSH production. The loss of these miRNAs in gonadotropes increased transcriptional suppressors and suppressed transcriptional activators: the net effect being severe suppression of gonadotropin subunit proteins, even after gonadectomy. Interestingly, Dicer deletion in females reduced basal mRNA levels of Lhb but not Fshb. This suggests a female-specific post-transcriptional mechanism of Fshb gene regulation. Whether this is dependent on the estrous cycle, and is specific to rodents remains to be seen. The next step will be to investigate which specific miRNAs are responsible for the regulation of gonadotropin subunit production and what their target RNAs are, and to assess their role in human physiology. This work may be a step towards the use of small interfering RNA molecules as drugs for fertility and pubertal disorders.

Leptin mediates the increase in blood pressure associated with obesity

Simonds SE, Pryor JT, Ravussin E, Greenway FL, Dileone R, Allen AM, Bassi J, Elmquist JK, Keogh JM, Henning E, Myers MG, Jr, Licinio J, Brown RD, Enriori PJ, O'Rahilly S, Sternson SM, Grove KL, Spanswick DC, Farooqi IS, Cowley MA
Department of Physiology, Monash Obesity and Diabetes Institute, Monash University, Clayton, VIC, Australia
isf20@cam.ac.uk; michael.cowley@monash.edu
Cell 2014;159:1404–1416

Background: Obesity is associated with increased blood pressure, which in turn increases the risk of cardiovascular diseases. Leptin is synthesised by adipocytes. Humans with loss of function mutations in leptin or leptin receptor (LepR) have low blood pressure despite severe obesity. Rodents deficient for leptin also develop severe obesity without increased blood pressure. Leptin regulates food intake by stimulating POMC neurons in the hypothalamus and indirectly increase the sympathetic nerve activity.
Methods: The authors investigated the role of leptin, and particularly its actions on the hypothalamus, in the elevated blood pressure of diet-induced obesity (DIO) in mice.
Results: DIO increased weight, heart rate and blood pressure. Leptin signalling was required for the obesity-induced increase in blood pressure. The effect of leptin on blood pressure was independent of its effects on body weight. Leptin modulated blood pressure via neural circuits in the dorsomedial hypothalamus (DMH). In vivo inhibition of LepR DMH-expressing neurons decreased blood pressure.
Conclusion: The hypertensive effect of leptin in obese mice is mediated through activation of hypothalamic neurons located in the dorsomedial hypothalamus.

It has been well known for several years that intracerebroventricular injection of leptin increases sympathetic nerve activity to numerous organs. However, the characterisation of the link between leptin, high blood pressure in obese mice and the activation of dorsomedial hypothalamic (DMH) neurons represents a novelty. The main effect of leptin is to control body weight by activating POMC neurons in the arcuate nucleus of the hypothalamus. This well-described effect involves the melanocortin system. The implication of DMH neurons in the control of blood pressure is interesting, as the physiological role of these neurons is poorly understood. They have been implicated in the control of food intake. The authors here demonstrate that the inhibition of leptin action on DMH neurons reduced blood pressure in obese mice without affecting body weight or food intake. The role of melanocortin signalling in leptin's effect on blood pressure in obesity remains to be elucidated.

Homeodomain proteins SIX3 and SIX6 regulate gonadotrope-specific genes during pituitary development

Xie H, Hoffmann HM, Meadows JD, Mayo SL, Trang C, Leming SS, Maruggi C, Davis SW, Larder R, Mellon PL
Department of Reproductive Medicine and the Center for Reproductive Science and Medicine, University of California, San Diego, La Jolla, CA, USA
Mol Endocrinol 2015;29:842–855

Background: Sine oculis-related homeobox 3 (SIX3) and SIX6 are related homeodomain transcription factors that regulate neuroendocrine development. This study aimed to assess the separate roles of SIX3 and SIX6.
Methods: Expression patterns of *Six3* and *Six6* were assessed in vitro and in vivo. Six3 and Six6 gene expression was reduced by small interfering (si)RNA and by genetic deletion to create Six6 knockout mice. Cell lines and pituitaries of knockout mice were studied.
Results: Findings of both the siRNA cell lines and the genetic knockout model supported roles for SIX3 and SIX6 in regulation of gonadotrope gene expression and confirmed that SIX3 and SIX6 can functionally compensate for each other. *Six3* and *Six6* expression patterns in gonadotrope cell lines reflected the timing of the expression of pituitary markers they regulate; *Six3* is expressed in an immature gonadotrope cell line and represses transcription of the early lineage-specific pituitary genes (GnRHR and the common alpha-subunit). In contrast, *Six6* is expressed in a mature gonadotrope cell line and represses the specific beta-subunits of LH and FSH (LHb and FSHb) that are expressed later in development. *SIX6* repression requires interaction with transducin-like enhancer of split corepressor proteins and competition for DNA-binding sites with the transcriptional activator pituitary homeobox 1 (Pitx1). Estradiol and circadian rhythm regulated pituitary expression of *Six6* and *Six3* in adult females but not in males.
Conclusion: SIX3 and SIX6 play distinct but compensatory roles in regulating transcription of gonadotrope-specific genes as gonadotrope cells differentiate.

Mammalian sine oculis-related homeobox (SIX)6 and SIX3 are a closely related subfamily of the SIX proteins that are vertebrate homologues of Drosophila optix. While *Six1*, *Six2*, *Six4* and *Six5* show broad expression during embryogenesis, *Six3* and *Six6* are restricted to the developing eye, brain and pituitary. When compared with *Six6*, the expression pattern of *Six3* is highly similar, but with a generally broader distribution in both the brain and visual system during development. Six proteins have two highly conserved domains: a homeodomain (HD) for DNA-binding and a 'Six' domain for protein-protein interaction. *Six3* knockout (KO) mice die at birth, lacking most head structures anterior to the midbrain, although the rest of the body appears normal. In contrast, *Six6*-KO mice have hypoplastic pituitaries, may be blind and fail to progress through the estrous cycle and are infertile. Total GnRH mRNA and GnRH neuron numbers are severely reduced in the hypothalamus, showing the importance of Six6 for regulation of gonadotropins.

This paper describes the distinct functions of Six3 and Six6 in pituitary lineage specification. *Six3* is mostly expressed in immature gonadotrope cell lines and *Six6* in mature gonadotrope cell lines. During formation of Rathke's pouch, *Six3* and *Six6* expression are detectable, with *Six3* expressed at higher levels during early development, and both *Six3* and *Six6* are expressed in pituitary precursors. The authors showed that SIX3 and SIX6 exhibit differing effects in the transcriptional regulation of gonadotrope-specific genes (*Cga*, *GnRHR*, *LHb*, *FSHb*) in different stages of maturity.

This work further identifies the overlapping and distinct functions of SIX3 and SIX6 as pituitary transcription factors of importance for gonadotrope function, and helps to further elucidate the molecular and cellular mechanisms underlying puberty and reproduction.

Deletion of OTX2 in neural ectoderm delays anterior pituitary development

Mortensen AH, Schade V, Lamonerie T, Camper SA
Department of Human Genetics, University of Michigan, Ann Arbor, MI, USA
Hum Mol Genet 2015;24:939–953

Background: Heterozygous mutations in the *OTX2* gene have been linked to central nervous system abnormalities, developmental delay, endocrine deficiencies with abnormalities of the pituitary gland but the role of *Otx2* in development of the hypothalamus and pituitary is not clear. In mice, homozygous deletion of *Otx2* results in forebrain truncation, which complicates studies into the function of *Otx2*. Expression of *Otx2* overlaps transiently with *Hesx1* in forebrain and pituitary gland. The aim of this study was to understand the role of *Otx2* during HP-axis development.
Methods: *Otx2* was deleted in a tissue-specific manner in either the oral ectoderm that will develop into the anterior pituitary (AP), or neural ectoderm that will become the posterior pituitary (PP) and prospective hypothalamus. Foxg1-Cre or Pitx2-Cre was used to conditionally delete *Otx2* in the oral ectoderm. Nkx2.1-Cre was used to delete *Otx2* in the neural-ectoderm. In situ hybridisation, immunohistochemistry and RT-PCR were used to analyse the phenotype. BrdU labelling was used to assess cell proliferation in the hypothalamus.
Results: Deletion of *Otx2* in early head development using the *Foxg1-Cre* line resulted in craniofacial and forebrain abnormalities such as microphthalmia, anophthalmia, facial defects and exencephaly, reminiscent of defects in patients with heterozygous *OTX2* mutations. Pituitary hyperplasia and protrusion of the pituitary into the palate was seen but hormone-producing pituitary cells showed normal terminal differentiation. *Pitx2-Cre* mice, in which Cre is expressed in the oral ectoderm and Rathke's pouch, were used to delete *Otx2* in the AP. No pituitary phenotype was observed in these mutants, suggesting that *Otx2* expression and action in the neural ectoderm is required for normal HP-axis development. To verify this hypothesis, *Otx2* was deleted from neural ectoderm using *NKx2.1-Cre* mice. This resulted in very poor PP formation and small AP, and abnormal ventral diencephalic signalling with transient absence of Fgf10 signals and reduced cell proliferation. Intriguingly, the loss of *Otx2* in the ventral diencephalon did not result in absence of terminally differentiating hormone producing cells and disruption of HP-axis in postnatal life.
Conclusions: *Otx2* within the neural ectoderm is required for normal development of the pituitary stalk and infundibulum, at least in part by affecting Fgf10 signalling. The early expression of *Otx2* in the brain is required for development of craniofacial bones, brain, eyes and pituitary gland.

OTX2 is an important homeodomain transcription factor, which is required for the formation of anterior forebrain and craniofacial development. In this elegant paper, tissue-specific ablation of *Otx2* was used to understand the role of *Otx2* during development. Expression of *Otx2* in the oral ectoderm or Rathke's pouch is not required for the formation of the anterior pituitary or terminal differentiation of its hormone-producing cells. However, *Otx2* is needed in the ventral diencephalon for the formation of the pituitary stalk and posterior pituitary. The authors identified that down-regulation of Fgf10 signalling mediated the pituitary phenotype. Paradoxically, these effects were transient, and in postnatal life $Otx2^{Fl/Fl}$-Nkx2.1-Ce animals displayed a normal HP-axis. This work leads to novel questions: how does *Otx2* regulate Fgf10 signals from the ventral diencephalon? Which genes or genetic mediators are involved in the postnatal recovery of hypothalamic pituitary function? The authors suggest that *Emx1* and *Emx2* may compensate to re-establish Fgf10 signalling. Future studies that aim to resolve these questions will shed further light on the genetic aetiology of congenital hypopituitarism.

New technical strategies

Differentiation of hypothalamic-like neurons from human pluripotent stem cells

Wang L, Meece K, Williams DJ, Lo KA, Zimmer M, Heinrich G, Martin Carli J, Leduc CA, Sun L, Zeltser LM, Freeby M, Goland RS, Tsang SH, Wardlaw SL, Egli D, Leibel RL
Division of Molecular Genetics, Department of Pediatrics and Naomi Berrie Diabetes Center, Columbia University College of Physicians and Surgeons, New York, NY, USA
J Clin Invest 2015;125:796–808

Generation of neuropeptidergic hypothalamic neurons from human pluripotent stem cells

Merkle FT, Maroof A, Wataya T, Sasai Y, Studer L, Eggan K, Schier AF
Department of Stem Cell and Regenerative Biology, Harvard University, Cambridge, MA, USA
keggan@scrb.harvard.edu; schier@fas.harvard.edu
Development 2015;142:633–643

Background: Hypothalamic neurons orchestrate many physiological and behavioural processes via secreted neuropeptides, and are relevant to diseases such as obesity, narcolepsy and infertility. The differentiation of neuropeptidergic hypothalamic neurons from neural progenitors is not well described. Several transcription factors have been described, however, the induction of these differentiation pathways remains unknown. Pluripotent stem cells are emerging tools to study the differentiation of specific cell types and to the aetiopathogenic mechanisms of genetic disorders, particularly in cells that are not easily accessible, such as hypothalamic neurons. In the following papers, two protocols were described to differentiate hypothalamic neurons from human pluripotent stem cells (hPSC).
Methods: Cell cultures of hPSC in different conditions to induce hypothalamic neuron differentiation. Both groups used the expression of *NKX2.1* as the marker of hPSC differentiation into hypothalamic neurons. The identity of differentiated neurons has been established by immunohistochemistry and mRNA quantification.
Results: In the first paper, Wang et al combined SHH exposure followed by the inhibition of the Notch pathway. With this protocol, differentiated cells expressed several transcription factors found in hypothalamic progenitors. The addition of the brain-derived neurotrophic factor promoted differentiation toward neurons expressing POMC and NPY but also other neuropeptides expressed by hypothalamic neurons in the arcuate nucleus. In addition, the authors showed that neurons differentiated from induced-pluripotent stem cells with the same protocol displayed a similar signature of gene expression. In the second paper, Merkle et al observed that hypothalamic neurons can be generated using a 'self-patterning' strategy that yields a broad array of cell types, or via a more reproducible directed

differentiation approach. These stem cell-derived human hypothalamic neurons share characteristic morphological properties and gene expression patterns with their counterparts in vivo, and are able to integrate into the mouse brain.
Conclusion: Neuropeptide expressing neurons can be easily differentiated from pluripotent stem cells. These neurons could form the basis of cellular models, chemical screens or cellular therapies to study and treat common human diseases.

These two papers describe in vitro generation of human hypothalamic neurons from pluripotent stem cells. Although they mainly report technical protocols, these papers bring new perspectives to delineate monogenic disorders due to hypothalamic defects. They also open the opportunity to develop new therapeutic avenues by in vitro screening of pharmacological components. In addition to basic research aiming to characterise molecular processes governing hypothalamic neuron differentiation, these papers thus represent a real new perspective for translational research in neuroendocrinology. They report how it is easy to get neuropeptide-expressing neurons from PSC. They also show that early SHH stimulation of PSC followed by incubation with a Notch inhibitor and then stimulation by BDNF orient the differentiation of PSC towards neuropeptide-expressing neurons similar to those found in the arcuate nucleus. In contrast, the 'self-patterning' strategy developed by Merkle et al differentiated PSC into neurons which seem to be less specific of a certain type of hypothalamic nucleus. The protocol of Wang et al should interest research teams working on the mechanism of obesity and the development of new pharmacological components to treat obesity. Indeed, energy homeostasis is under the control of hypothalamic neurons located in the arcuate nucleus. Although this protocol opens the possibility to investigate the control of the expression of neuropeptides involved in the control of food intake, further work is needed to assess whether these neurons form neuronal networks similar to those described in vivo. In addition, to express specific neuropeptides, we know that the capacity of hypothalamic neurons to interact with each other is primordial to control energy homeostasis. The assessment of these neurons to form such neuronal networks will be the next step in the development of this in vitro strategy.

Review of the year

Isolated growth hormone deficiency (GHD) in childhood and adolescence: recent advances

Alatzoglou KS, Webb EA, Le Tissier P, Dattani MT
Developmental Endocrinology Research Group, Clinical and Molecular Genetics Unit, UCL Institute of Child Health, London, UK
Endocr Rev 2014;35:376–432

Background: The diagnosis of growth hormone deficiency (GHD) in childhood is far from simple and involves clinical history, examination with detailed auxology, biochemical testing and pituitary imaging. There is an increasing contribution from genetics in patients with congenital GHD.
Methods and results: This review describes our increasing understanding of the factors involved in the development of somatotropes and the somatotrope network. Mutations in known genes such as those encoding GH (*GH1*), GHRH receptor (*GHRHR*), or transcription factors involved in pituitary development, are identified in a relatively small percentage of patients, suggesting the involvement of other, yet unidentified, factors. Genome-wide association studies point toward an increasing number of genes involved in the control of growth, but their role in the aetiology of IGHD remains unknown. Controversies on the aetiology, diagnosis and management of IGHD in children are discussed. Recent data suggest that childhood IGHD may have a wider impact on the health and neurodevelopment of children, but it is yet unknown to what extent treatment with recombinant human GH can reverse this effect. Finally, the safety of recombinant human GH is discussed, and the need for long-term controlled studies to clarify the consequences of childhood IGHD and the long-term safety of its treatment.

This is an excellent review for both clinicians and basic scientists. It describes the physiology of pituitary GH production and secretion and its control, all known molecular causes for isolated GHD but also all natural and genetically manipulated mice that have been developed as models of human GH deficiency, or as tools to investigate the hypothalamic-pituitary-GH axis.

Important for clinical practice

Hormone modeling in preterm neonates: establishment of pituitary and steroid hormone reference intervals

Greaves RF, Pitkin J, Ho CS, Baglin J, Hunt RW, Zacharin MR
School of Medical Sciences and School of Mathematical and Geospatial Sciences, RMIT University, VIC, Australia
J Clin Endocrinol Metab 2015;100:1097–1103

Background: Differences in serum hormone concentrations are likely to exist between extremely preterm compared with late preterm and full-term infants. The aim of this study was to develop reference intervals for three pituitary hormones and five steroid hormones in the serum of preterm infants.
Methods: Blood samples were collected from 248 (128 male and 120 female) preterm neonates born between 24 and 32 weeks' gestation, recruited from three neonatal intensive care wards. No infant had ambiguous genitalia or other endocrine abnormalities. All infants included in the RI determination survived beyond the equivalent of term. Automated electrochemiluminescence immunoassay (Roche Cobas 8000-e601) was used to analyse prolactin, FSH and LH. Liquid chromatography coupled with tandem mass spectrometry was used for analysis of 17-hydroxyprogesterone, androstenedione, cortisol, cortisone and testosterone. Robust statistical analyses were performed.
Results: Reference intervals were defined for LH, FSH, testosterone, cortisone, 17 OH progesterone, androstenedione, cortisol and prolactin. Gender-specific intervals were identified for FSH, LH and testosterone. Cortisone and 17- hydroxyprogesterone levels required division by gestational age: neonates born at <30 weeks' gestation had higher levels than later-born neonates. Androstenedione, cortisol and prolactin did not require any division within this cohort for RI assignment.
Conclusions: This report provides the first characterisation of serum steroids measured by mass spectrometry in preterm neonates, with the additional characterisation of three pituitary hormones in infants born ≤32 weeks' gestation. These data inform the interpretation of clinical data in very preterm neonates and reduce the risk of misinterpretation leading to incorrect diagnosis.

Five to 18% of babies are born preterm. Over the last decades survival has increased remarkably. The lack of normative endocrine data in these babies limits accurate diagnosis and decision making. Understanding endocrine physiology in the extreme preterms and establishment of reference ranges therefore has significant clinical value.

The authors established a biobank for blood samples from 248 extremely and very preterm infants, born between 24 and 32 weeks' gestation, at two to three-week intervals, to 36 weeks' gestational age. They used validated techniques with good reproducibility for hormone measurements (chemiluminescence immunoassays and liquid chromatography/mass spectroscopy), and took great care to describe the methods and quality controls, appropriate for determination of reference ranges. Only the first sample drawn, at a mean age of two days, was analysed. This is important as hormone concentrations often depend on postnatal age and clinical stability of the baby. Normal ranges are presented as 95% reference intervals (2.5^{th} and 97.5^{th} percentile lines). In general, LH, FSH, testosterone and adrenal steroids were at higher concentrations in extremely premature infants compared with later premature infants. Interestingly, a sexual divergence in mean LH and FSH was observed, with girls having much higher concentrations than boys (median FSH: 1.1 in boys versus 57.0 in girls, median LH: 1.9 in boys versus 13.3 mu/L in girls).

This work is a good start for the development of normal ranges in neonates, gives additional insight into neonatal physiology and informs the investigation of pituitary disease, adrenal disease and differences in sexual differentiation in premature neonates.

Required enhancer-matrin-3 network interactions for a homeodomain transcription program

Skowronska-Krawczyk D, Ma Q, Schwartz M, Scully K, Li W, Liu Z, Taylor H, Tollkuhn J, Ohgi KA, Notani D, Kohwi Y, Kohwi-Shigematsu T, Rosenfeld MG
Howard Hughes Medical Institute, Department of Medicine, School of Medicine, University of California, San Diego, La Jolla, CA, USA
Nature 2014;514:257–261

Background: Homeodomain proteins were described 30 years ago. They act as regulators of target gene expression and play essential roles in development; however, the molecular mechanisms underlying transcriptional activity of homeodomain factors remain poorly understood. The aim of this study was to investigate Pit1 (also called Pou1f1), a developmentally required POU-homeodomain transcription factor.
Methods: Mass spectrometry was used to identify interacting proteins with immunoprecipitated HA-tagged Pit1 from 293T cells, which identified matrin-3 and hnRNPU as interacting proteins. ChIP-Seq with a specific alpha-matrin-3 antibody was subsequently used, followed by immuno-FISH experiments with DNA-FISH probes specific to the growth hormone locus and alpha-matrin-3 antibodies, finding that >65% of the FISH signals co-localised with matrin-3.
Results: Unexpectedly, Pit1-occupied enhancers were found to bind to a nuclear matrin-3-rich network and this was a key event in activation of the Pit1-regulated enhancer/coding gene transcriptional program. Pit1 association with Satb1 and beta-catenin is required for this tethering event. A naturally occurring, dominant negative, point mutation in human *PIT1* (R271W), causing combined pituitary hormone deficiency, resulted in loss of Pit1 association with beta-catenin and Satb1 and therefore the matrin-3-rich network, blocking Pit1-dependent enhancer/coding target gene activation. When the R271W Pit1 mutant protein was artificially tethered to the matrin-3 network, the association with beta-catenin and Satb1 was bypassed and Pit1-dependent gene activation was rescued.
Conclusion: These studies reveal an unanticipated homeodomain factor/beta-catenin/Satb1-dependent localisation of target gene regulatory enhancer region to a subnuclear architectural structure that serves as an underlying mechanism by which an enhancer-bound homeodomain factor effectively activates developmental gene transcriptional programs.

This fundamental paper characterises the transcriptional activity of Pit1 (or Pouf1). Unexpectedly, Pit1 does not bind to transcriptional start sites, but instead is located to specific enhancers that form a 3D network. Pit1 is localised to these specific enhancers through interaction with the novel identified Pit1 protein partner, Matrin3. Matrin3 forms part of the nuclear scaffold and directs the homeodomain transcriptional complex formed by Pit1, beta-catenin and Satb1 to enhancer elements. These results suggest a novel model by which transcription factors are located in subnuclear structure via the 'nuclear Matrin3 rich-network'. This biological phenomenon could be similar for other pituitary transcription factors such as Lhx3, Prop1 or Oct1, and could therefore help in future studies of how the highly complex transcriptional regulatory control of the HP-axis is accomplished.

Postoperative copeptin concentration predicts diabetes insipidus after pituitary surgery

Winzeler B, Zweifel C, Nigro N, Arici B, Bally M, Schuetz P, Blum CA, Kelly C, Berkmann S, Huber A, Gentili F, Zadeh G, Landolt H, Mariani L, Muller B, Christ-Crain M
Departments of Endocrinology, Diabetology and Metabolism and Neurosurgery, University Hospital of Basel, Basel, Switzerland
J Clin Endocrinol Metab 2015;100:2275–2282

Background: Copeptin is a stable surrogate marker of arginine vasopressin (AVP) secretion; the peptides are stoichiometrically secreted from the posterior pituitary in response to elevated plasma osmolality or non-osmotic stress. The authors hypothesised that following stress from pituitary surgery, patients with neurohypophyseal damage and eventual diabetes insipidus (DI) would not exhibit the expected pronounced copeptin elevation. The objective of this study was to evaluate the accuracy of copeptin to predict DI following pituitary surgery.
Methods: A prospective multicenter observational cohort study of consecutive pituitary surgery patients was performed. Post-surgery, copeptin was measured daily until discharge. Logistic regression models and diagnostic performance measures were calculated to assess relationships between postoperative copeptin concentrations and DI.
Results: Of 205 patients, 50 (24.4%) developed postoperative DI. Initial post-surgical copeptin concentrations were lower in patients developing DI versus those not: 2.9 [1.9–7.9] pmol/L versus 10.8 [5.2–30.4] pmol/L; P<0.001. Logistic regression analysis revealed strong association between copeptin concentrations and DI even after adjustment for known predisposing factors: adjusted odds ratio (95% CI) 1.41 (1.16–1.73). DI occurred in 22/27 patients with copeptin <2.5 pmol/L (positive predictive value, 81%; specificity, 97%), but only 1/40 with copeptin >30 pmol/L (negative predictive value, 95%; sensitivity, 94%) on postoperative day one. Limitations of the study: Lack of standardised DI diagnostic criteria; postoperative blood samples for copeptin obtained during everyday care versus at fixed time points.
Conclusions: In patients undergoing pituitary procedures, low copeptin concentrations reflect postoperative DI, whereas high levels virtually exclude it. Copeptin may become a novel tool for early goal-directed management of postoperative DI.

Copeptin is a stable, reliable and rapidly measurable blood biomarker of AVP release. This peptide comprises the C-terminal portion of preprovasopressin, and is co-secreted with AVP in an equimolar ratio. The main stimulus for copeptin release is therefore the same as for AVP release, that is, raised osmolarity. The major advantage of measuring copeptin is that a result could be available the same day, whereas AVP is less stable and notoriously difficult to measure. This study shows that median copeptin concentrations doubled after cranial surgery, and that low copeptin concentration, as early as within 12 hours postoperatively, predicts the development of DI with a positive predictive value of 81% (95% CI: 62–94%) with 97% specificity. Conversely, high copeptin concentration, occurring in 34% of the cases, virtually ruled out DI (negative predictive value of 95% with a specificity of 95%). Therefore, copeptin seems to represent a single new, early and reliable marker to predict postoperative DI. Measurement of copeptin may thus be a very useful clinical tool in the assessment of the postoperative patient with midline tumours. Unfortunately, it was not possible to use copeptin concentrations to predict the development of SIADH.

Novel lethal form of congenital hypopituitarism associated with the first recessive LHX4 mutation

Gregory LC, Humayun KN, Turton JP, McCabe MJ, Rhodes SJ, Dattani MT
Developmental Endocrinology Research Group, Genetics and Epigenetics in Health and Disease Unit, Genetic and Genomic Medicine Programme, UCL Institute of Child Health, London, UK
J Clin Endocrinol Metab 2015;100:2158–2164

Background: Two LIM homeodomain (LIM-HD) transcription factors, Lhx3 and Lhx4, are critical in the development of the nervous system and pituitary gland in mice. *Lhx4* null mice die shortly after birth and exhibit incomplete pituitary gland development. Autosomal dominant negative *LHX4* mutations in humans have been associated with variable penetrant combined hormone pituitary deficiency (CHPD). The authors describe the first homozygous missense mutation in *LHX4* in a patient with a lethal form of congenital hypopituitarism.

Methods: DNA was extracted from 97 patients with an ectopic posterior pituitary, of whom 62 had CHPD, 22 isolated GH deficiency and 13 septo-optic-dysplasia. Western blotting and luciferase assays using the prolactin promoter were used to assess functional effects of the variants.

Results: Sanger sequencing identified homozygous *LHX4* mutations (c.377C>T) in a non-consanguineous Pakistani family with one daughter and two sons. The girl had mid-facial hypoplasia and died in the first week of life. The first boy presented at birth with ACTH and TSH deficiency and the second son had ACTH, TSH and GH deficiency, and facial abnormalities, small genitalia and bilateral undescendent testes. Both had anterior pituitary aplasia and ectopic posterior pituitary. Despite immediate treatment with hydrocortisone and thyroxin, both died within one week after birth. The parents are heterozygotes and are unaffected. Gene activation assays using alpha-GSU and prolactin promoter upstream of luciferase, failed to show a difference on the activation ability between hLHX4 (p.T126M) variant and wild-type. Moreover, synergistic experiments between LHX4 and PIT1 showed that LHX4 increased the activity of PIT transcriptional activation at the same fashion to the LHX4 mutant counterpart. These data indicate that this mutation in the LIM2 domain does not affect transcriptional activating genes, however, it may affect interaction with yet unknown protein partners.

Conclusions: Previously identified heterozygous *LHX4* mutations result in haplo-insufficiency and cause CHPD with variable penetrance. The authors describe the first recessive mutation of *hLHX4* linked to a lethal congenital form of congenital hypopituitarism.

The authors report for the first time a recessive *LHX4* mutation in a pedigree with a lethal form of congenital hypopituitarism. Interestingly, the mutation seems not to affect transcriptional transactivation or synergistic action with PIT1. Rather, the mutation is found in the LIM2 domain, and therefore the binding to other partner proteins could be affected. It remains important to identify the network of protein partners of LHX4 and to delineate the LHX4 transcriptional programme that controls HP-axis development. This article opens the door to further investigation of genetic variants of LHX4 to assess how such variants affect the transcriptional programme and lead to congenital hypopituitarism.

Antenatal and Neonatal Endocrinology

Khalid Hussain

Clinical and Molecular Genetics Unit, The Developmental Endocrinology Research Group, Institute of Child Health, University College London, London, UK

Neonatal glucose and insulin physiology

Sulfonylurea treatment before genetic testing in neonatal diabetes: pros and cons

Carmody D, Bell CD, Hwang JL, Dickens JT, Sima DI, Felipe DL, Zimmer CA, Davis AO, Kotlyarevska K, Naylor RN, Philipson LH, Greeley SA

Departments of Medicine and Pediatrics, Section of Adult and Pediatric Endocrinology, Diabetes, and Metabolism, The University of Chicago, Chicago, IL, USA

J Clin Endocrinol Metab 2014;99:E2709–E2714

Background: Diabetes in neonates nearly always has a monogenic aetiology. Earlier sulfonylurea therapy can improve glycaemic control and potential neurodevelopmental outcomes in children with KCNJ11 or ABCC8 mutations, the most common gene causes.
Objective: To assess the risks and benefits of initiating sulfonylurea therapy before genetic testing results become available.
Methods: Observational retrospective study of subjects with neonatal diabetes within the University of Chicago Monogenic Diabetes Registry.
Main outcome: Response to sulfonylurea was determined by whether insulin could be discontinued and treatment side effects in those treated empirically.
Results: 154 infants were diagnosed with diabetes before six months of age. A genetic diagnosis had been determined in 118 (77%), with 73 (47%) having a mutation in KCNJ11 or ABCC8. The median time from clinical diagnosis to genetic diagnosis was 10.4 weeks (range, 1.6 to 58.2 weeks). In nine probands, an empiric sulfonylurea trial was initiated within 28 days of diabetes diagnosis. A genetic cause was subsequently found in eight cases, and insulin was discontinued within 14 days of sulfonylurea initiation in all of these cases.
Conclusions: Sulfonylurea therapy appears to be safe and often successful in neonatal diabetes patients before genetic testing results are available; however, larger numbers of cases must be studied. Given the potential beneficial effect on neurodevelopmental outcome, glycaemic control and the current barriers to expeditious acquisition of genetic testing, an empiric inpatient trial of sulfonylurea can be considered. However, obtaining a genetic diagnosis remains imperative to inform long-term management and prognosis.

There have been major advances in the last 10 years in understanding the genetic mechanisms of neonatal diabetes mellitus [1–3]. Currently, mutations in at least 18 different genes have been described that lead to neonatal diabetes mellitus. The most common genetic cause is mutations in the genes *KCNJ11/ABCC8* which encode the KIR6.2/SUR components, respectively of the pancreatic beta-cell K_{ATP} channel. Finding a mutation in one of these genes has enormous implications for patient management. The vast majority of patients with neonatal diabetes mellitus due to mutations in the *KCNJ11/ABCC8* genes can be treated with oral sulphonylureas thus avoiding the need for insulin injections. However, not all clinicians have access to rapid genetic testing. This study assessed the suitability and safety of treating children with neonatal diabetes mellitus before a genetic diagnosis was possible. In nine patients treatment with oral sulfonylurea trial was initiated without a genetic diagnosis. In eight of these patients insulin therapy could be stopped. Subsequent genetic testing showed that eight of these patients had a genetic diagnosis due to mutations in the *KCNJ11/ABCC8* genes. This study therefore suggests that oral sulfonylurea treatment appears to be safe in a clinical setting in patients with neonatal diabetes patients before a genetic diagnosis is possible. These findings are especially important in those settings globally where there is limited access for rapid genetic testing. However, a lager cohort of patients needs to be studied and the side effects of oral sulfonylurea monitored.

Age at the time of sulfonylurea initiation influences treatment outcomes in KCNJ11-related neonatal diabetes

Thurber BW, Carmody D, Tadie EC, Pastore AN, Dickens JT, Wroblewski KE, Naylor RN, Philipson LH, Greeley SA, United States Neonatal Diabetes Working Group
Departments of Pediatrics and Medicine, Section of Adult and Pediatric Endocrinology, Diabetes, and Metabolism, University of Chicago, Chicago, IL, USA
Diabetologia 2015;58:1430–1435

Background: Individuals with heterozygous activating mutations of the *KCNJ11* gene encoding a subunit of the ATP-sensitive potassium channel (KATP) can usually be treated with oral sulfonylurea (SU) pills in lieu of insulin injections. This study tested the hypothesis that younger age at the time of initiation of SU therapy is correlated with lower required doses of SU therapy, shorter transition time and decreased likelihood of requiring additional diabetes medications.
Methods: This was a retrospective cohort study using data on 58 individuals with neonatal diabetes due to KCNJ11 mutations identified through the University of Chicago Monogenic Diabetes Registry (http://monogenicdiabetes.uchicago.edu/registry). The authors assessed the influence of age at initiation of SU therapy on treatment outcomes.
Results: HbA_{1c} fell from an average of 8.5% (69mmol/mol) before transition to 6.2% (44mmol/mol) after SU therapy (P<0.001). Age of initiation of SU correlated with the dose (mg/kg/day) of SU required at follow-up (r=0.80, P<0.001). Similar associations were observed across mutation subtypes. Ten participants required additional glucose-lowering medications and all had initiated SU at age 13 years or older. No serious adverse events were reported.
Conclusion: Earlier age at initiation of SU treatment is associated with improved response to SU therapy. Declining sensitivity to SU may be due to loss of beta-cell mass over time in those treated with insulin. These data support the need for early genetic diagnosis and appropriate personalised treatment in all cases of neonatal diabetes.

Heterozygous activating mutations of the *KCNJ11* gene which encodes the KIR6.2 component of the pancreatic K_{ATP} channel are the most common cause of permanent neonatal diabetes mellitus. Mutations in *KCNJ11* can disrupt the K_{ATP} channel to varying degrees and result in a broad range of phenotypes. In patients the clinical severity can range from isolated transient neonatal diabetes to the most severe cases permanent neonatal diabetes affected by neurodevelopmental disability, seizures and insensitivity to sulfonylurea treatment. This retrospective study suggests that therapy with oral sulfonylureas should be started as early as possible in patients with neonatal diabetes mellitus. The younger the age of starting oral sulfonylurea therapy, the lower the dose of sulfonylurea will be required and there is decreased likelihood of patients requiring additional diabetes medications when they are older. Interestingly, those patients who started oral sulfonylurea late (age 13 years) all required additional medications to lower their blood glucose. The early treatment with oral sulfonylureas might have a protective effect on the beta-cell. These observations have important clinical implications for those patients with neonatal diabetes mellitus. Thus early genetic diagnosis and starting treatment as early as possible with oral sulfonylureas in patients with neonatal diabetes mellitus due to mutations in the *KCNJ11/ABCC8* genes seems to be the optimal management of these patients.

GATA4 mutations are a cause of neonatal and childhood-onset diabetes

Shaw-Smith C, De Franco E, Lango Allen H, Batlle M, Flanagan SE, Borowiec M, Taplin CE, van Alfen-van der Velden J, Cruz-Rojo J, Perez de Nanclares G, Miedzybrodzka Z, Deja G, Wlodarska I, Młynarski W, Ferrer J, Hattersley AT, Ellard S
Institute of Biomedical and Clinical Science, University of Exeter Medical School, Exeter, UK
sian.ellard@nhs.net
Diabetes 2014;63:2888–2894

Background: The GATA family zinc finger transcription factors GATA4 and GATA6 are known to play important roles in the development of the pancreas. In mice, both Gata4 and Gata6 are required for pancreatic development. In humans, GATA6 haploinsufficiency can cause pancreatic agenesis and heart defects. Congenital heart defects also are common in patients with GATA4 mutations and deletions, but the role of GATA4 in the developing human pancreas is unproven.

Methods/Results: This study reports five patients with deletions (n=4) or mutations of the *GATA4* gene who have diabetes and a variable exocrine phenotype. Four cases presented with diabetes in the neonatal period (age at diagnosis, one to seven days old). A de novo *GATA4* missense mutation (p.N273K) was identified in a patient with complete absence of the pancreas confirmed at post-mortem. This mutation affects a highly conserved residue located in the second zinc finger domain of the GATA4 protein. In vitro studies showed reduced DNA binding and transactivational activity of the mutant protein.
Conclusions: *GATA4* mutations/deletions are a cause of neonatal or childhood-onset diabetes with or without exocrine insufficiency. These results confirm a role for *GATA4* in normal development of the human pancreas.

GATA transcription factors broadly regulate embryogenesis and influence survival of several cell types including pancreatic beta-cells. GATA factors are known to be expressed in a wide variety of tissues where they act as critical regulators of cell-specific gene expression. This includes multiple endocrine organs such as the pituitary, pancreas, adrenals and especially the gonads. GATA4 (GATA-binding factor 4) is a zinc finger transcription factor. It plays important roles in the development of multiple organs. In human embryos, GATA4 is detected in the area of the developing pancreas at 29–31 dpc, at the same time of the early transcription factor PDX1, suggesting a role of GATA4 in human pancreas development. Mouse studies have suggested a role for Gata4 in pancreatic development. Gata4 -/- mice die prior to pancreas formation because of defective extra-embryonic tissue development, but investigation of Gata4 -/- mice rescued from embryonic lethality showed agenesis of the pancreas. Gata4 +/- mice are phenotypically normal. Mutations in GATA4 have recently been described to cause pancreatic hypoplasia and neonatal diabetes mellitus in association with congenital heart disease [4,5]. In this study the phenotype of patients with GATA4 mutations is expanded to include not only neonatal diabetes mellitus but also late-onset diabetes mellitus. In these patients there was also variable degree of pancreatic developmental abnormalities (ranging from agenesis to hypoplasia of the pancreas) and pancreatic exocrine involvement. Thus GATA4 mutations can also cause childhood-onset diabetes with or without exocrine insufficiency.

Recessive mutations in a distal PTF1A enhancer cause isolated pancreatic agenesis

Weedon MN, Cebola I, Patch AM, Flanagan SE, De Franco E, Caswell R, Rodriguez-Segui SA, Shaw-Smith C, Cho CH, Lango Allen H, Houghton JA, Roth CL, Chen R, Hussain K, Marsh P, Vallier L, Murray A, International Pancreatic Agenesis Consortium, Ellard S, Ferrer J, Hattersley AT
Institute of Biomedical and Clinical Science, University of Exeter Medical School, Exeter, UK
Nature Genetics 2014;46:61–64

Background: The contribution of cis-regulatory mutations to human disease remains poorly understood. Whole-genome sequencing can identify all non-coding variants, yet the discrimination of causal regulatory mutations represents a formidable challenge.
Methods and Results: This study used epigenomic annotation in human embryonic stem cell (hESC)-derived pancreatic progenitor cells to guide the interpretation of whole-genome sequences from individuals with isolated pancreatic agenesis. This analysis uncovered six different recessive mutations in a previously uncharacterised ~400-bp sequence located 25kb downstream of PTF1A (encoding pancreas-specific transcription factor 1a) in 10 families with pancreatic agenesis. This region acts as a developmental enhancer of PTF1A and that the mutations abolish enhancer activity. These mutations are the most common cause of isolated pancreatic agenesis.
Conclusions: Integrating genome sequencing and epigenomic annotation in a disease-relevant cell type can thus uncover new non-coding elements underlying human development and disease.

Pancreas transcription factor 1a (PTF1a) plays a crucial role in the early development of the pancreas and in the maintenance of the acinar cell phenotype. Studies in mouse embryos have shown that PTF1a is expressed as early as embryonic day 8.5 in the region of the future pancreas and in neural cell progenitors. Homozygous coding mutations in the PTF1A gene were first reported in two families with pancreatic agenesis, microcephaly and cerebellar hypoplasia/agenesis [6–8]. Only a few mutations in regulatory elements that cause human disease have been identified thus far. In this elegant study patients with pancreatic agenesis were found to have homozygous mutations in a distal regulatory element (an enhancer) of PTF1A. Using epigenomic annotation from human embryonic stem cell (hESC)-derived pancreatic progenitor cells in combination with whole genome sequencing, the authors identified cis-regulatory mutations comprising an allelic repertoire involving not only a 7.6kb deletion but also five independent point mutations located in an element highly conserved in mammals. This region is located 25kb downstream of PTF1A and recent studies have shown that it is selectively active during development of the pancreas. Mutations in this region cause a milder phenotype than mutations in the coding region of PTF1A (pancreatic agenesis but not cerebellar agenesis). The absence of a neurological phenotype is likely due to tissue specificity of the enhancer region. Recessively inherited mutations of the PTF1A enhancer are the most common cause of pancreatic agenesis among patients born to consanguineous parents. This study demonstrates the importance of using epigenomic annotation in combination with whole exome sequencing of the human genome to uncover tissue-specific functional elements relevant to gene regulation.

Lactate, rather than ketones, may provide alternative cerebral fuel in hypoglycaemic newborns

Harris DL, Weston PJ, Harding JE
Newborn Intensive Care Unit, Waikato District Health Board, Hamilton, New Zealand and Liggins Institute, University of Auckland, Auckland, New Zealand
Arch Dis Child Fetal Neonatal Ed 2015;100:F161–F164

Background: Alternative cerebral fuels are reputed to provide neuroprotection during hypoglycaemia, particularly in breastfed babies. Concentrations of alternative cerebral fuels in hypoglycaemic babies in the first 48 hours were measured.
Patients and methods: Babies were ≥35 weeks, ≤48 hours old and at risk of hypoglycaemia (infant of diabetic, preterm, small or large) were recruited. Plasma glucose, beta-hydroxybutyrate, lactate and insulin concentrations were measured in babies who had been hypoglycaemic (<2.6mM) for longer than one hour.
Results: Blood samples were taken from 35 hypoglycaemic babies at 3.7; 1.8–39.6 (median; range) hours after birth. Concentrations of glucose and beta-hydroxybutyrate were low (2.03; 0.19–3.39mM and 0.06; 0.00–1.20mM), but lactate concentrations varied widely (3.06; 0.02–7.96mM). Infants of diabetics had lower beta-hydroxybutyrate and higher insulin concentrations, but mode of feeding did not influence plasma concentrations of alternative cerebral fuels.
Conclusions: Hypoglycaemic babies within the first 48 hours after birth are unlikely to receive neuroprotection from ketones. However, lactate may provide an alternative cerebral fuel for many. Lactate, rather than ketones, may provide alternative cerebral fuel in hypoglycaemic newborns.

Hypoglycaemia is common in some newborns (preterm, infant of diabetic mother, large for gestational age, IUGR and infant of diabetic mother). Traditionally, ketone bodies (mainly beta-hydroxybutyrate) were thought to be the alternative fuel for brain function at the time of hypoglycaemia in newborns [9–11]. The process of glycolysis in the cytoplasm produces the intermediate metabolite pyruvate. Under aerobic conditions, pyruvate is then converted to acetyl-CoA to enter the Kreb's cycle. However, when there is lack of oxygen, pyruvate is converted by the enzyme lactate dehydrogenase (LDH) to lactic acid (lactate). In this study, the authors measured plasma glucose, beta-hydroxybutyrate, lactate and insulin concentrations in at-risk babies who were hypoglycaemic (blood glucose <2.6mmol/L) for longer than hour. The results showed that the levels of beta-hydroxybutyrate were low whereas the serum lactate levels were higher. The mode of feeding did not affect the concentration of the alternative cerebral fuels. Thus serum lactate might have a more important role as an alternative cerebral fuel in babies with hypoglycaemia in the first few days of life. Further biochemical studies are required to understand what causes the elevation in the serum lactate in these babies and how lactate might be used at a cellular level as a metabolic fuel.

Recommendations from the Pediatric Endocrine Society for evaluation and management of persistent hypoglycemia in neonates, infants, and children

Thornton PS, Stanley CA, De Leon DD, Harris D, Haymond MW, Hussain K, Levitsky LL, Murac MH, Rozance PJ, Simmons RA, Sperling MA, Weinstein DA, White NH, Wolfsdorf JI
Division of Endocrinology, Cook Children's Medical Center, Fort Worth, TX, USA
J Pediatr 2015;167:238–245

Re-evaluating "transitional neonatal hypoglycemia": mechanism and implications for management

Stanley CA, Rozance PJ, Thornton PS, De Leon DD, Harris D, Haymond MW, Hussain K, Levitsky LL, Murad MH, Simmons RA, Sperling MA, Weinstein DA, White NH, Wolfsdorf JI
Division of Endocrinology, Children's Hospital of Philadelphia, Philadelphia, PA. USA
J Pediatr 2015;166:1520–1525.e1

Hypoglycaemia is one of the most common biochemical abnormalities observed in paediatric practice. However, despite its high frequency, there is no consensus on the diagnostic and management approach in newborns and infants with persistent hypoglycaemia. In order to address some of the controversial issues on the topic of hypoglycaemia a panel of experts were convened. These two manuscripts describe the recent recommendations by a Committee of the Pediatric Endocrine Society (PES) for the diagnosis and management of neonates, infants and children with persistent hypoglycaemia. These guidelines have been developed to aid clinicians in recognising those infants who have a genetic cause of their persistent hypoglycaemia and to prevent these patients from developing hypoglycaemic brain injury. To aid in formulating recommendations for neonates, the available data were analysed on the brief period of hypoglycaemia (now referred to as transitional neonatal hypoglycaemia), which is commonly observed in normal newborns during the transition from fetal to extrauterine life. The goal was to try and better understand the mechanism/s underlying this phenomenon in order to formulate recommendations for recognising neonates requiring diagnosis and treatment during the first days of life for disorders causing severe and persistent hypoglycaemia.

During the period of transitional neonatal hypoglycaemia (the first 24–48 hours of life) it is not possible to know if this will be transient or persistent hypoglycaemia. For this reason, the PES guidelines recommend that the focus for the first 24–48 hours of life should be on stabilisation of glucose levels; whereas after 48 hours, neonates whose glucose values remain low or who have other risk factors should be evaluated to determine the aetiology of hypoglycaemia and to ensure their safety prior to discharge. These guidelines should aid clinicians in picking up those infants who might have a genetic form of persistent hypoglycaemia before discharge and thus preventing brain injury form hypoglycaemia.

Impact of maternal obesity and gestational diabetes on neonatal adiposity

Effect of maternal obesity with and without gestational diabetes on offspring subcutaneous and preperitoneal adipose tissue development from birth up to year

Uebel K, Pusch K, Gedrich K, Schneider KT, Hauner H, Bader BL
PhD Graduate School 'Nutritional adaptation and epigenetic mechanisms', ZIEL – Research Center for Nutrition and Food Sciences, Technische Universitat Munchen, Freising-Weihenstephan, Germany
BMC Pregnancy Childbirth 2014;14:138

Background: Maternal obesity and gestational diabetes mellitus (GDM) may independently influence offspring fat mass and metabolic disease susceptibility. In this pilot study, body composition and fat distribution in offspring from obese women with and without GDM and lean women were assessed within the first year of life, and maternal and newborn plasma factors were related to offspring adipose tissue distribution.

Methods: Serum and plasma samples from pregnant obese women with (n=16) or without (n=13) GDM and normoglycaemic lean women (n=15) at third trimester and offspring cord plasma were used for analysing lipid profiles, insulin and adipokine levels. At week-one and six, month-four and year-one, offspring anthropometrics and skinfold thickness (SFT) were measured, and abdominal subcutaneous (SCA) and preperitoneal adipose (PPA) tissue were determined by ultrasonography.
Results: Cord insulin was higher in the GDM group, whereas levels of cord leptin, total and high molecular weight (HMW) adiponectin were similar between the groups. Neonates of the GDM group showed higher SFT and fat mass until week-six and higher SCA at week-one compared with the lean group that persisted as strong trend at week-six. Interestingly, PPA in neonates of the GDM group was elevated at week-one compared with both the lean and obese group. At month-four and year-one, differences in adipose tissue growth between the groups were not observed. Multiple linear regression analyses revealed that cord insulin levels were independently related to neonatal PPA and were related to PPA development at year-one. Maternal fasting C-peptide and HMW adiponectin levels at third trimester emerged to be determinants for PPA at week-one.
Conclusions: Maternal pregravid obesity combined with GDM leads to newborn hyperinsulinaemia and increased offspring fat mass until week-six, whereas pregravid obesity without GDM does not. This strongly suggests the pivotal role of GDM in adverse offspring outcomes. Maternal C-peptide and HMW adiponectin levels in pregnancy were predictive for elevated PPA in newborns and might be indicative for the obesity risk at later life.

Childhood obesity is leading to rising incidences of type 2 diabetes mellitus and metabolic syndrome in children. Maternal obesity and gestational diabetes mellitus (GDM) may independently influence offspring fat mass and metabolic disease susceptibility. Besides maternal age, ethnicity and family history of diabetes, pregravid obesity is also a major predictor for GDM. Importantly, maternal obesity and GDM are independent risk factors for fetal hyperinsulinaemia, elevated weight and body fat at birth, suggesting that both GDM and pregravid obesity influence fetal development through a similar mechanism [12–14]. Children born to obese and/or diabetic mothers are at a higher risk for developing obesity and insulin resistance and diabetes from the childhood period into adolescence. The distribution of fat depots is a stronger predictor for the metabolic and cardiovascular risk than the total amount of fat. Visceral fat has been associated with insulin resistance, decreased adiponectin and hypertriglyceridaemia in children and adolescents. Ultrasonography is a valid method for measuring infant abdominal fat distribution in clinical research. Preperitoneal adipose (PPA) tissue assessed by ultrasonography has been proposed as a surrogate for visceral/intra-abdominal fat. However, there is missing information about metabolic markers, such as insulin, leptin and adiponectin, associated with the distribution of abdominal subcutaneous adipose (SCA) and PPA tissues in neonates and early infancy.

This study shows that that offspring of obese GDM mothers have higher cord blood insulin levels associated with higher fat mass than offspring of euglycaemic lean and obese mothers. The major novel findings are that abdominal SCA and PPA in infants from obese GDM mothers were higher at week-one and SFT was elevated at week-one and week-six compared with offspring of lean mothers. The neonatal PPA was highly related to PPA development at year-one. There was a positive relationship between maternal C-peptide levels for adipose tissue growth and obesity risk, and an inverse relationship for adiponectin with infant PPA at week one. However, these associations did not persist in the first year of life. The limitations of this pilot study are its small size, imbalanced offspring sex distribution and short observational follow-up period. However, the study does show that ultrasound can be used to characterise longitudinal adipose tissue growth and distribution and their association to blood markers and obesity risk.

Antepartum determinants of rapid early-life weight gain in term infants born to women with and without gestational diabetes

Kramer CK, Hamilton JK, Ye C, Hanley AJ, Connelly PW, Sermer M, Zinman B, Retnakaran R
Leadership Sinai Centre for Diabetes, Mount Sinai Hospital, Toronto, ON, Canada
Clinical Endocrinology 2014;81:387–394

Background: Rapid weight gain in the first three months of life has been associated with an unfavourable cardiometabolic phenotype in adulthood. However, little is known about the antepartum determinants of this rapid weight gain, which may reflect key developmental exposures that programme metabolic

pathways. The authors aimed to characterise the antepartum determinants of rapid weight gain in the first three months of life in infants exposed to gestational diabetes mellitus (GDM), a patient population at risk for early cardiometabolic disease.
Methods and patients: Prospective observational cohort study. Pregnant women with (n=90) and without (n=250) GDM underwent detailed antepartum metabolic characterisation, followed by assessment of their term offspring at age three months. Rapid infant weight gain in the first three months was defined as weight gain ≥0.5 SD.
Results: No features of maternal metabolic function in pregnancy (including insulin sensitivity, lipid profile, adiponectin, leptin and C-reactive protein) were associated with infant weight gain in either the GDM or non-GDM group. Interestingly, although all infants were born at term (≥37 weeks), length of gestation was inversely associated with weight gain at three months in the infants of women with GDM (beta=-148.5, P=0.01). In these infants, length of gestation <39 weeks was an independent predictor of rapid weight gain (OR=7.9, 95% CI 1.7–38, P=0.009) in the fully adjusted model. These associations were not observed in infants of women without GDM.
Conclusions: Delivery before 39 weeks was independently associated with rapid weight gain in the first three months of life in term infants of women with GDM and hence may be an antepartum marker of future cardio-metabolic risk.

Early life exposures play an important role in the later development of the metabolic syndrome. According to the Developmental Origins of Health and Disease paradigm, the risk of adult-onset metabolic syndrome is thought to originate as early as fetal development in utero. Exposure to an abnormal intrauterine environment might lead to reprogramming of fetal/infant metabolic pathways via epigenetic mechanisms [15,16]. Birthweight was initially considered a marker of developmental exposure that may relate to later metabolic syndrome. However, recent studies emphasise the importance of rapid early-life weight gain. Rapid weight gain (defined as weight gain ≥0.5 SD) in the first three months of life (as opposed to any other three-month interval in the first year) specifically predicts an unfavourable phenotype in early adulthood consisting of insulin resistance, increased waist circumference and adverse lipid profile. The findings of this study suggest that length of gestation was the major antepartum determinant of weight gain in the first three months of life in term infants of women with GDM. Specifically, those infants born before 39 weeks exhibited a robust independent association with rapid weight gain. Given the emergence of rapid infant weight gain as a predictor of future metabolic syndrome, these findings suggest that there may be long-term benefit in reaching 39 weeks' gestation before delivery, especially in women with GDM. Furthermore, children of women with GDM delivered before 39 weeks may represent a high-risk patient population that warrants closer surveillance for the early development of metabolic syndrome.

Fetal growth and metabolic syndrome

Fetal and infant growth patterns associated with total and abdominal fat distribution in school-age children

Gishti O, Gaillard R, Manniesing R, Abrahamse-Berkeveld M, van der Beek EM, Heppe DH, Steegers EA, Hofman A, Duijts L, Durmus B, Jaddoe VW
The Generation R Study Group, Erasmus University Medical Center, Rotterdam, The Netherlands
J Clin Endocrinol Metab 2014;99:2557–66

Background: Higher infant growth rates are associated with an increased risk of obesity in later life.
Objectives: The associations of longitudinally measured fetal and infant growth patterns with total and abdominal fat distribution in childhood were examined.
Study design, setting and patients: A population-based prospective cohort study among 6,464 children was performed. Growth characteristics in the second and third trimesters of pregnancy, at birth and at six, 12 and 24 months were undertaken.
Main outcome measures: Body mass index (BMI), fat mass index (body fat mass/height^2), lean mass index (body lean mass/height^2), android/gynoid fat ratio measured by dual-energy X-ray absorptiometry and

subcutaneous and preperitoneal abdominal fat measured by ultrasound at the median age of 6.0 years (90% range, 5.7–7.4).
Results: Weight gain in the second and third trimesters of fetal life and in early, mid and late infancy were independently and positively associated with childhood BMI (P<0.05). Only infant weight gain was associated with higher fat mass index, android/gynoid fat ratio and abdominal fat in childhood (P<0.05). Children with both fetal and infant growth acceleration had the highest childhood BMI, fat mass index and subcutaneous abdominal fat, whereas children with fetal growth deceleration and infant growth acceleration had the highest value for android/gynoid fat ratio and the lowest value for lean mass index (P<0.05).
Conclusion: Growth in both fetal life and infancy affects childhood BMI, whereas only infant growth directly affects measured total body and abdominal fat. Fetal growth deceleration followed by infant growth acceleration may lead to an adverse body fat distribution in childhood.

Fetal life and infancy are critical periods for the development of overweight and cardiometabolic diseases. Both children with high birthweight and those with low birthweight followed by infant growth acceleration have an increased risk of overweight in later life. Although higher infant weight gain is a well-established risk factor of childhood overweight, studies relating directly measured fetal growth to later adiposity are scarce. Also, BMI is a widely accepted outcome measure, but more detailed body fat distribution measures might be more strongly related to cardiometabolic risk factors.

The authors aimed to identify critical periods during fetal life and infancy that might be important for the development of an adverse total and abdominal fat profile in childhood. In 6,464 children participating in a population-based prospective cohort study from early fetal life onward, the authors examined the associations of repeatedly measured fetal and infant growth characteristics with childhood BMI and fat mass index, and abdominal fat distribution measured by dual-energy X-ray absorptiometry and abdominal ultrasound at the age of six years. The findings suggest that both fetal growth and infant growth affect childhood BMI, whereas only infant growth directly affects measured fat mass index, android fat (in areas such as the abdomen, chest, shoulder and nape of neck), gynoid fat mass (around the hips and bottom) and subcutaneous and preperitoneal abdominal fat. Fetal growth deceleration followed by infant growth acceleration may lead to an adverse body fat distribution. Further studies are needed to explore whether these growth patterns affect body fat distribution and risk of diseases later in life.

Genetic risk score for prediction of newborn adiposity and large-for-gestational-age birth

Chawla R, Badon SE, Rangarajan J, Reisetter AC, Armstrong LL, Lowe LP, Urbanek M, Metzger BE, Hayes MG, Scholtens DM, Lowe WL Jr
Division of Pediatric Endocrinology, Ann & Robert H. Lurie Children's Hospital of Chicago, IL, USA
J Clin Endocrinol Metab 2014;99:E2377–E2386

Background: Macrosomic infants are at increased risk for adverse metabolic outcomes. Prediction of large-for-gestational-age (LGA) birth may help prevent these outcomes.
Objective: To determine whether genes associated with obesity-related traits in adults are associated with newborn size, and whether a genetic risk score (GRS) predicts LGA birth.
Methods: Single nucleotide polymorphisms (SNPs) in 40 regions associated with adult obesity-related traits were tested for association with newborn size. GRSs for birthweight and sum of skinfolds (SSF) specific to ancestry were calculated using the most highly associated SNP for each ancestry in genomic regions with one or more SNPs associated with birth weight and/or SSF in at least one ancestry group or meta-analyses.
Patients: Newborns from the Hyperglycemia Adverse Pregnancy Outcomes Study were studied (942 Afro-Caribbean, 1,294 Northern European, 573 Mexican-American and 1,182 Thai).
Outcome measures: Birthweight >90th percentile (LGA) and newborn SSF >90th percentile were primary outcomes.
Results: After adjustment for ancestry, sex, gestational age at delivery, parity, maternal genotype, maternal smoking/alcohol intake, age, BMI, height, blood pressure and glucose, 25 and 23 SNPs were associated (P<0.001) with birthweight and newborn SSF, respectively. The GRS was highly associated with

both phenotypes as continuous variables across all ancestries ($P \leq 1.6 \times 10^{-19}$) and improved prediction of birthweight and SSF >90th percentile when added to a baseline model incorporating the covariates listed above.
Conclusions: A GRS comprised of SNPs associated with adult obesity-related traits may provide an approach for predicting LGA birth and newborn adiposity beyond established risk factors.

Infants born large for gestational age (LGA) (birthweight for gestational age >90th percentile) are at increased risk of adverse perinatal outcomes and infant mortality. High birthweight is also associated with adverse metabolic outcomes during childhood and adulthood, including higher risk of metabolic diseases such as obesity, dyslipidaemia, hypertension and type 2 diabetes. In addition, former LGA mothers themselves are at increased risk for having LGA offspring, perpetuating the cycle of adverse metabolic health outcomes. The incidence of LGA birth has increased over the last three decades, likely due, in part, to environmental changes in the setting of an underlying genetic predisposition. Fetal growth and adiposity are influenced by complex interactions between fetal genes and the intra-uterine environment, with maternal glucose having a significant effect on birthweight and adiposity. Limited information is available on fetal genetic variation that influences size at birth, although recent genome-wide association data have identified several loci associated with birthweight or newborn adiposity. These loci have generally not demonstrated associations with adult obesity.

The present study tested whether genetic variation within genes associated with adult obesity-related traits is associated with newborn size. These studies were performed using genome-wide single nucleotide polymorphism (SNP) data collected from four different ancestry groups by the Hyperglycaemia and Adverse Pregnancy Outcome Study, an observational study that examined associations of levels of glucose intolerance during pregnancy and risks of adverse newborn outcomes. Genetic risk scores (GRSs) comprised of SNPs with ancestry-specific associations created to ascertain whether a greater burden of adult obesity susceptibility alleles is associated with higher birthweight and greater newborn adiposity and whether application of the GRS improves prediction of LGA birth and greater newborn adiposity beyond traditional risk factors. The results showed that 25 and 23 SNPs were associated with birthweight and newborn SSF, respectively. Limitations of the study were the lack of data on gestational weight gain and maternal nutrition, both of which can affect fetal size at birth.

Association of cord blood leptin, soluble leptin receptor, insulin-like growth factor-I and insulin-like growth factor-binding protein-1 on birth indices in healthy full-term newborns

Tennekoon KH, Poopalapillai J, Karunanayake AG, Jayasinghe HD, Kumarasiri JM, De SWAP, Karunanayake EH
Institute of Biochemistry, Molecular Biology and Biotechnology, University of Colombo, Colombo, Sri Lanka
Horm Res Paediatr 2014;81:232–238

Background: Leptin and insulin-like growth factor-I (IGF-I) promote fetal growth. Their availability is modulated by soluble leptin receptor (SLR) and insulin-like growth factor-binding proteins (IGFBP). Studies that accounted for SLR levels when investigating the association of leptin, IGF-I and IGFBPs on birth indices are scarce.
Methods: Cord blood leptin, SLR, IGF-I, IGFBP-1 and their association with birth indices were studied in term newborns (n=110; males=60). Univariate correlations and multiple regression analyses were performed to identify variables that influence birth indices.
Results: Birth indices were comparable between male and female newborns. Females had a lower SLR (P=0.014), a higher leptin/Ponderal Index (P=0.033) and a higher free leptin index (leptin/SLR) (P=0.008). Leptin and male gender positively and IGFBP-1 negatively influenced birthweight (P=0.0005, P=0.02 and P=0.005, respectively) and head circumference (P=0.005, P=0.0098 and P=0.018, respectively), accounting for other variables. In a different multiple regression model, the free leptin index positively influenced crown–heel length (P=0.0016) in addition to birthweight (P<0.0001) and head circumference (P=0.0016).
Conclusions: In healthy full-term pregnancies, cord blood leptin and IGFBP-1 exert independent and opposing effects on fetal growth.

Leptin and insulin-like growth factor-I (IGF-I) are known to promote fetal growth and some studies have suggested their growth regulatory effects to be independent of each other. Bioavailability of leptin is modulated by soluble leptin receptor (SLR) and that of IGF-I by IGF-binding proteins (IGFBP). SLR is devoid of transmembrane and cytoplasmic domains and hence is secreted and binds to circulating leptin. SLR is generated either by alternative splicing or by shedding of the ectodomain of membrane-bound receptor isoforms. Cord blood SLR has been shown to exert a negative effect on birthweight and SLR levels may be elevated in the absence of a difference in leptin levels in intrauterine growth restriction compared with appropriate for gestational age newborns.

The present study examined cord blood levels of leptin, SLR and the free leptin index in a cohort of full-term newborns to identify the effects of these on birth indices while accounting for the possible effects exerted by IGF-I and IGFBP-1. The authors observed that cord blood leptin and male gender independently increased birthweight and head circumference, whereas cord blood IGFBP-1 independently decreased birthweight and head circumference. SLR, IGF-I and maternal parity had no effect on birthweight or head circumference. Cord blood IGF-I levels were not associated with any of the birth indices whereas IGBBP-1 showed significant negative correlations and the IGF-I/IGFBP-1 ratio showed significant positive correlations with birthweight, crown-heel length and head circumference.

Maternal glucose homeostasis and its impact on fetal growth

Fetal growth is associated with maternal fasting plasma glucose at first prenatal visit

Liu B, Chen H, Xu Y, An C, Zhong L, Wang X, Zhang Y, Chen H, Zhang J, Wang Z
Department of Obstetrics and Gynecology, The First Affiliated Hospital of Sun Yat-sen University, Guangzhou, PR China
PloS One 2014;9:e116352

Background: Fasting plasma glucose (FPG) concentration measured at the first prenatal visit is a predictor of gestational diabetes mellitus (GDM); however, whether this test is indicative of fetal growth has not been clarified. This study aimed to determine whether birthweight and birth length are related to FPG concentration at the first prenatal visit.
Methods: Research samples were collected from pregnant women who took an FPG test at their first prenatal visit (10–24 gestational weeks), received regular prenatal care and delivered in one centre. FPG value, maternal pregravid BMI, weight gain before FPG test, before and after oral glucose tolerance test (OGTT), neonatal birthweight, birth length, Ponderal Index and birthing method were recorded for analysis. Data were analysed by independent sample t-test, Pearson correlation and Chi-square test, followed by partial correlation or logistic regression to confirm differences.
Results: 2,284 pregnant women, including 462 GDM and 1,822 with normal glucose tolerance (NGT) were recruited for the present study. FPG concentration at the first prenatal visit was associated with neonatal birthweight (partial correlation coefficient $r'=0.089$, $P<0.001$) and birth length ($r'=0.061$, $P=0.005$), but not with Ponderal Index or birthing method. Maternal pregravid BMI was associated with FPG value ($r'=0.113$, $P<0.001$). FPG concentration at the first prenatal visit (OR=2.945, $P<0.001$), weight gain before OGTT test (OR=1.039, $P=0.010$) and age (OR=1.107, $P<0.001$) were independent related factors of GDM.
Conclusions: FPG at the first prenatal visit is associated with fetal growth. Maternal pregravid BMI and weight gain are related to glucose metabolism.

Gestational diabetes mellitus (GDM) is common all over the world and is associated with several adverse fetal consequences, including macrosomia, respiratory distress syndrome and hypoglycaemia. Moreover, offspring of GDM mothers are more likely to develop diabetes, obesity and metabolic disorder in childhood and adulthood. A recent study reported that hyperglycaemia at the first prenatal visit was an early indicator of subsequent GDM and demonstrated the importance of a fasting plasma glucose (FPG) test during the early stages of pregnancy [17].

The current study aimed to investigate the relationship between FPG in early pregnancy and fetal growth, and to look at the possible correlations between maternal BMI, weight gain and glycaemic metabolism. The main findings were that basal glucose concentration (at first prenatal visit and at oral glucose tolerance test) is associated with neonatal birth weight and length, while maternal pre-gravid BMI and gestational weight gain is related to glycaemic metabolism. The clinical relevance of this study is the importance of the FPG test in the early stages of pregnancy, not only as an indicator of GDM, but also a predictor of fetal growth [18].

Elevated FGF21 leads to attenuated postnatal linear growth in preterm infants through GH resistance in chondrocytes

Guasti L, Silvennoinen S, Bulstrode NW, Ferretti P, Sankilampi U, Dunkel L
Centre for Endocrinology, William Harvey Research Institute, Barts and the London, Queen Mary University of London, London, UK
J Clin Endocrinol Metab 2014;99:E2198–E2206

Background: The hormone fibroblast growth factor 21 (FGF21) is a key metabolic regulator in the adaptation to fasting. In food-restricted mice, inhibition of skeletal growth is mediated by the antagonistic effect of FGF21 on growth hormone (GH) action in the liver and growth plate.
Objective: To assess the role of FGF21 in growth regulation in humans using postnatal growth failure of very preterm infants as a model.
Methods: FGF21 levels were measured serially in very preterm infants, and their linear growth evaluated from birth to term-equivalent age. Primary chondrocytes obtained from paediatric donors were used to test whether FGF21 can directly interfere with GH signalling.
Results: A negative association (beta=-0.415, P<0.005, linear regression model) of FGF21 levels with the change in SD score for length was found. In primary chondrocytes, FGF21 upregulated basal and GH-induced SOCS2 expression and inhibited GH-induced signal transducer and activator of transcription 5 phosphorylation as well as GH-induced COLII and ALP expression. Finally, FGF21 inhibited GH-induced IGF-1 expression and cell proliferation, indicating GH resistance. However, FGF21 did not affect IGF-1-induced cell proliferation.
Conclusions: Elevated FGF21 serum levels during the first weeks of life are independently associated with postnatal growth failure in preterm infants. Furthermore, these data provide mechanistic insights into GH resistance secondary to prematurity and may offer an explanation for the growth failure commonly seen in chronic conditions of childhood.

Fibroblast growth factor 21 (FGF21) is predominantly produced by the liver, but is also expressed in adipocytes and the pancreas. It regulates glucose and lipid metabolism through pleiotropic actions in these tissues and the brain. In mice, fasting leads to increased PPAR-alpha mediated expression of FGF21 in the liver where it stimulates gluconeogenesis, fatty acid oxidation and ketogenesis as an adaptive response to fasting and starvation. In the fed state, FGF21 acts as an autocrine factor in adipocytes, regulating the activity of PPAR-gamma through a feed-forward loop mechanism. During calorie restriction in mice, increased expression of FGF21 causes growth attenuation and growth hormone (GH) insensitivity. Increased expression of FGF21 during chronic food restriction is associated with reduced bone growth and growth hormone (GH) insensitivity. Increased expression of FGF21 during food restriction causes growth attenuation by antagonising the GH stimulatory effects on chondrogenesis directly at the growth plate. In addition, high concentrations of FGF21 may directly suppress growth plate chondrocyte proliferation and differentiation [19–21].

In the current study plasma FGF21 levels were measured serially in very preterm infants and their linear growth was evaluated from birth to term-equivalent age. A negative correlation was found between the level of FGF21 and linear growth. High levels of FGF21 were associated with growth failure in these preterm infants. The mechanism might involve GH resistance. GH signalling is negatively regulated by the Suppressor of Cytokine Signaling-2 (SOCS2) and increased FGF21 leads to GH resistance by GH-induced SOCS2 expression and inhibiting GH-induced signal transducer and activator of transcription 5 (STAT5) phosphorylation. This provides further mechanistic insights into the interaction between FGF21 and GH.

In utero undernutrition in male mice programmes liver lipid metabolism in the second-generation offspring involving altered Lxra DNA methylation

Martinez D, Pentinat T, Ribo S, Daviaud C, Bloks VW, Cebria J, Villalmanzo N, Kalko SG, Ramon-Krauel M, Diaz R, Plosch T, Tost J, Jimenez-Chillaron JC
Hospital Sant Joan de Deu, Pediatric Endocrinology, Esplugues de Llobregat, Barcelona, Spain
jjimenezc@fsjd.org
Cell Metab 2014;19:941-951

Background: Obesity and type 2 diabetes have heritable components that are not fully attributable to genetic factors. Instead, epigenetic mechanisms may play a role.
Methods: The authors developed a mouse model of intrauterine growth restriction (IUGR) by in utero malnutrition.
Results: IUGR mice developed obesity and glucose intolerance with ageing. Strikingly, offspring of IUGR male mice also developed glucose intolerance. In utero malnutrition of F1 (first generation) males influenced the expression of lipogenic genes in livers of F2 (second generation) mice, partly due to altered expression of the liver X receptor-alpha (Lxra). In turn, Lxra expression is attributed to altered DNA methylation of its 5' UTR region. The same epigenetic signature in the sperm of their progenitors, F1 males was found.
Conclusion: In utero malnutrition results in epigenetic modifications in germ cells (F1) that are subsequently transmitted and maintained in somatic cells of the F2, thereby influencing health and disease risk of the offspring.

Among early environmental exposures, nutrition plays a key role in predisposition to type 2 diabetes mellitus (T2DM), not only to directly exposed individuals, but also to their offspring and, in a few striking examples, their grand-offspring. Offspring of people exposed to malnutrition in utero have increased prevalence of cardiovascular disease and T2DM risk. Likewise, increased grand-paternal food supply during the prepubertal growth period augmented the risk of cardiovascular and diabetes-related death in their grandchildren. In agreement, in rodent models, nutritional imbalance during fetal and/or early neonatal development also increased the risk of obesity, glucose intolerance, insulin resistance and T2DM in the following generation. It has been proposed that transmission of such environmentally acquired phenotypes may be mediated by epigenetic mechanisms, which is conceptually termed as transgenerational epigenetic inheritance. This refers to the transmission of a specific phenotype to the next generation offspring via epigenetic modifications in the germline [22–24].

The authors tested the hypothesis that epigenetic modifications, namely DNA methylation, contribute to the development of metabolic dysfunction in the second-generation offspring through the paternal lineage. To evaluate this, the authors analysed global gene expression profile and specific DNA methylation signatures in livers from IUGR-F2 mice. They then determined whether the epigenetic signatures identified in the liver were already present in the sperm of their progenitors (IUGR-F1). They found that the in utero malnutrition altered the patterns of DNA methylation of the liver X receptor-alpha (Lxra) locus in sperm samples of IUGR-first generation males and liver samples of their offspring (IUGR-second generation). These data suggest that in utero under nutrition may reprogramme the epigenome of cells from the germline/mature gametes that can be inherited into the next generation offspring, thereby influencing health and disease risk.

Hypotension following patent ductus arteriosus ligation: the role of adrenal hormones

Clyman RI, Wickremasinghe A, Merritt TA, Solomon T, McNamara P, Jain A, Singh J, Chu A, Noori S, Sekar K, Lavoie PM, Attridge JT, Swanson JR, Gillam-Krakauer M, Reese J, DeMauro S, Poindexter B, Aucott S, Satpute M, Fernandez E, Auchus RJ, Patent Ductus Arteriosus Ligation/Hypotension Trial Investigators
Department of Pediatrics, Cardiovascular Research Institute, University of California San Francisco, San Francisco, CA, USA
clymanr@peds.ucsf.edu
J Pediatr 2014;164:1449–1455.e1

Background: To test the hypothesis that an impaired adrenal response to stress might contribute to the hypotension that follows patent ductus arteriosus (PDA) ligation.
Methods: A multicentre study of infants born at <32 weeks' gestation who were about to undergo PDA ligation. Serum adrenal steroids were measured three times: before and after a cosyntropin (1.0 microgram/kg) stimulation test (performed before the ligation), and at 10–12 hours after PDA ligation. A standardised approach for diagnosis and treatment of postoperative hypotension was followed. A modified inotrope score (1 x dopamine [microgram/kg/min] + 1 x dobutamine) was used to quantify catecholamine support. Infants were considered to have catecholamine-resistant hypotension if their greatest inotrope score was >15.
Results: Of 95 infants enrolled, 43 (45%) developed hypotension and 14 (15%) developed catecholamine-resistant hypotension. Low postoperative cortisol levels were not associated with the overall incidence of hypotension after ligation. However, low cortisol levels were associated with the refractoriness of the hypotension to catecholamine treatment. In a multivariate analysis the risk for catecholamine-resistant hypotension was OR 36.6 (95% CI 2.8–476, P=0.006). Low cortisol levels (in infants with catecholamine-resistant hypotension) were not attributable to adrenal immaturity or impairment; their cortisol precursor concentrations were either low or unchanged, and their response to cosyntropin was similar to infants without catecholamine-resistant hypotension.
Conclusion: Infants with low cortisol concentrations after PDA ligation are likely to develop postoperative catecholamine-resistant hypotension. It is speculated that decreased adrenal stimulation, rather than an impaired adrenal response to stimulation, may account for the decreased production.

Some 25–35% of preterm infants having surgical ligation of the patent ductus arteriosus (PDA) develop systemic hypotension and haemodynamic deterioration approximately eight to 14 hours after the procedure. The underlying factors are unclear. Retrospective studies have not identified differences in the surgical, anaesthetic or intraoperative fluid management. Indices of impaired myocardial performance are often observed before the development of hypotension and prophylactic administration shortly after surgery of milrinone (a phosphodiesterase 3 inhibitor that increases the heart's contractility and decreases pulmonary vascular resistance) appears to reduce the incidence of cardiorespiratory instability.

Preterm infants have an altered adrenal response to hypotension and postnatal stress during the first week of life: in 30%, the cortisol levels are increased with postnatal stress but in 70% the levels are either similar to or lower than those of healthy infants. Infants at risk for perioperative hypotension may have depressed cortisol responses to (ACTH1-24) stimulation [25–27].

This study was designed to test the following hypotheses: 1) infants who develop hypotension after PDA ligation have a diminished postoperative cortisol response compared with normotensive infants; 2) infants who develop catecholamine-resistant hypotension have the most diminished cortisol response and have a limited ability to convert cortisol precursors to cortisol (or a more rapid conversion of cortisol to cortisone); and 3) preoperative measurements of cortisol precursors or metabolites (before and after ACTH stimulation) predict which infants develop post-ligation cardiopulmonary deterioration. The authors found that low postoperative cortisol concentrations were not associated with the incidence of postoperative hypotension. They were, however, associated with the severity of hypotension when it occurred and its resistance to catecholamine treatment. Decreased adrenal stimulation, rather than adrenal immaturity or impairment, may be responsible for the decreased cortisol concentrations in these hypotensive infants. The authors suggest a prospective controlled trial to elucidate the contribution of low cortisol production to the severity of postoperative hypotension.

Neonatal estrogen exposure results in biphasic age-dependent effects on the skeletal development of male mice

Connelly KJ, Larson EA, Marks DL, Klein RF
Department of Pediatrics, Oregon Health and Science University, Doernbecher Children's Hospital, Portland, OR, USA
Endocrinology 2015;156:193–202

Background: Peak bone mass, one of the most important predictors for fracture risk later in life, is attained during puberty and adolescence, and is influenced by neonatal and pubertal sex-specific gonadal hormones and GH-IGF-I secretion patterns.
Methods: This study examined the effects of brief neonatal estrogen (NE) exposure on growth and skeletal development in C57BL/6J mice. A single injection of 100 microgram estradiol or vehicle was administered on the first day of life. Growth parameters were monitored and skeletal phenotyping performed at 16 weeks in female mice and at four and 16 weeks in male mice.
Results: NE exposure negatively impacted adult femoral length in both sexes, but adult body weight, areal bone density and bone strength in female mice were unaffected. In contrast, somatic growth was attenuated in estrogen-exposed male mice throughout the study period. At the prepubertal time point, the estrogen-exposed males exhibited higher bone mineral density, cortical volume and cortical thickness compared with controls. However, by the time of peak bone mass acquisition, the early skeletal findings had reversed; estrogen-exposed mice had lower bone density with reduced cross-sectional area, cortical volume and cortical thickness, resulting in cortical bones that were less resistant to fracture. NE exposure also resulted in reduced testicular volume and lower circulating IGF-I.
Conclusions: Male mice exposed to estrogen on the first day of life experience age-dependent changes in skeletal development. Prepubertal animals experience greater endocortical bone acquisition as a result of estrogen exposure. However, by adulthood, continued developmental changes result in overall reduced skeletal integrity.

Estrogens have important effects on bone turnover in both humans and animal models. The presence of the estrogen receptor on both osteoblasts and osteoclasts has suggested a direct role of these steroid hormones on bone. Thus, this tissue is now regarded as a specific estrogen target tissue [28–30]. Exposure to estrogens during various stages of development irreversibly influences the responsive target organs. During early (days one to five of life) development, transient exposure to estrogen of female mice results in an augmented bone density in the adult animals. Alterations in the maternal estrogenic levels during pregnancy can influence early phases of fetal bone tissue development and subsequently result in permanent changes in the skeleton. The effect of this short-term estrogen treatment can be seen in the fetal skeleton, suggesting an estrogen-imprinting effect on bone cell-programming in fetal life because treatment effects on bone cell turnover can be observed later in adult life. This study suggests that brief neonatal estrogen has marked age-specific effects on male mice compared with female mice. However, it is not clear what the underlying mechanisms are of these observations.

References

1. Mak CM, Lee CY, Lam CW, Siu WK, Hung VC, Chan AY. Personalized medicine switching from insulin to sulfonylurea in permanent neonatal diabetes mellitus dictated by a novel activating ABCC8 mutation. Diagn Mol Pathol 2012;21:56–59.
2. Pearson ER, Flechtner I, Njølstad PR, Malecki MT, Flanagan SE, Larkin B, et al. Switching from insulin to oral sulfonylureas in patients with diabetes due to Kir6.2 mutations. N Engl J Med 2006;355:467–477.
3. Rafiq M, Flanagan SE, Patch AM, Shields BM, Ellard S, Hattersley AT; Neonatal Diabetes International Collaborative Group. Effective treatment with oral sulfonylureas in patients with diabetes due to sulfonylurea receptor 1 (SUR1) mutations. Diabetes Care 2008;31:204–209.
4. Minami K. GATA transcription factors: New key regulators in pancreas organogenesis. J Diabetes Investig 2013;4:426–427.

5. Viger RS, Guittot SM, Anttonen M, Wilson DB, Heikinheimo M. Role of the GATA family of transcription factors in endocrine development, function, and disease. Mol Endocrinol 2008;22:781–798.
6. Demirbilek H, Arya VB, Ozbek MN, Houghton JA, Baran RT, Akar M, et al. Clinical characteristics and molecular genetic analysis of 22 patients with neonatal diabetes from the South-Eastern region of Turkey: predominance of non-KATP channel mutations. Eur J Endocrinol 2015;172:697–705.
7. Sellick GS, Barker KT, Stolte-Dijkstra I, Fleischmann C, Coleman RJ, Garrett C, et al. Mutations in PTF1A cause pancreatic and cerebellar agenesis. Nat Genet 2004;36:1301–1305.
8. Masui T, Swift GH, Hale MA, Meredith DM, Johnson JE, Macdonald RJ. Transcriptional autoregulation controls pancreatic Ptf1a expression during development and adulthood. Mol Cell Biol 2008;28:5458–5468.
9. Fanelli C, Di Vincenzo A, Modarelli F, Lepore M, Ciofetta M, Epifano L, et al. Post-hypoglycaemic hyperketonaemia does not contribute to brain metabolism during insulin-induced hypoglycaemia in humans. Diabetologia 1993;36:1191–1197.
10. Maayan-Metzger A, Lubin D, Kuint J. Hypoglycemia rates in the first days of life among term infants born to diabetic mothers. Neonatology 2009;96:80–85.
11. Harris DL, Weston PJ, Harding JE. Incidence of neonatal hypoglycemia in babies identified as at risk. J Pediatr 2012;161:787–791.
12. Boney CM, Verma A, Tucker R, Vohr BR. Metabolic syndrome in childhood: association with birth weight, maternal obesity, and gestational diabetes mellitus. Pediatrics 2005;115(3):e290–e296.
13. Gillman MW, Rifas-Shiman S, Berkey CS, Field AE, Colditz GA. Maternal gestational diabetes, birth weight, and adolescent obesity. Pediatrics 2003;111(3):e221–e226.
14. Catalano PM, Farrell K, Thomas A, Huston-Presley L, Mencin P, de Mouzon SH, et al. Perinatal risk factors for childhood obesity and metabolic dysregulation. Am J Clin Nutr 2009;90:1303–1313.
15. Retnakaran R, Ye C, Hanley A, Sermer M, Connelly P, Zinman B, et al. Effect of maternal gestational diabetes on the cardiovascular risk factor profile of infants at 1 year of age. Nutr Metab Cardiovasc Dis 2013;23:1175–1181.
16. Black MH, Sacks DA, Xiang AH, Lawrence JM. The relative contribution of prepregnancy overweight and obesity, gestational weight gain, and IADPSG-defined gestational diabetes mellitus to fetal overgrowth. Diabetes Care 2013;36:56–62.
17. Zhu WW, Yang HX, Wei YM, Yan J, Wang ZL, Li XL, et al. Evaluation of the value of fasting plasma glucose in the first prenatal visit to diagnose gestational diabetes mellitus in china. Diabetes Care 2013;36:586–590.
18. Mello G, Parretti E, Cioni R, Lucchetti R, Carignani L, Martini E, et al. The 75-gram glucose load in pregnancy: relation between glucose levels and anthropometric characteristics of infants born to women with normal glucose metabolism. Diabetes Care 2003;26:1206–1210.
19. Wu S, Grunwald T, Kharitonenkov A, Dam J, Jockers R, De Luca F. Increased expression of fibroblast growth factor 21 (FGF21) during chronic undernutrition causes growth hormone insensitivity in chondrocytes by inducing leptin receptor overlapping transcript (LEPROT) and leptin receptor overlapping transcript-like 1 (LEPROTL1) expression. J Biol Chem 2013;288:27375–27383.
20. Kubicky RA, Wu S, Kharitonenkov A, De Luca F. Role of fibroblast growth factor 21 (FGF21) in undernutrition-related attenuation of growth in mice. Endocrinology 2012;153:2287–2295.
21. Inagaki T, Lin VY, Goetz R, Mohammadi M, Mangelsdorf DJ, Kliewer SA. Inhibition of growth hormone signaling by the fasting-induced hormone FGF21. Cell Metab 2008 Jul;8(1):77–83.
22. Jimenez-Chillaron JC, Isganaitis E, Charalambous M, Gesta S, Pentinat-Pelegrin T, Faucette RR, et al. Intergenerational transmission of glucose intolerance and obesity by in utero undernutrition in mice. Diabetes 2009;58:460–468.
23. Ding GL, Wang FF, Shu J, Tian S, Jiang Y, Zhang D, et al. Transgenerational glucose intolerance with Igf2/H19 epigenetic alterations in mouse islet induced by intrauterine hyperglycemia. Diabetes 2012;61(5):1133–1142.
24. Radford EJ, Ito M, Shi H, Corish JA, Yamazawa K, Isganaitis E, et al. In utero effects. In utero undernourishment perturbs the adult sperm methylome and intergenerational metabolism. Science 2014;345:1255903.
25. EL-Khuffash A, McNamara PJ, Lapointe A, Jain A. Adrenal function in preterm infants undergoing patent ductus arteriosus ligation. Neonatology 2013;104:28–33.
26. Naik-Mathuria B, Chang S, Fitch ME, Westhoff J, Brandt ML, Ayres NA, et al. Patent ductus arteriosus ligation in neonates: preoperative predictors of poor postoperative outcomes. J Pediatr Surg 2008;43:1100–1105.
27. Moin F, Kennedy KA, Moya FR. Risk factors predicting vasopressor use after patent ductus arteriosus ligation. Am J Perinatol 2003;20:313–320.
28. Venken K, Schuit F, Van Lommel L, Tsukamoto K, Kopchick JJ, Coschigano K, et al. Growth without growth hormone receptor: estradiol is a major growth hormone-independent regulator of hepatic IGF-I synthesis. J Bone Miner Res 2005;20:2138–2149.
29. Kennedy OD, Sun H, Wu Y, Courtland HW, Williams GA, Cardoso L, et al. Skeletal response of male mice to anabolic hormone therapy in the absence of the Igfals gene. Endocrinology 2014;155:987–999.
30. Migliaccio S, Newbold RR, Bullock BC, Jefferson WJ, Sutton FG Jr, McLachlan JA, et al. Alterations of maternal estrogen levels during gestation affect the skeleton of female offspring. Endocrinology 1996;137:2118–2125.

Thyroid

Gabor Szinnai[a], Athanasia Stoupa[b,c], Dulanjalee Kariyawasam[b,d], Sanjay Gawade[a], Aurore Carré[c,d] and Michel Polak[b–d]

[a]Pediatric Endocrinology, University Children's Hospital Basel, and Department of Biomedicine, University of Basel, Basel, Switzerland

[b]Pediatric Endocrinology, Gynecology and Diabetology, Necker Enfants-Malades Hospital, Assistance Publique-Hôpitaux de Paris, IMAGINE Institute, Université Paris Descartes, Sorbonne Paris Cité, Paris, France

[c]Imagine Institute, Paris Descartes-Sorbonne Paris Cité University, France

[d]INSERM U1016, Université Paris Descartes, Faculté de Médecine, Hôpital Cochin, Paris, France

To present the last year's clinically and experimentally most relevant and innovative manuscripts in the field of thyroid disease is the task when preparing the Yearbook. During the year, a large number of papers are saved in the folder 'Yearbook 2015', however, only a few finally make it into this chapter. We picked out a range of papers covering clinical, translational and fundamental work that in our opinion could either change our clinical approach to patients or open new avenues in the molecular understanding of thyroid diseases from congenital hypothyroidism to thyroid cancer. We hope you enjoy reading this year's selection.

Clinical aspects of hypothyroidism

Systematic appraisal of lactose intolerance as cause of increased need for oral thyroxine

Cellini M, Santaguida MG, Gatto I, Virili C, Del Duca SC, Brusca N, Capriello S, Gargano L, Centanni M

Department of Medico-Surgical Sciences and Biotechnologies, «Sapienza» University of Roma, and Endocrinology Unit, Azienda Unita Sanitaria Locale Latina, Latina, Italy

J Clin Endocrinol Metab 2014;99:E1454–E1458

Background: There is a lack of systematic studies assessing the need for T4 dose modification in hypothyroid patients with lactose intolerance, a widespread and often occult disorder.
Methods: The authors assessed the dose required in hypothyroid patients with lactose intolerance and non-compliance with lactose-free diet in a monocentre cohort study.
Results: In all patients with isolated Hashimoto's thyroiditis, target TSH (median TSH 1.02mU/L) was obtained at a median T4 dose of 1.31 microgram/kg/d. In patients also with both Hashimoto's thyroiditis and lactose intolerance, only 5/34 patients reached the desired TSH (median TSH 0.83mU/L) with a similar T4 dose (1.29 microgram/kg/d). In 29/34 patients, the T4 dose was progressively increased and the target TSH (median TSH 1.21mU/L) was only attained at a median T4 dose of 1.81 microgram/kg/d (+38%, P<0.0001). In the 23/29 patients with isolated lactose intolerance, a median T4 dose of 1.72 microgram/kg/d (+31%, P<0.0001) was required to attain normal thyroid function, while in 6/29 patients, other gastrointestinal disorders were diagnosed, and their median T4 requirement was even higher (2.04 microgram/kg/d; +55%; P=0.0032).
Conclusions: Lactose intolerance increased the necessary oral LT4 dose to reach normal TSH levels in hypothyroid patients.

An increased need for T4 has been described in patients with various gastrointestinal disorders, due to the reduced resorptive capacity of the intestine. Besides coeliac disease, lactose intolerance should be considered if unusually high doses of LT4 substitution are necessary to reach euthyroidism, and in patients with known lactose intolerance higher doses should be prescribed.

The severity of congenital hypothyroidism of central origin should not be underestimated

Zwaveling-Soonawala N, van Trotsenburg AS, Verkerk PH
Department of Pediatric Endocrinology, Emma Children's Hospital, Academic Medical Center, University of Amsterdam, Amsterdam, The Netherlands
J Clin Endocrinol Metab 2015;100:E297–E300

Background: Only a few screening programmes measure total or free T4 and TSH simultaneously or stepwise, enabling detection of congenital hypothyroidism of thyroidal (CHT) as well as congenital hypothyroidism of central origin (CHC). The authors aimed to assess disease severity of CHC compared with CHT in a Dutch cohort of CH patients.
Methods: Pretreatment FT4 concentrations were analysed in all children with CH detected by the Dutch neonatal T4+TSH+T4-binding-globulin (TBG) screening between 1995 and 2011. Disease severity was classified using the FT4-based ESPE classification.
Results: 1,288 children were diagnosed with CH between 1995 and 2011. Data of 1,200 (143 CHC and 1,057 CHT) were available for analysis. Based on FT4 concentrations, four children with CHC (2.8%) had severe, 75 (52.4%) had moderate and 64 (44.8%) had mild CH. In the CHT group, 280 children (26.5%) had severe, 341 (32.3%) moderate and 436 (41.2%) mild CH.
Conclusion: Based on initial FT4 values, severe CH was much more prevalent in CHT compared with CHC. However, more than half of CHC patients have moderate CH with initial FT4 below 10pmol/L (0.78ng/dL).

Systematic detection of central congenital hypothyroidism is only possible by combined TSH and T4 based screening programs. A frequently used argument against screening for central congenital hypothyroidism by combined TSH and T4 screening is its presumed mild hypothyroid character. However, the article presented here systematically reviewed the severity of central congenital hypothyroidism in the Netherlands, where neonatal screening is based on T4+TSH+T4-binding globulin measurements. Central congenital hypothyroidism occurred in 12% of all patients. Two messages are important: the severity of central hypothyroidism should not be underestimated; and the policy of neonatal screening should be re-evaluated with these data.

Pregnancy outcomes and relationship to treatment adequacy in women treated early for congenital hypothyroidism: a longitudinal population-based study

Léger J, dos Santos S, Larroque B, Ecosse E
Assistance Publique-Hopitaux de Paris, Hopital Robert Debre, Service d'Endocrinologie Diabetologie Pediatrique, Centre de Reference des Maladies Endocriniennes Rares de la Croissance, Paris, France
J Clin Endocrinol Metab 2015;100:860–869

Background: Hypothyroidism during pregnancy is well known to be associated with adverse outcomes in the mother and her children. So far no data are available on pregnancy outcomes in mothers diagnosed and treated for congenital hypothyroidism (CH) and on the outcome of their children.
Methods: In a cohort of 1,158 women with CH, 207 singleton pregnancies ending >22 weeks were identified retrospectively by questionnaire, and 174 pregnancies were studied prospectively in the three years following the initial questionnaire survey. The reference group comprised 7,245 subjects from the French National Perinatal Survey.
Results: In both the overall and prospective analyses, CH was associated with gestational hypertension, emergency caesarean delivery, induced labour for vaginal delivery and prematurity. In the prospective study, the adjusted odds ratios (aOR) (95% confidence intervals [CI]) were 2.19 (1.26–3.81), 1.88 (1.17–3.02), 1.58 (1.12–2.24) and 1.85 (1.06–3.25), respectively. TSH concentrations at least 10mIU/L during the first three or six months of pregnancy were associated with a higher risk of preterm delivery (aOR, 5.6; 95% CI 1.6–20.0) and fetal macrosomia (aOR, 4.5; 95% CI 1.03–20.1), respectively, whereas no such relationship was observed for TSH concentrations of 5.0–9.9mIU/L.
Conclusion: Adverse pregnancy outcomes in patients with CH treated early in life, can be documented especially when thyroid supplementation is not adequate.

Maternal perchlorate levels in women with borderline thyroid function during pregnancy and the cognitive development of their offspring: data from the Controlled Antenatal Thyroid Study

Taylor PN, Okosieme OE, Murphy R, Hales C, Chiusano E, Maina A, Joomun M, Bestwick JP, Smyth P, Paradice R, Channon S, Braverman LE, Dayan CM, Lazarus JH, Pearce EN
Thyroid Research Group, Institute of Molecular and Experimental Medicine, Cardiff University School of Medicine, Cardiff, UK
J Clin Endocrinol Metab 2014;99:4291-4298

Background: Thyroid dysfunction in the mother is associated with impaired cognitive development of the offspring. Perchlorate decreases thyroidal iodine uptake, potentially reducing thyroid hormone production. The authors investigated the effect of perchlorate exposure in early life on neurodevelopment. *Methods:* The authors studied an historical cohort of 21,846 women at gestational age <16 weeks and identified 487 mother–child pairs whose mothers were hypothyroid/hypothyroxinaemic during pregnancy. In these 487 mothers, they analysed whether first trimester maternal perchlorate levels in the highest 10% of the study population were associated with risk of offspring IQ being in the lowest 10% at three years of age. *Results:* Urine perchlorate was detectable in all women (median 2.58 microgram/L); iodine levels were low (median 72 microgram/L). Maternal perchlorate levels in the highest 10% of the population increased the risk of offspring IQ being in the lowest 10%; OR=3.14 (95% CI 1.38–7.13), P=0.006, with a greater negative impact observed on verbal OR=3.14 (95% CI 1.42–6.90), P=0.005 than performance IQ. Maternal levothyroxine therapy did not reduce the negative impact of perchlorate on offspring IQ. *Conclusions:* High maternal urine perchlorate concentrations were associated with a negative impact on neurocognitive development in the offspring. This effect was independent of maternal levothyroxine therapy.

These two studies underline the importance of an intact thyroid axis in pregnant women for the health of their offspring. The French nationwide study provides the first evidence that maternal congenital hypothyroidism might expose the mother as well as the child to important pregnancy complications such as gestational hypertension, emergency caesarean delivery and prematurity. The study results suggest that better thyroid disease management is required, particularly during the first two trimesters of pregnancy, together with vigilant monitoring of the pregnant woman. These data are in accordance with data from mothers with autoimmune thyroid disease, however, they provide a clearer view on the isolated effect of hypothyroidism versus the combined effect of hypothyroidism and positive thyroid antibodies in studies of pregnancy outcomes in women with autoimmune thyroid disease.

The second study using individual-level patient data to study maternal perchlorate exposure and offspring neurocognitive development suggests that high maternal perchlorate levels in hypothyroid/hypothyroxinaemic pregnant women had an adverse effect on offspring cognitive development at three years of age. However, due to the study protocol, not all questions could be answered definitively. Whether the negative perchlorate effect is due to maternal hypothyroidism or a direct effect on the thyroid function of the fetus, remains open. As stated by the authors, these results require replication in additional studies, including in euthyroid mothers.

Paediatric thyroid nodules and cancer

Ultrasound characteristics of the thyroid in children and adolescents with goiter: a single center experience

Kambalapalli M, Gupta A, Prasad UR, Francis GL
Department of Pediatrics, Children's Hospital of Richmond at Virginia Commonwealth University, Richmond, VA, USA
Thyroid 2015;25:176-182

Background: The authors aimed to evaluate the ultrasound characteristics of the thyroid parenchyma and the prevalence of thyroid nodules in children and adolescents presenting with goitre of autoimmune and non-autoimmune origin.

Methods: Retrospective review of ultrasound exams of the thyroid in 154 children with goitre. Ultrasound characteristics were analysed according to the patient's age, sex, TSH level and thyroid peroxidase antibody titre (TPOAb). Heterogeneity and nodule prevalence were compared between antibody-positive and -negative goitres.
Results: First, heterogeneity was more common in TPOAb-positive (59/71, 83%) compared with TPOAb-negative goitre (24/46, 52%; P<0.001). Second, nodules were equally prevalent in children with (17%) and without (17.4%) TPOAb, and there was no correlation between the serum TSH level or TPOAb titre and the presence of nodules. Third, papillary thyroid cancer (PTC) was diagnosed in 3/71 TPOAb positive patients compared with 1/46 TPOAb negative patients. Finally, pseudonodules were identified in 11/71 TPOAb positive and 0/46 TPOAb negtive patients. However, during follow-up, two pseudonodules were later identified as nodules and one was PTC.
Conclusions: The majority of children and adolescents with goitre had positive TPOAb (71/117). Sonographic heterogeneity was more common among TPOAb-positive patients. Thyroid nodules and PTC were equally common in both groups.

Goitre may appear as a common paediatric condition, especially during adolescence. The data presented support the utility of thyroid ultrasound to detect unsuspected thyroid nodules and papillary thyroid cancer in children with goitre. Only 15% of the nodules and none of the papillary thyroid cancer were palpable. Interestingly, the frequency of thyroid cancer was not decreased in the context of thyroiditis. Therefore a thyroid nodule even in the context of thyroiditis should be investigated as thyroid nodules in patients without autoimmune thyroiditis. Prospective follow-up studies of children with goitre are needed to define recommendations for evaluation with ultrasound and fine-needle aspiration.

Therapeutic effectiveness of screening for multiple endocrine neoplasia type 2A

Machens A, Dralle H
Department of General, Visceral and Vascular Surgery, Martin-Luther-University Halle-Wittenberg, Halle (Saale), Germany
J Clin Endocrinol Metab 2015;100:2539–2545

Background: Genetic screening for mutations in the RET gene allows us to detect patients at risk of hereditary medullary thyroid cancer in the context of multiple endocrine neoplasia type 2A (MEN 2A). The authors aimed to assess the achievements of screening for MEN 2A and identify the challenges and limits.
Methods: Retrospective analysis of 455 carriers at risk of MEN 2A screened and operated between 1963 and 2014. The study comprised 175 carriers of American Thyroid Association (ATA) level C mutations (codon 634); 116 carriers of ATA level B mutations (codons 609, 611, 618, 620 and 630); and 164 carriers of ATA level A mutations (codons 768, 790, 791, 804 and 891) who underwent thyroidectomy. The outcome measures were: 1) percentage of index patients among all carriers, and 2) percentage of MTC, node-positive MTC and biochemical cure among non-index patients.
Results: The percentage of index patients among all carriers fell from 50% (ATA level C) and 100% (ATA level B and A) to 16, 29 and 31%, respectively. Among non-index patients, the percentage of MTC fell for ATA levels C and B but not for ATA level A mutations. The corresponding percentage of node-positive MTC declined since 1963 from 100 to 0% (ATA level C) and since 1995 from 67 to 33% (ATA level B) and from 11 to 10% (ATA level A), whereas biochemical cure increased from 0 to 100% since 1963 (ATA level C), and since 1995 from 0 to 78% (ATA level B) and from 95 to 100% (ATA level A).
Conclusions: Genetic screening clearly improved the outcome in ATA level C patients. More efforts are needed for the less aggressive ATA level B and ATA level A mutations.

Genetic screening for *RET* gene mutations has completely changed the approach in affected families allowing preclinical thyroidectomy in mutation carriers. The authors show clearly a shift to less aggressive stages in patients affected by the ATA C level mutation (c634) with no nodal positive patients at thyroidectomy and 100% biochemical cure nowadays. This is an enormous success bearing in mind the high penetrance of the medullary thyroid carcinoma caused by mutations in codon 634. In contrast, the authors also detect limitations of screening. Based on their results, the focus must now shift to the less aggressive mutations (ATA level B and A). Although improved by use of genetic testing, the rate of nodal positive patients and biochemical cure after thyroidectomy could be improved by more efforts in identifying and testing family members of index patients with ATA level B and A mutations earlier.

Management guidelines for children with thyroid nodules and differentiated thyroid cancer: The American Thyroid Association Guidelines Task Force on Pediatric Thyroid Cancer

Francis GL, Waguespack SG, Bauer AJ, Angelos P, Benvenga S, Cerutti J, Dinauer CA, Hamilton JK, Hay ID, Luster M, Parisi MT, Rachmiel M, Thompson G, Yamashita S
Virginia Commonwealth University, Pediatric Endocrinology, Richmond, VA, USA
Thyroid 2015;25:716–759

Background: Due to the scarcity of thyroid cancer in children, previous guidelines for the management of thyroid nodules and cancers were focused on adults. However, thyroid neoplasms in the paediatric population exhibit differences in pathophysiology, clinical presentation and long-term outcomes compared with thyroid cancer biology in adults. Furthermore, therapy that may be recommended for an adult may not be appropriate for a child who is at low risk for death but at higher risk for long-term harm from overaggressive treatment. For these reasons, unique guidelines for children and adolescents with thyroid tumours were needed.
Methods: An expert panel commissioned by the American Thyroid Association (ATA) developed clinically relevant questions on the management of children with thyroid nodules and differentiated thyroid cancer. Using an extensive literature search, primarily focused on studies that included subjects ≤18 years of age, the task force identified and reviewed relevant articles through to April 2014. Recommendations were made based upon evidence and expert opinion and were graded using a modified schema from the United States Preventive Services Task Force.
Results: The authors present the first paediatric-specific guidelines for evaluation and management of thyroid nodules and differentiated thyroid cancer, including specific management algorithms for papillary and follicular thyroid cancers.
Conclusions: The ATA task force developed recommendations based on scientific evidence and expert opinion for the management of thyroid nodules and differentiated thyroid cancer in children and adolescents.

These guidelines were long awaited, and provide for the first time specific recommendations for paediatric thyroid cancer diagnosis, treatment and follow-up independently of adult medicine. These represent the current optimal care for children and adolescents with these conditions and are an important tool for critical discussions with adult healthcare providers also involved in treatment of children.

Experiences from Fukushima and Chernobyl

The thyroid status of children and adolescents in Fukushima Prefecture examined during 20–30 months after the Fukushima nuclear power plant disaster: a cross-sectional, observational study

Watanobe H, Furutani T, Nihei M, Sakuma Y, Yanai R, Takahashi M, Sato H, Sagawa F
Radiation Countermeasures Research Institute for Earthquake Disaster Recovery Support, Hirata, Fukushima, Japan; Kasukabe Kousei Hospital, Kasukabe, Saitama, Japan
PLoS One 2014;9:e113804

Background: The authors aimed to: 1) screen for early development of thyroid cancer in children exposed to the Fukushima nuclear accident in 2011; and 2) search for associations between thyroid ultrasonographic findings, thyroid-relevant biochemical markers and iodine-131 ground deposition in the locations of residence during very early days after the accident.

Methods: Cross-sectional study of Fukushima residents <19 years (including fetuses) at the time of the accident including 1) a questionnaire, 2) thyroid ultrasonography, 3) thyroid-related blood tests and 4) urinary iodine measurements. The authors analysed a possible relationship among thyroid ultrasonographic findings (n=1,137), serum hormonal data (n=731), urinary iodine concentrations (n=770) and iodine-131 ground deposition (n=1,137).
Results: No patient with thyroid cancer was identified. Further, no association between thyroid ultrasound anomalies (nodules, cysts) with iodine-131 ground deposits or other parameters were found.
Conclusions: At the early timepoint of 20–30 months after the accident, the authors did not confirm any discernible deleterious effects of the emitted radioactivity on the thyroid of young Fukushima residents.

Initial presentation and late results of treatment of post-Chernobyl papillary thyroid carcinoma in children and adolescents of Belarus

Fridman M, Savva N, Krasko O, Mankovskaya S, Branovan DI, Schmid KW, Demidchik Y
Department of Pathology, Republican Centre for Thyroid Tumors, Minsk, Belarus
J Clin Endocrinol Metab 2014;99:2932–2941

Background: The authors aimed to evaluate the clinical and pathological characteristics and outcome of papillary thyroid carcinoma (PTC) that have arisen in children in Belarus exposed to the radioactive fallout from the Chernobyl accident over a long-term period.
Methods: The long-term treatment results were investigated in 1,078 children and adolescents (<19 years) with PTC who were surgically treated during the years 1990 to 2005.
Results: At presentation, patients suffered from high rates of metastatic PTC, with 73.8% of cases having lymph node involvement and 11.1% having distant spread. The overall survival was 96.9% ± 0.9% with a median follow-up of 16.21 years, and 20-year event-free survival and relapse-free survival were 87.8% ± 1.6% and 92.3% ± 0.9%, respectively. Patients had lower probability of both loco-regional (P<0.001) and distant relapses (P=0.005) after total thyroidectomy and radioactive iodine therapy. For loco-regional relapses after total thyroidectomy, only radioactive iodine therapy influenced the prognosis (P<0.001). For distant relapses after total thyroidectomy, the refusal to treat with radioactive iodine (hazard ratio [HR]=9.26), vascular invasion (HR=8.68) and age at presentation (HR=6.13) were risk factors.
Conclusions: The outcome of PTC both in children and in adolescents exposed to the post-Chernobyl radioiodine fallout was favourable. Total thyroidectomy in combination with radioactive iodine therapy was succesful in minimising loco-regional or distant relapses.

A possible increase in thyroid cancer in the young represents the most critical health problem to be considered after the nuclear accident in Fukushima, Japan (March 2011), which is an important lesson from the Chernobyl disaster (April 1986). Although it was reported that childhood thyroid cancer had started to increase three to five years after the Chernobyl accident, the Japanese authors of the first study speculated that the actual period of latency might have been shorter than reported, considering the delay in initiating thyroid surveillance in the former Soviet Union and also the lower quality of ultrasonographic technology in the 1980s. Fortunately, the thyroid status of young Fukushima residents after the nuclear disaster was normal 20–30 months after the accident. Longer-term follow-up studies are of course necessary to monitor thyroid function and possible thyroid cancer in that population, as the experience of Chernobyl has taught us.

The second study, presenting long-term follow-up data from children and adolescents exposed to the Chernobyl fallout, show rather favourable outcomes of patients with papillary thyroid carcinoma after total thyroidectomy in combination with radioactive iodine treatment, again a key result for a better understanding of the risks of childhood exposure to radiation.

Mutations of the thyroid hormone transporter MCT8 cause prenatal brain damage and persistent hypomyelination

Lopez-Espindola D, Morales-Bastos C, Grijota-Martinez C, Liao XH, Lev D, Sugo E, Verge CF, Refetoff S, Bernal J, Guadano-Ferraz A
Instituto de Investigaciones Biomedicas Alberto Sols, Consejo Superior de Investigaciones Cientificas-Universidad Autonoma de Madrid, Madrid, Spain
J Clin Endocrinol Metab 2014;99:E2799–E2804

Background: The nature of the central nervous system damage is unknown in patients affected with MCT8 mutations. The authors aimed to describe the neuropathology of Allan-Herndon-Dudley syndrome by analysing brain tissue sections from MCT8-deficient subjects.
Methods: They analysed brain sections from a 30th gestational week male fetus and an 11-year-old boy and as controls, brain tissue from a 30th and 28th gestational week male and female fetuses, respectively, a 10-year-old girl and a 12-year-old boy. Staining with haematoxylin-eosin and immunostaining with brain development markers were performed. Thyroid hormone determinations and quantitative PCR for deiodinases were also performed.
Results: The MCT8-deficient fetus showed a delay in cortical and cerebellar development and myelination, impaired axonal maturation and diminished biochemical differentiation of Purkinje cells. The 11-year-old boy showed altered cerebellar structure and deficient myelination. The MCT8-deficient fetal cerebral cortex showed 50% reduction of thyroid hormones and increased type 2 deiodinase and decreased type 3 deiodinase mRNAs.
Conclusions: Brain damage in patients with MCT8 deficiency was diffuse, without evidence of focal lesions and present from fetal stages despite apparent normality at birth. Deficient hypomyelination persisted up to 11 years of age. The neuropathological findings were compatible with the deficient action of thyroid hormones in the developing brain caused by impaired transport to the target neural cells.

Placenta passage of the thyroid hormone analog DITPA to male wild-type and Mct8-deficient mice

Ferrara AM, Liao XH, Gil-Ibanez P, Bernal J, Weiss RE, Dumitrescu AM, Refetoff S
Departments of Medicine and Pediatrics and the Committee on Genetics, The University of Chicago, Chicago, IL, USA
Endocrinology 2014;155:4088–4093

Background: The thyroid hormone (TH) analogue diiodothyropropionic acid (DITPA) corrected thyroid function test (TFT) abnormalities and hypermetabolism of MCT8-deficient children but did not improve the neurological phenotype. The latter result was attributed to the late initiation of treatment. Therefore, the authors gave DITPA to pregnant mice carrying Mct8-deficient embryos to determine whether DITPA, when given prenatally, crosses the placenta and affects the serum TFTs and cerebral cortex of embryos.
Methods: After depletion of the endogenous TH, Mct8-heterozygous pregnant dams carrying both wild-type (Wt) and Mct8-deficient (Mct8KO) male embryos were given DITPA. Effects were compared with those treated with levothyroxine (L-T4).
Results: With DITPA treatment, serum DITPA concentration was not different in the two genotypes, which produced equal effects on serum TSH levels in both groups of pups. In contrast, with L-T4 treatment, TSH did not normalise in Mct8KO pups whereas it did in the Wt littermates and dams despite a higher concentration of serum T4.
Conclusions: DITPA is a candidate for intrauterine treatment of MCT8 deficiency due to: its ability to cross the placenta; its better accessibility of the thyrothrophs in the pituitary gland as shown by negative feedback compared with T4 alone; and its ability to modulate the gene expression of TH-dependent genes in the brain.

In vitro and mouse studies support therapeutic utility of triiodothyroacetic acid in MCT8 deficiency

Kersseboom S, Horn S, Visser WE, Chen J, Friesema EC, Vaurs-Barriere C, Peeters RP, Heuer H, Visser TJ
Erasmus University Medical Center, Rotterdam, The Netherlands
Mol Endocrinol 2014;28:1961–1970

Background: Mutations in MCT8 cause Allan-Herndon-Dudley syndrome and result in severe psychomotor retardation and elevated serum T3 levels. As the neurological symptoms are most likely caused by a lack of thyroid hormone (TH) transport into the CNS, the administration of a TH analogue that does not require MCT8 for cellular uptake may represent a therapeutic strategy. The authors investigated the therapeutic potential of the biologically active T3 metabolite Triac (triiodothyroacetic acid; TA3) by studying TA3 transport, metabolism and action both in vitro and in vivo.
Methods: TA3 uptake and metabolism were studied in neuronal cell lines, fibroblasts of affected patients and in Pax8 and MCT8/Oatp1c1 double knockout mice.
Results: First, fibroblasts from MCT8 patients showed an impaired T3 uptake compared with controls, whereas TA3 uptake was similar in patient and control fibroblasts. Second, in neuronal cell lines, TA3 induced T3-like gene expression. Finally, treatment of athyroid Pax8 knockout mice and Mct8/Oatp1c1 double knockout mice between postnatal day one and 12 with TA3 restored T3-dependent neural differentiation in the cerebral and cerebellar cortex, indicating that TA3 can replace T3 in promoting brain development.
Conclusions: The authors demonstrated uptake of TA3 in neuronal cells and in fibroblasts of MCT8 patients, and similar gene responses to T3 and TA3 in vitro as in vivo.

Monocarboxylate transporter 8 (MCT8; SLC16A2) deficiency causes severe X-linked intellectual and neuropsychological impairment associated with abnormal thyroid function tests producing thyroid hormone deprivation in brain and excess in peripheral tissues (Allan-Herndon-Dudley syndrome, AHDS; OMIM #300523). The time course of brain damage and the pathology of the brain of affected patients was unknown. In the first paper, the authors describe in human fetuses and children neuropathological features of the disease in detail and show that the lesions are compatible with the effects of thyroid hormone deficiency on the brain.

Treatment options for patients with MCT8 deficiency are limited. The administration of propylthiouracil, which blocks thyroid hormone production and inhibits T4 to T3 conversion, combined with L-T4 has shown some metabolic benefits, but no effect on the neurological phenotype. To treat patients with MCT8 deficiency, substances with thyroid hormone effect but alternative cellular uptake mechanisms than by MCT8 are necessary. So far, two thyromimetics, diiodothyropropionic acid (DITPA) and triiodothyroacetic acid (Triac) are under investigation, DIPTA already being used in four patients from nine months of age. The following two papers provide detailed insights into the actions and metabolism of DIPTA and Triac in vitro and in vivo, and pave the way for more effective treatment of affected patients.

In an attempt to treat affected patients as early as in utero, the authors of the second study provided evidence that DIPTA crosses the placenta and reaches the neuronal target cells (neurons, thyrothrophs) in the mice model inducing a T3-like effect. The approach to treat affected patients as early as in utero is even more relevant in the context of the data presented in the first paper showing that brain damage in the human fetus is already induced in utero. In the third study in mice, the authors show new insights into the uptake and action of Triac, and provide further evidence in the mouse model, that Triac fulfils criteria to be used therapeutically in MCT8 patients: MTC8 independent cellular uptake, T3-like effects in neuronal cells and T3-like response in the hypothyroid brain. More clinical research is necessary to confirm these encouraging translational data.

Effects of early thyroxine treatment on development and growth at age 10.7 years: follow-up of a randomized placebo-controlled trial in children with Down's syndrome

Marchal JP, Maurice-Stam H, Ikelaar NA, Klouwer FC, Verhorstert KW, Witteveen ME, Houtzager BA, Grootenhuis MA, van Trotsenburg AS
Department of Pediatric Endocrinology, and Psychosocial Department, Academic Medical Center/Emma Children's Hospital, Amsterdam, The Netherlands
J Clin Endocrinol Metab 2014;99:E2722–E2729

Background: The authors aimed to determine the long-term effects of early T4 treatment on development and growth in children with Down's syndrome (DS) with either an elevated or normal neonatal TSH concentration.
Methods: 123/196 patients participating in a first randomised placebo-controlled study comparing T4 and placebo treatment during the first two years of life were reassessed for mental development and growth parameters at a mean age of 10.7 years. Outcomes were compared between T4- and placebo-treated children, and between treatment groups with either a normal (<5mIU/L), or elevated (≥5mIU/L) TSH concentration at original trial entry.
Results: No differences were found in mental or motor development, communication skills or fine-motor co-ordination between T4-treated (n=64) and placebo-treated children (n=59). T4-treated children had a larger head circumference (HC) (50.4 versus 49.8cm, P=0.04) and tended to be taller (133.2 versus 131.1cm, P=0.06). These differences were somewhat greater in children with TSH ≥5mIU/L (HC: T4, 50.5 versus placebo, 49.7cm; P=0.01; height: T4, 133.8 versus placebo, 130.8cm; P=0.02), but were not found in children with TSH <5mIU/L (HC: T4, 50.1 versus placebo, 50.0cm; P=0.75; height: T4, 132.1 versus placebo, 131.6cm; P=0.22).
Conclusions: Early T4 treatment of children with Down's syndrome did not result in improved mental or motor development at 10 years of age. However, the positive effect on growth was still measurable, especially in children with an elevated plasma TSH concentration in the neonatal period.

In the original study, analysing the effect of early T4 treatment during the first two years of life in children with Down's syndrome, at the end of the intervention at two years of age, the authors found a slightly better motor development and growth. In this unique long-term follow-up study, this effect was not sustained when these children were re-evaluated almost nine years after the initial trial. Whether this is due to a lack of major effect of thyroxine on neurocognitive development in children with Down's syndrome or whether thyroxine treatment should be maintained throughout childhood to obtain favourable results should be tested in further clinical trials.

DYRK1A BAC transgenic mouse: a new model of thyroid dysgenesis in Down syndrome

Kariyawasam D, Rachdi L, Carré A, Martin M, Houlier M, Janel N, Delabar JM, Scharfmann R, Polak M
Inserm U1016, Paris, France
Endocrinology 2015;156:1171–1180

Background: The molecular basis of mild thyroid dysgenesis in children with Down's syndrome is unknown. Transgenic Dyrk1A mice, obtained by bacterial artificial chromosome engineering (mBACTgDyrk1A), have three copies of the *Dyrk1A* gene and are a model of Down's syndrome. The authors aimed to determine whether this transgenic Dyrk1A (Dyrk1A(+/++)) mouse is an adequate murine model for the study of thyroid dysgenesis in Down's syndrome.
Methods: Embryonic thyroid development was analysed in wild-type (WT) and Dyrk1A(+/++) mice by immunofluorescence with markers of early thyroid development, hormonogenesis and final differentiation. The adult phenotype was compared at eight to 12 weeks in Dyrk1A(+/++) and WT mice for T4 and TSH levels, thyroidal weight and histological analysis.
Results: During development at E17.5, thyroglobulin stained surface in Dyrk1A(+/++) thyroids was less than a third as large and their differentiated follicular surface half the size (P=0.004) compared with WT. In adult mice, Dyrk1A(+/++) mice had lower plasma T4 levels (2.4ng/mL versus WT,

3.7ng/mL; P=0.019) while plasma TSH (114mUI/L versus WT, 73mUI/L; P=0.09) were not different. Dyrk1A(+/++) thyroid glands were heavier (P=0.04) and exhibited large disorganised regions.
Conclusions: Dyrk1A overexpression caused functional and morphological impairment of thyroid development. The Dyrk1A(+/++) mouse can be considered a suitable study model for thyroid dysgenesis in Down's syndrome.

The most common abnormalities of thyroid function and morphology in children with Down's syndrome are: mildly elevated TSH, with normal or slightly decreased T4; and thyroid hypoplasia. In contrast, severe congenital hypothyroidism is less frequent at birth, and autoimmune thyroiditis occurs beyond infancy. This paper: 1) provides insight into the disordered development of the thyroid possibly involved in Down's syndrome associated mild thyroid hypothyroidism; 2) confirms earlier results of the group analysing fetal thyroids of children with Down's syndrome, and finally establishes the model of transgenic mice with three copies of the *Dyrk1A* gene as an accurate model of Down's syndrome associated thyroid dysgenesis. Further work should aim at determining the precise molecular mechanism linking *Dyrk1A* and thyroid development.

New insights into molecular mechanisms of congenital hypothyroidism

The paired box transcription factor Pax8 is essential for function and survival of adult thyroid cells

Marotta P, Amendola E, Scarfo M, De Luca P, Zoppoli P, Amoresano A, De Felice M, Di Lauro R
IRGS, Biogem, Ariano Irpino, Avellino, Italy
mario.defelice@unina.it
Mol Cell Endocrinol 2014;396:26–36

Background: The transcription factor Pax8 is known to be essential at very early stages of mouse thyroid gland development, before the onset of thyroid hormone production. The authors aimed to determine the role of Pax8 in late thyroid development.
Methods: Detailed analysis of a mouse line with late embryonic conditional inactivation of Pax8.
Results: The removal of the Pax8 protein at late stages in thyroid gland development resulted in severe hypothyroidism, consequent to a reduced gland size and a deranged differentiation.
Conclusions: These results demonstrate that Pax8 is not only relevant for thyroid gland morphogenesis, but also an essential player in controlling survival and differentiation of adult thyroid follicular cells.

The observation that a transcription factor may control embryonic development as well as maintenance and survival has earlier been shown for Nkx2-1 in the thyroid gland. So far, no data were available on the role of Pax8 in the adult thyroid. The authors nicely show in a conditional knockout model that Pax8 is crucial for normal differentiation and inhibits apoptosis of thyroid follicular cells.

Extreme phenotypic variability of thyroid dysgenesis in six new cases of congenital hypothyroidism due to PAX8 gene loss-of-function mutations

Ramos HE, Carré A, Chevrier L, Szinnai G, Tron E, Cerqueira TL, Léger J, Cabrol S, Puel O, Queinnec C, De Roux N, Guillot L, Castanet M, Polak M
INSERM U1016, Universite Paris Descartes, Sorbonne Paris Cite, Paris, France
Eur J Endocrinol 2014;171:499–507

Background: The authors searched for PAX8 mutations in a cohort of patients with congenital hypothyroidism (CH) and various types of thyroid gland defects.
Methods: The French neonatal screening programme was used for recruiting patients.
Results: 118 patients with CH, including 45 with familial and 73 with sporadic diseases, were studied. The thyroid gland was normal in 23 patients, 28 had hypoplasia, 25 had hemithyroid agenesis, 21 had athyreosis and 21 had ectopy. The authors identified four different PAX8 mutations (p.R31C, p.R31H, p.R108X

and p.I47T) in 10 patients (six patients with CH and four family members), two with sporadic and eight with familial diseases. Imaging studies performed in the index cases showed ectopic thyroid gland (n=2), hypoplasia (n=2), eutopic lobar asymmetry (n=1) and eutopic gland compatible with dyshormonogenesis (n=1). The previously reported p.R31C and the novel p.I47T PAX8 mutations are devoid of activity.
Conclusion: The novel p.I47T PAX8 mutation presented loss of function leading to CH. Thyroid ectopy was observed in two cases of PAX8 (p.R31H) mutation, a finding that has not been reported previously.

In the last two decades, heterozygous loss-of-function *PAX8* mutations have been reported in patients with a range of hypothyroidism and thyroid morphology despite the presence of identical mutations. Thyroid ectopy is the most prevalent phenotype of thyroid dysgenesis, however, genetic defects have not been found in known thyroid transcription factors. First, the presented study extends current knowledge on the variability of thyroid function and type of dysgenesis even within families. Second, the study reports for the first time of molecular defects in known genes causing thyroid ectopy. As a consequence, *PAX8* mutations have to be considered as molecular cause of thyroid ectopy.

Functional zebrafish studies based on human genotyping point to netrin-1 as a link between aberrant cardiovascular development and thyroid dysgenesis

Opitz R, Hitz MP, Vandernoot I, Trubiroha A, Abu-Khudir R, Samuels M, Desilets V, Costagliola S, Andelfinger G, Deladoey J
Institute of Interdisciplinary Research in Molecular Human Biology, Universite Libre de Bruxelles, Brussels, Belgium
Endocrinology 2015;156:377–388

Background: Congenital heart disease is the most frequent associated malformation in patients with thyroid dysgenesis. The authors aimed to identify common genetic or epigenetic factors causing the combination of congenital hypothyroidism and congenital heart disease.
Methods: Genome-wide single-nucleotide polymorphism array and Sanger sequencing to analyse blood DNA samples from three selected patients with co-occurring congenital hypothyroidism caused by thyroid dysgenesis and congenital heart disease to search for de novo copy number variants and coding mutations in candidate genes.
Results: Rare variants were identified in all three patients. The Netrin-1 gene was selected as the biologically most plausible contributory factor for functional studies. In zebrafish, ntn1a and ntn1b were not expressed in thyroid tissue, but ntn1a was expressed in pharyngeal arch mesenchyme, and ntn1a-deficient embryos displayed defective aortic arch artery formation and abnormal thyroid morphogenesis. The functional activity of the thyroid in ntn1a-deficient larvae was, however, preserved. Phenotypic analysis of affected zebrafish indicates that abnormal thyroid morphogenesis resulted from a lack of proper guidance exerted by the dysplastic vasculature of ntn1a-deficient embryos.
Conclusions: Clinical and genetic data in humans and developmental studies in zebrafish identified Netrin-1 as a potential candidate gene for thyroid dysgenesis in the context of congenital heart disease.

Up to 8% of individuals with congenital hypothyroidism caused by thyroid dysgenesis have co-occurring congenital heart disease. The authors conducted careful phenotyping of patients without *NKX2-5* mutations combined with molecular and functional studies in zebrafish and identified Netrin-1 as a potential shared genetic factor for cardiac and thyroid congenital defects. In analogy with other transcription factors associated with thyroid dysgenesis in animal models, in netrin-1 deficiency the primary defect is not within the thyroid precursor cells but within the surrounding mesenchyme. Netrin-1 is proposed as a new candidate gene for thyroid dysgenesis and congenital heart disease.

When an intramolecular disulfide bridge governs the interaction of DUOX2 with its partner DUOXA2

Carré A, Louzada RA, Fortunato RS, Ameziane-El-Hassani R, Morand S, Ogryzko V, de Carvalho DP, Grasberger H, Leto TL, Dupuy C
Universite Paris-Sud, Orsay, France
Antioxid Redox Signal 2015 (Epub ahead of print) Apr 20

Background: Mutations in dual oxidase 2 (DUOX2) and dual oxidase activator 2 (DUOXA2) cause thyroid dyshormonogenesis. DUOX2 forms with DUOXA2 a stable complex at the cell surface that

is crucial for the H_2O_2-generating activity. However, the mechanism of their interaction is unknown. The contribution of some cysteine residues located in the N-terminal ectodomain of DUOX2 in a surface protein–protein interaction is suggested.
Methods: The authors investigated in vitro the involvement of different cysteine residues in the formation of covalent bonds possibly critical for the function of the complex.
Results: The authors report the identification and the characterisation of an intramolecular disulphide bond between cys-124 of the N-terminal ectodomain and cys-1162 of an extracellular loop of DUOX2. This disulphide bridge has important functional implications in both export and activity of DUOX2; and provides structural support for the formation of interdisulphide bridges between the N-terminal domain of DUOX2 and the two extracellular loops of its partner, DUOXA2.
Conclusions: The oxidative folding of DUOX2 that takes place in the endoplasmic reticulum appears to be a key event in the trafficking of the DUOX2/DUOXA2 complex as it promotes an appropriate conformation of the N-terminal region, which is propitious to subsequent covalent interactions with the maturation factor, DUOXA2.

The dual oxidase 2 (DUOX2) protein belongs to the NADPH oxidase (NOX) family. As a H_2O_2 generator, it plays a key role in both thyroid hormone biosynthesis and innate immunity. Both stability and function of the maturation factor, DUOXA2, are dependent on the oxidative folding of DUOX2, indicating that DUOX2 displays a chaperone-like function with respect to its partner. This basic structure/function study provides clues to better understand the impact of different mutations of these enzymes identified in patients with congenital hypothyroidism.

Mechanism of the year: new arguments in an old discussion

Differences in hypothalamic type 2 deiodinase ubiquitination explain localized sensitivity to thyroxine

Werneck de Castro JP, Fonseca TL, Ueta CB, McAninch EA, Abdalla S, Wittmann G, Lechan RM, Gereben B, Bianco AC
Division of Endocrinology, Diabetes and Metabolism, University of Miami School of Medicine, Miami, FL, USA
J Clin Invest 2015;125:769–781

Background: Patients with hypothyroidism are routinely treated with L-T4, which aims to normalise the thyroid stimulating hormone (TSH) level. However, normalisation of serum TSH with L-T4 monotherapy results in relatively low serum 3,5,3′-triiodothyronine (T3) and high serum thyroxine/T3 (T4/T3) ratio. In the hypothalamus–pituitary dyad as well as the rest of the brain, the majority of T3 present is generated locally by T4 deiodination via the type 2 deiodinase (D2); this pathway is self-limited by ubiquitination of D2 by the ubiquitin ligase WSB-1.
Methods: Investigations in WT and astrocyte-specific Wsb-1 knockout mice.
Results: Tissue-specific differences in D2 ubiquitination accounted for the high T4/T3 serum ratio in adult thyroidectomised rats chronically implanted with subcutaneous L-T4 pellets. Whole-body D2-dependent T4 conversion to T3 was decreased by L-T4 treatment. In contrast, D2 activity in the hypothalamus was only minimally affected by L-T4. In vivo studies in Wsb1 knockout mice as well as in vitro analysis of D2 ubiquitination driven by different tissue extracts indicated that D2 ubiquitination in the hypothalamus was relatively less. As a result, in contrast to other D2-expressing tissues, the hypothalamus had increased sensitivity to T4.
Conclusions: Tissue-specific differences in D2 ubiquitination are an inherent property of the TRH/TSH feedback mechanism and indicate that only constant delivery of L-T4 and L-T3 fully normalises T3-dependent metabolic markers and gene expression profiles in thyroidectomised rats.

The type 2 iodothyronine deiodinase (D2) is essential for feedback regulation of TSH by T4. Monotherapy with L-T4 in hypothyroid patients normalises TSH and T4 levels, while in 15% of patients T3 remains below the lower limit of reference. Further, 5–10% of L-T4 treated patients experience persistent symptoms of hypothyroidism despite normalisation of TSH and T4.

The authors investigated in an extensive and elegant animal study the role of D2 activity at different levels and under different substitution regimens in thyroidectomised rats. First, they confirm their own earlier results concerning the benefits of combined L-T4 and L-T3 treatment for normalisation of all thyroid function parameters, providing further arguments for clinical re-evaluation of combined L-T3 and L-T4 treatment regimens in patients experiencing hypothyroid symptoms despite adequate TSH and T4 levels. Second, they add important insights into the differences of L-T4 and L-T3 feedback mechanisms by revealing that deiodination in peripheral tissues as well as in most brain regions is very sensitive to T4-induced D2 ubiquitination in contrast to the hypothalamus, where T4-induced D2 inactivation is not present. As a consequence, TSH is normalised based on adequate T3 conversion from T4 in the hypothalamus, while in the peripheral tissues the conversion of T4 to T3 is blocked by T4 sensitive ubiquitination causing tissue-specific hypothyroidism in the context of normalised TSH and T4 levels. Whether these data are valid in the subgroup of patients experiencing hypothyroid symptoms despite adequate TSH and T4 values remains to be shown in new clinical studies.

Human thyroid stem cells

Human embryonic stem cells form functional thyroid follicles

Ma R, Latif R, Davies TF
Thyroid Research Unit, Department of Medicine, Icahn School of Medicine at Mount Sinai and the James J. Peters VA Medical Center, New York, NY, USA
Thyroid 2015;25:455–461

Background: Overexpression of the regulatory transcription factors PAX8 and NKX2-1 directs murine embryonic stem cells to differentiate into thyroid follicular cells subsequently organised into three-dimensional follicular structures. The authors studied human embryonic stem (hES) cells with the aim of recapitulating this scenario and producing functional human thyroid cell lines.
Methods: Reporter gene tagged pEZ-lentiviral vectors were used to express human PAX8-eGFP and NKX2-1-mCherry in the H9 hES cell line followed by differentiation into thyroid cells directed by Activin A and thyrotropin (TSH).
Results: Both transcription factors were expressed efficiently in hES cells expressing either PAX8 or NKX2-1, or in combination in the hES cells. Further differentiation of the double transfected cells showed the expression of thyroid-specific genes, including thyroglobulin (TG), thyroid peroxidase, the sodium/iodide symporter and the TSH receptor as assessed by qPCR and immunostaining. Activin and TSH-induced differentiation resulted in thyroid follicle formation and abundant TG protein expression within the follicular lumens. On stimulation with TSH, these hES-derived follicles were also capable of dose-dependent cAMP generation and radioiodine uptake, indicating functional thyroid epithelial cells.
Conclusion: In analogy with the murine model, this study provides proof of principle that hES cells can be committed to thyroid cell speciation under appropriate conditions.

After induction of murine embryonic stem cells into functional follicular cells, the authors successfully reproduced the directed differentiation of human embryonic stem cells to follicular cells expressing specific differentiation markers and capable of iodine uptake. These are important technical achievements in the manipulation of human stem cells. However, as also stated by the authors, more research is necessary to replace lentiviral overexpression of NKX2-1 and PAX8 by optimised growth and differentiating protocols avoiding the genetic manipulation of the stem cells.

Growth and Growth Factors

Elena Inzaghi[a] and Stefano Cianfarani[a,b]

[a]DPUO 'Bambino Gesù' Children's Hospital – 'Tor Vergata' University, Rome Italy

[b]Department of Women's and Children's Health, Karolinska Institutet, Stockholm, Sweden

Our selection of papers first describes a series of studies with potential relevance to clinical practice, such as the impact of new IGF-I assays in the work-up and monitoring of children with short stature, and the effect of combined rhGH + IGF-I therapy to stimulate bone and growth plate. In the same section, a paper from the French SAGHE cohort reports a higher risk of cerebrovascular morbidity in young adults treated with rhGH during childhood, and a systematic review evaluates the long-term efficacy of rhGH therapy in children with Noonan syndrome. Among the clinical trials, we have selected a study reporting promising effects of rhGH in children with hypochondroplasia, and the benefits of early rhGH therapy in infants with Prader-Willi syndrome. New mechanisms have been elucidated in experimental models, such as the growth hormone (GH) effect on the distribution of immune cells in white adipose tissue, the IGF-1 dependent stabilisation of nascent blood vessels, the direct IGF-1 independent GH stimulation of growth plate chondrogenesis and longitudinal bone growth, and the IGF-2 effects on beta-cell dedifferentiation and dysfunction. New physiological and clinical perspectives are provided by papers reporting the optimal early growth pattern in children born small for gestational age; the common genetic background linking short stature and risk of coronary artery disease; the role of vitamin B12 in growth and bone mass; and the value of serum IGF-1 levels as a marker of beta-cell function and metabolic homeostasis. In this genomics era, the finding that environment rather than genes regulates critical growth periods is, in our opinion, food for thought. Finally, evidence that insulin and IGF-1 receptors modulate the expression of many imprinted genes through epigenetic changes independently of their ligand binding is the breakthrough mechanism of the year. Our hope is that the reading of these digested cutting-edge papers may be as enjoyable and stimulating for you as it was for us.

Important for clinical practice

The introduction of the IDS-iSYS total IGF-I assay may have far-reaching consequences for diagnosis and treatment of GH deficiency

Varewijck AJ, Lamberts SWJ, van der Lely AJ, Neggers SJ, Hofland LJ, Janssen JA
Department of Internal Medicine, Division of Endocrinology, Erasmus Medical Center, Rotterdam, The Netherlands
j.a.m.j.l.janssen@erasmusmc.nl
J Clin Endocrinol Metab 2015;100:309–316

Background: The assessment of serum IGF-1 levels is used for the investigation of growth disorders and for monitoring of therapy in growth hormone deficiency (GHD) and acromegaly. The aim of this study was to define the reliability of the recently developed IGF-1 immunoassay (IDS-iSYS) in diagnosis and monitoring of patients affected by GHD or acromegaly.
Methods: IGF-1 levels were assessed in 121 patients by both Immulite (IM) and IDS-iSYS (ID) assays. 106 patients with GHD (84 diagnosed as adult-onset GHD and 22 as childhood-onset GHD) were evaluated before and during GH treatment. Fifteen acromegalic subjects were studied at baseline and after 12 months of therapy.
Results: In GHD subjects, the two assays gave different absolute IGF-1 levels at baseline ($P<0.001$) but not during GH therapy ($P=0.32$). Mean Z-scores for IGF-1 differed both before (IM: -2.23 versus ID: -1.43, $P<0.001$) and after (IM: -0.6 versus ID: +0.21, $P<0.001$) the beginning of the treatment. 62.5% of untreated GHD patients had IGF-1 Z-score < -2SD by IM and 24.5% by ID assay. On therapy, 81.2% of GHD patients reached normal IGF-1 range by IM and 94.7% by ID assay. In acromegalic patients, differences between the two assays were not found before treatment ($P=0.18$) but were found after GH

treatment (P=0.009). But no differences in mean Z-scores for IGF-1 were found at baseline (IM: 10.93 versus ID: 10.78, P=0.41) or on treatment (IM: 3.6 versus ID: 3.18, P=0.23).
Conclusions: In GHD patients, IGF-1 Z-scores were lower when assessed by IM assay and differences were detectable both at baseline and during treatment. By contrast, in acromegalic patients, IGF-1 values were similar in the two assays. Replacing IM with ID assay could impact the management of GHD subjects with potential clinical consequences.

Serum IGF-1 evaluation is an important tool used for the screening and management of diseases characterised by altered growth hormone (GH) secretion and action. For instance, in GH deficient (GHD) subjects, GH replacement dose is adjusted according to IGF-1 value, and IGF-1 monitoring is used for testing the adherence to therapy as well as being a safety marker for avoiding overtreatment. Different assays give different IGF-1 values [1]. These differences are mainly attributed to the interference of IGF binding proteins, the use of international reference reagents and the different antibody specificity. Therefore, the results obtained by different assays are often not comparable and this generates confusion in the management of GH secretion disorders [2]. Recently, a new IGF-1 immunoassay calibrated against new recommended National Institute for Biological Standards and Control has been developed and validated in a large cohort of more than 15,000 subjects, aged 0 to 64 years [3]. This study aimed to test the usability of the new assay to monitor GHD and acromegalic patients, by comparing its values to the most commonly used assay, Immulite. Whereas in acromegalic patients the two assays gave overlapping data, in GHD subjects IGF-1 Z-scores were lower when measured by the Immulite assay than by IDS-iSYS, before as well as after starting GH treatment. About 40% of GHD patients may show IGF-1 levels within the normal range at baseline. Here, 37.5% of GHD patients had IGF-1 within the normal range when measured by Immulite and 75.5% by IDS-iSYS. Nevertheless, before and after starting GH treatment, there was good agreement in mean absolute IGF-1 concentrations between both assays. This finding suggests that differences observed in GHD patients may be due to the different assay-specific normative data. One potential bias is that IDS-iSYS measurements were performed three to four years after the Immulite measurements. Overlapping results between the two assays in acromegaly patients reflect the small size of that cohort. These findings may have important clinical implications and strongly argue for the use of this new assay to investigate growth disorders and monitor GH therapy.

Combined treatment with GH and IGF-I: additive effects on cortical bone mass but not on linear bone growth in female rats

Sundström K, Cedervall T, Ohlsson C, Camacho-Hübner C, Sävendahl L
Pediatric Endocrinology Unit, Department of Women's and Children Health, Karolinska Institutet, Stockholm, Sweden
katja.sundstrom@ki.se
Endocrinology 2014;155:4798–4807

Background: Both growth hormone (GH) and IGF-1 are important regulators of longitudinal bone growth and are involved in the maintenance of bone homeostasis. The aim of this study was to define the effects of rhGh and rhIGF-1 alone or in a combined therapy on longitudinal bone growth and mass.
Methods: Intact female Sprague-Dawley rats were divided into six groups: control, rhIGF-1 2.2mg/kg/d, rhIGF-1 4.4mg/kg/d, rhIGF-1 2.2mg/kg/d + rhGH 5mg/kg/d, rhIGF-1 4.4mg/kg/d + rhGH 5mg/kg/d, or rhGH 5mg/kg/d alone. During the four treatment weeks, GH was administered twice a day subcutaneously while rhIGF-1 was continuously infused subcutaneously. Each animal underwent weekly radiographs to assess tibial length. Nose–anus lengths were evaluated as further assessment of longitudinal bone growth. Cortical bone parameters were measured by quantitative computed tomography at the completion of treatment. Histomorphometry was performed in the tibial growth plate. Serum levels of IGF-1, GH and bone formation markers were measured, as well as the IGF-1/IGFBP-3/ALS 150-kDa ternary complex formation. Western blot analyses of IGFBP-3 and ALS in serum samples were performed.
Results: The highest doses of rhIGF-1 increased nose–anus length but were less effective than rhGH monotherapy (P<0.001). The combination therapy did not further increase tibia or nose–anus length than rhGH monotherapy. Growth plate length, proliferative and hypertrophic zone heights and cell numbers in these zones were not further increased by the combination therapy as compared with single rhGH therapy. By contrast, combined treatment with rhGH and rhIGF-1 (4.4mg/kg/d) increased

cortical bone area, cortical bone thickness, cortical bone mineral content and periosteal circumference compared with rhGH monotherapy. No treatment influenced endosteal circumference and bone mineral density. Serum levels of fragmented collagen type I were lower on combined therapy than on rhGH alone, whereas osteocalcin levels were similar across treatment regimens. Compared with rhGH monotherapy, combined therapy produced higher IGF-1 levels. No difference in pituitary weights, GH, ALS levels or 150-kDa ternary complex formation was found across treatment groups, whereas IGFBP-3 levels were higher in all groups receiving IGF-1. Combined therapy increased bodyweight and organ growth more than rhGH monotherapy. No changes in glucose levels were found in the different groups. *Conclusions:* The addition of rhIGF-1 to rhGH was ineffective in further increasing longitudinal bone growth but had an additive stimulatory effect on cortical bone mass in female rats.

The GH-IGF-1 axis regulates bone growth by stimulating differentiation and accretion of cartilage cells in the epiphyseal growth plate. Both GH and IGF-1 also act on bone resorption and formation, influencing bone metabolism [4]. Although IGF-1 has long been considered the mediator of GH growth-promoting effects in peripheral tissues, increasing evidence indicates an IGF-1 independent action of GH on both cartilage and bone growth, thus suggesting that their combined administration may have an additive effect on both of these target tissues. Nevertheless, previous studies of combined therapy have reported conflicting findings on longitudinal bone growth and bone mass accrual. In healthy adults, combined administration of rhGH and rhIGF-1 stimulated bone formation [5,6], while in normal rats it did not augment bone mineral content [7]. Interestingly, a randomised, open-label controlled trial evaluating rhGH and rhIGF-1 in short prepubertal children reported a greater increase in first year height velocity compared with rhGH monotherapy [8]. In hypophysectomised or undernourished rats, combined therapy had additive effects on bodyweight and longitudinal bone growth.

Here, the authors describe, in healthy non-GH-deficient female rats, additive effects of combined rhGH–rhIGF-1 therapy on bone cortical mass, but no additional stimulation of the growth plate or longitudinal bone growth. rhGH was more effective than rhIGF-1 in stimulating longitudinal bone growth. Consistent with previous reports, the additive effect on cortical bone mass was mostly due to increased periosteal apposition [5,6]. It is unlikely that the lack of additive effect of combined treatment is due to reduced endogenous GH/IGF-1 production as there were no differences in IGF-1, GH and ALS levels between GH alone or combination therapy groups. An explanation could lie in the differential responsiveness in growth plate chondrocytes versus bone cells. In conclusion, these findings show that combined GH–IGF-1 therapy has no additive effect on bone longitudinal growth compared with GH monotherapy, and increases organ growth in rats.

Growth hormone treatment for childhood short stature and risk of stroke in early adulthood

Poidvin A, Touzé E, Ecosse E, Landier F, Béjot Y, Giroud M, Rothwell PM, Carel JC, Coste J
Biostatistics and Epidemiology Unit and APEMAC Equipe d'Accueil, Assistance Publique-Hôpitaux de Paris, Université de Lorraine and University Paris Descartes, Paris, France
Neurology 2014;83:780–786

Background: Increased cardiac and cerebrovascular mortality in young adults treated with growth hormone (GH) in childhood was reported in a French cohort. The aim of this study was to evaluate the morbidity for cerebrovascular diseases in the same cohort of French patients.
Methods: An initial cohort of 10,332 patients treated with GH during childhood was evaluated. According to their clinical condition, patients were subdivided into three risk groups and the final analysis was performed in the low-risk group of 6,874 children treated with GH between 1985 and 1996 for idiopathic isolated GH deficiency and short stature either idiopathic or associated with being born small for gestational age. Adult morbidity data were obtained in 2008–2010. Medical reports and imaging data were evaluated by a single neurologist to detect cerebrovascular events which were classified, using standard definitions, as subarachnoid haemorrhage, intracerebral haemorrhage or ischaemic stroke. Capture–recapture analysis was used to estimate the number of missed cases. Reference data from the stroke registries of Dijon and Oxford were used to compare the incidence rates between the study cohort and the general population.
Results: Patients who were treated with GH during childhood showed a higher risk of stroke than the reference population. This was largely attributable to higher risks of haemorrhagic stroke (standardised

incidence ratios ranged from 3.5 to 7.0 by the different registries) and subarachnoid haemorrhage (5.7 to 9.3).
Conclusions: A higher morbidity for haemorrhagic stroke in subjects treated with GH during childhood was found. The authors propose that patients treated with GH worldwide should be informed about this long-term potential risk.

Over the last two decades the long-term safety of childhood GH treatment has been extensively investigated, the main focus being on the risk of cancer. The SAGhE project (safety and appropriateness of growth hormone treatments in Europe) was initiated to define mortality and morbidity in young adults who received rhGH therapy as children. The first report from the SAGhE French cohort showed higher cardiac and cerebrovascular mortality in rhGH-treated subjects [9]. That finding was consistent with the notions that acromegalic patients have higher risks of these diseases [10]; and the GH–IGF-1 axis may be implicated in the pathogenesis of cardiovascular disease [11]. However, another SAGhE group did not find one single case of death from cardiovascular or cerebrovascular disease [12].

In the current SAGhE study, the authors analysed a population-based French cohort of patients treated in childhood with GH for short stature. They describe higher risks of haemorrhagic stroke associated with childhood GH treatment for isolated GH deficiency or childhood short stature. These findings persisted when the estimation of the potentially missed cases was evaluated. This is the first industry-independent investigation in a large patient cohort, with strict inclusion criteria and long-term follow-up. The methods used to define and classify stroke cases were rigorous [13]. Nevertheless, the study has several limitations. The absolute number of reported events, though statistically significant, was small (11 cases out of 6,874 patients). The two population-based registries used for comparison are known to underestimate the incidence of cerebrovascular diseases, thus potentially leading to fictitiously higher incidences in the study cohort [14]. The lack of a control group of untreated patients with the same conditions is another important but unavoidable weakness. Finally, the lack of information about other potential confounders such as family history (that is, genetic predisposition), lifestyle, smoking, diabetes, dyslipidaemia or hypertension further curtails the impact of this study. This study provoked contrasting opinions among paediatric endocrinologists and led all adult and paediatric endocrine societies to release reassuring statements claiming that the available evidence is too weak to change the standard worldwide accepted management of patients undergoing GH therapy [15,16]. Despite all these caveats, this study raises new concern about a potential increased risk of haemorrhagic stroke in young adults who received rhGH therapy in childhood and will hopefully prompt us to conduct long-term prospective studies aimed at rigourously testing the long-term safety of GH therapy by addressing the effect of all potential confounding factors.

The impact of growth hormone therapy on adult height in Noonan syndrome: a systematic review

Giacomozzi C, Deodati A, Shaikh MG, Ahmed SF, Cianfarani S
Dipartimento di Medicina Pediatrica, Bambino Gesù Children's Hospital, Rome, Italy
dr.giacomozzi@gmail.com
Horm Res Paediatr 2015;83:167–176

Background: Noonan syndrome is a genetic disorder associated with short stature in about 70% of cases. The efficacy of recombinant-human growth hormone (rhGH) is still debated, this indication being approved in the US but not in Europe. This systematic review aimed to evaluate the available evidence on the long-term impact of childhood rhGH treatment on adult height in Noonan syndrome.
Methods: The authors systematically reviewed all studies available in the Cochrane Central Register of Controlled Trials, ISI Web of Science, MEDLINE and the references from all articles published up to April 2014. The final analysis included all papers reporting adult height or near adult height in patients with Noonan syndrome who received rhGH treatment. Clinical trials with at least three years follow-up were also assessed. A mean difference in AH between treated and untreated patients >0.9 SDS was considered as a satisfactory response to rhGH treatment. In non-randomised trials, rhGH efficacy was defined by height gain expressed as SDS. The Endocrine Society criteria were used to measure the quality and strength of evidence.

Results: Of 23 published studies assessing the impact of childhood rhGH therapy in Noonan syndrome, 17 were excluded because they did not satisfy the inclusion criteria. One further study had no control group and no information about adult height or near adult height. Among the included studies, two were longitudinal prospective trials and three were longitudinal retrospective studies. Not a single randomised controlled trial was identified. Extreme inter-individual variability in the responses to rhGH treatment was observed. Mean height gains ranged from 0.6 to 1.4 SDS when compared with national references and from 0.6 to 2.0 when compared with the Noonan reference. Low quality of evidence and weak recommendations were assigned to all selected studies.
Conclusions: To date, no high-quality randomised controlled trials into the effect of rhGH on adult height in patients with Noonan syndrome are available. More robust data are needed to ascertain the efficacy and the cost/benefit ratio of rhGH therapy in this condition.

Noonan syndrome is a genetic disorder belonging to the family of RASopathies, caused by mutations altering the RAS-MAPK pathway, with an estimated prevalence of one in 1,000–2,500 [17]. The wide spectrum of clinical features includes feeding difficulties, dysmorphic facial features, auditory deficits, heart defects, chest and spinal deformities, mild mental retardation and short stature. Average adult height is 169.2cm in males (range 153–188.7cm) and 154.4cm in females (range 146.1–167.8cm) [18]. Children with Noonan syndrome show normal responses on GH stimulation tests but may have reduced circulating IGF-1 levels, more pronounced in patients with *PTPN11* mutations. GH treatment increased short-term growth velocity, but no conclusive data are available on adult height [18]. This systematic review highlights the urgent need for well-designed clinical trials to assess the effect of rhGH therapy on adult height because the available data are insufficient to recommend such therapy in children with Noonan syndrome. The authors also raise doubts about the interpretation of efficacy when height gains are compared with national references in normal children. A common feature of children with Noonan syndrome is the delay in puberty that might confound interpretation of the catch-up growth associated with rhGH therapy when it occurs in late adolescence because a spontaneous pubertal growth spurt may account for the observed height gain. Patients with Noonan syndrome are genetically susceptible to cancer. The available data do not show any further increased risk in children undergoing rhGH therapy. However, the assessment of risk requires long-term surveillance even after discontinuation of treatment. In conclusion, these findings show that the available data on the efficacy of rhGH therapy on adult height in patients with Noonan syndrome do not fulfil the evidence-based medicine criteria to allow strong recommendations to be made.

Clinical trials

Efficacy and safety of growth hormone treatment in children with hypochondroplasia: comparison with an historical cohort

Pinto G, Cormier-Daire V, Le Merrer M, Samara-Boustani D, Baujat G, Fresneau L, Viaud M, Souberbielle JC, Pineau JC, Polak M
Pediatric Endocrinology, Gynecology and Diabetes, Centre des Maladies Endocriniennes Rares de la Croissance, Hôpital Universitaire Necker-Enfants Malades, Paris, France
graziella.pinto@nck.aphp.fr
Horm Res Paediatr 2014;82:355–363

Background: Hypochondroplasia (HCH) is an autosomal dominant skeletal dysplasia with a heterogeneous phenotype associated with disproportionate short stature. The objective of this study was to define the efficacy and safety of recombinant human growth hormone (rhGH) treatment in subjects affected by HCH.
Methods: A three-year open-label interventional study was conducted in 19 HCH patients (11 females; mean age at start 9.3 ± 3.1 years). The patients received rhGH at a mean dose of 0.053mg/kd/day for three years. Both weight and IGF-1 levels were used to adjust doses. For comparison, a historical cohort of 40 untreated patients was used to design suitable reference growth charts.
Results: The treated children showed a height increase of +0.62 ± 0.81 SDS compared with the general population, and +1.39 ± 0.9 SDS compared with an untreated historical HGH cohort. The mean height

gain was 7.4 ± 6.6cm compared with the untreated cohort. The effect of the treatment was inversely correlated with age at the start of therapy (P=0.04) but not with the presence of fibroblast growth factor receptor 3 (FGF3) mutations. During therapy approximately 20% of the patients showed insulin resistance as suggested by a HOMA-IR value above 3.16, but none showed glucose intolerance and HbA_{1c} remained in the normal range. The therapy was well tolerated.
Conclusions: rhGH therapy increases short-term height gains of children with HCH. It is safe and its efficacy is higher when started early. There was wide between-individual variability in treatment responses, suggesting the need for personalised evaluation during treatment in order to establish appropriate management.

Hypochondroplasia (HCH) is an autosomal dominant skeletal dysplasia, mostly due to mutations in the *FGFR3 (fibroblast growth factor receptor 3)* gene. Clinically, HCH shows a wide spectrum of disease severity. Short stature is already present in childhood but tends to worsen during puberty, due to the lack of pubertal spurt. Male HCH patients achieve adult heights ranging from 145cm to 165cm, whereas female adult height varies from 133cm to 151cm [19]. Nowadays, GH administration is not limited only to subjects with GH deficiency but is also used in syndromes characterised by short stature, such as Turner and Prader-Willi syndrome. The few available studies on the effectiveness of GH treatment in HCH patients report a wide range of height gain [20,21], overall suggesting a positive impact on height velocity [22]. The present study reports the efficacy and safety of 3-year GH therapy in a cohort of HCH children, compared with a historical cohort of untreated patients. GH therapy showed good safety and efficacy. No serious adverse effects were reported and the treated cohort showed an increase of 7.4 ± 6.6cm compared with the untreated cohort. As GH may also improve bone mineral density, dual-energy X-ray absorptiometry was performed, revealing a moderate, though non-significant, increase of bone lumbar spine mineralometry. These results should be interpreted with caution as a short-term improvement in height velocity is not necessarily associated with an improvement of adult height. In the only seven treated patients who reached adult height, the mean height SDS (compared with the French general population reference) was the same as at baseline (-3.1 at baseline and -3.0 at adult height), but compared with the untreated historical cohort the mean height gain was +1.39 SDS. Another limitation was the small size of the historical HCH cohort (n=40) used for anthropometric comparisons. Furthermore, the historical cohort was not genotyped. It is also important to note that treated HCH patients showed a wide variation in the response to treatment, thus raising the need for a more accurate clinical, laboratory, radiological and genetic characterisation of patients in order to identify the responders. In conclusion, further collaborative prospective clinical trials, ideally randomised and controlled, are warranted to confirm these promising results that would open a new avenue for the management of patients with HCH.

Growth hormone therapy, muscle thickness, and motor development in Prader-Willi syndrome: an RCT

Reus L, Pillen S, Pelzer BJ, van Alfen-van der Velden JAAEM, Hokken-Koelega ACS, Zwarts M, Otten BJ, Nijhuis-van der Sanden MWG
Department of Rehabilitation, Pediatric Physical Therapy, Scientific Institute for Quality of Healthcare, Radboud University Medical Center, Nijmegen, The Netherlands
lin.reus@gmail.com
Pediatrics 2014;134:e1619–e1627

Background: Infants with Prader-Willi Syndrome (PWS) show neuromotor alterations such as hypotonia, muscle weakness and motor developmental delay. This study aimed to define the ability of growth hormone (GH) therapy on a background of physical training to improve muscle thickness, muscle strength and motor development in infants with PWS.
Methods: A two-year randomised, single-blind controlled trial was performed in 22 infants with PWS (mean age at start 12.9 ± 7.1 months). Both treatment (n=10) and control groups (n=12) received physical training and underwent a follow-up of two years. The treatment group received GH 1mg/m^2/day. Ultrasonography was used to assess the muscle thickness of four different muscle groups (left biceps brachii, right forearm flexors, right quadriceps and left tibialis anterior muscle). Muscle strength and motor performance were evaluated by Infant Muscle Strength meter and Gross Motor Function Measurements, respectively.

Results: Baseline muscle strength was 58% of the normal reference. After six months, GH increased muscle thickness of the biceps brachii, forearm flexors and tibialis anterior compared with baseline, whereas in the control group muscle thickness increased only in the tibialis anterior. After 12 months of GH treatment, muscle thickness improved in all four muscle groups but only in the forearm flexors and quadriceps in the control group. Muscle thickness positively correlated with muscle strength ($P<0.001$) and motor performance ($P<0.001$).
Conclusions: GH treatment combined with physical training increased muscle thickness in infants with PWS. GH-independent catch-up growth was faster in muscles used for the early motor development suggesting a training effect.

Infants with Prader-Willi syndrome (PWS) show neuromotor alterations, motor developmental delay and increased fat at the expense of muscle mass [23,24]. Hypotonia and muscular weakness further contribute to muscle anomalies. Early GH therapy improves lean body mass [24] and motor function [25]. This study confirms that infants with PWS have reduced muscle thickness, which is strongly related to muscle strength and motor performance. The early start of GH treatment improves muscle thickness which, in turn, associates with increased muscle strength and motor performance. Different muscle groups showed different growth patterns. In muscles that are largely used in the acquisition of fundamental early motor skills, there was a naturally occurring catch-up growth independent of GH treatment, thus suggesting a training effect. Another strength of this study is the evaluation of very early start of GH therapy, which in PWS patients is more commonly started in childhood. As suggested by the recent Consensus Guidelines for rhGH therapy in patients with PWS, an early start of GH therapy may be more beneficial even though the exact optimal age has not yet been established [26]. The main limitations of this study are the small size that makes it more like a pilot study and the short follow-up period. In conclusion, these findings suggest that early start of GH treatment improves muscle strength and motor performance by stimulating muscle thickness in infants with PWS.

New mechanisms

Male bovine GH transgenic mice have decreased adiposity with an adipose depot-specific increase in immune cell populations

Benencia F, Harshman S, Duran-Ortiz S, Lubbers ER, List EO, Householder L, Al-Naeeli M, Liang X, Welch L, Kopchick JJ, Berryman DE
Department of Biomedical Sciences, Heritage College of Osteopathic Medicine; Russ College of Engineering and Technology; Diabetes Institute; Edison Biotechnology Institute; Ohio University, Athens, OH, USA
berrymad@ohio.edu
Endocrinology 2015;156:1794–1803

Background: White adipose tissue (WAT) comprises adipocytes as well as a complex stromal vascular fraction (SVF), containing a variety of immune cells. Different WAT depots show different patterns of resident immune cells and different impact on metabolic homeostasis. The factors involved in the distribution of immune cell types in the different WAT depots have not yet been fully elucidated. Growth hormone (GH) is a candidate factor as it has potent lipolytic and antilipogenic effects on adipocytes, and the GH receptor is expressed in a wide range of innate and adaptive immune cells. This study aimed to characterise the GH-dependent and depot-specific differences in WAT immune cells.
Methods: Bovine GH (bGH) transgenic mice, an animal model mimicking acromegaly, were compared with wild-type (WT) mice. bGH mice showed higher bodyweight with decreased adiposity and increased lean mass, impaired glucose metabolism and shortened lifespan. Three different WAT depots were collected: inguinal SC, epididymal (EPI) and mesenteric (MES). Flow cytometry was used to define the immune cell subsets. RNA sequencing was performed to assess the activation of T-cell pathways.
Results: bGH mice showed a higher number of total SVF cells compared with WT mice in both SC and MES depots. Leucocyte infiltration was higher in MES and lower in EPI depots in bGH compared with controls. In bGH SC and MES depots macrophages represented a larger proportion of total SVF cells.

Increased levels of macrophages expressing M2 markers were found in all depots of bGH mice with the highest levels in SC and MES. T helper cells were more abundant in the SC depot of bGH compared with controls. Regulatory T cells were higher in both SC and MES depots in bGH mice. Higher levels of cytotoxic T cells were found in the bGH EPI depot. RNA sequencing revealed significant alterations in pathways related to T-cell infiltration and activation in the SC depots with fewer significant changes in the EPI bGH WAT depots.
Conclusions: GH affects the distribution of immune cells in WAT and its influence depends on the location of WAT depot.

White adipose tissue (WAT) is an active endocrine organ, which functions not only as a fat store, but also regulates several metabolic pathways [27]. It is composed of both adipocytes and a stromal vascular fraction consisting of several types of cells, including immune cells, which differ by degree of adiposity as well as by the type of adipose depot [28,29]. A proinflammatory phenotype is more commonly found in visceral depots [28,30]. Visceral and non-visceral WAT influence metabolism in different ways, which might partially reflect their differences in local immune cell compositions. GH promotes lipolysis and regulates pre-adipocyte proliferation, differentiation and senescence [31], but also exerts actions on the immune system. In addition, in obese patients, GH deficiency could favour the inflammation and the metabolic alterations of WAT by affecting adipokine and cytokine expression [32].

Here, the authors describe the influence of GH on immune cells in different WAT depots by studying an animal model mimicking acromegaly. The main findings were the differences in the total amount of stromal vascular fraction cells among WAT depots as well as macrophage polarisation towards an anti-inflammatory phenotype and changes in T-cell proportions. Despite the anti-inflammatory properties exhibited by the WAT of these mice, these animals had a shortened lifespan [33], suggesting that other factors may affect their lifespan. Functional analysis of WAT macrophages was not performed and it was impossible to confirm that the cells were functional anti-inflammatory M2 macrophages. Another interesting finding was the detection of depot-specific modifications in the proportions of distinct T-cell subsets. Different T-cells have been associated with obesity-related alterations [30,34], but their role in obesity is not yet clear. Unfortunately, T-cells were not characterised in this study thus leaving unanswered the question about the GH-dependent modulation of different T-cell subtypes such as TH1, TH2, NK and cytotoxic. These findings suggest that GH influences the immune cell pattern in WAT with potential clinical implications in the management of metabolic disorders.

Insulin-like growth factor 1 (IGF-1) stabilizes nascent blood vessels

Jacobo SM, Kazlauskus A
Department of Ophthalmology, Harvard Medical School, The Schepens Eye Research Institute and Massachusetts Eye and Ear Infirmary, Boston, MA, USA
andrius_kazlauskas@meei.harvard.edu
J Biol Chem 2015;290:6349-6360

Background: IGF-1 has been proposed as a promoter of angiogenesis, but it is unclear whether this phenomenon results from formation of new vessels versus stabilising existing vessels. The aim of this study was to clarify the role of IGF-1 in the stabilisation of neovessels.
Methods: Primary endothelial cells were derived from different vascular beds (human microvascular retinal endothelial cells, human umbilical vein endothelial cells, human choroidal endothelial cells), as well as from mouse retinal explants. Destabilisation/regression of the different culture systems was induced by means of lysophosphatidic acid (LPA).
Results: Treatment of human microvascular retinal endothelial cells with vascular endothelial cell growth factor (VEGF) induced tube formation. The addition of LPA caused tube regression by stimulating the migration and subsequent disorganisation of tubes organised from primary endothelial cells. IGF-1 prevented LPA-stimulated regression of tubes stabilising both endothelial cell tubes and retinal neovessels. These findings were confirmed by the analysis of different vascular beds. The IGF-1-mediated stabilisation was dependent on Erk activity and associated with prolonged Erk activation. Similar findings were confirmed on vessels sprout from mouse retinal explants.

Conclusions: IGF-1 stabilises nascent vessels whose formation is driven by VEGF. The underlying mechanism of IGF-1-mediated stabilisation involves prolonged activation of Erk, which antagonises LPA-driven regression.

Angiogenesis is a complex process involving an interplay between endothelial cells and several regulatory factors leading to the formation of new blood vessels. Several lines of evidence suggest a key role of IGF-1 in angiogenesis. The IGF-1 receptor is present on endothelial cells of both large and small vessels [35], and IGF-1 is known to exert a chemotactic action on vascular endothelial cells [36]. In vitro IGF-1 induces endothelial tube-forming activity [37]. IGF-1 also induces the expression of hypoxia-inducible factors which in turn regulate the transcription of key angiogenic genes [35]. The deletion of IGF-1 receptor impairs neovascularisation [38]. All these findings support a critical role for IGF-1 in angiogenesis. Here, the authors show that IGF-1 stabilises endothelial cell tubes and retinal neovessels formed in response to VEGF. They further analysed the mechanism by which IGF-1 contrasts regression and identified Erk as the key pathway. Most actions of IGF-1 are mediated by the IGF-1 receptor and the downstream activation of different signalling pathways such as Ras/Raf/ERK and PI3 kinase/Akt [35]. As angiogenesis is important in both physiological and pathological processes, such as cancer and diabetic retinopathy, it is extremely useful to have a better knowledge of these mechanisms. This study clarifies the IGF-1 contribution to angiogenesis and opens avenues for new therapeutic approaches based on the modulation of the IGF system in the management of diseases characterised by alterations in vessel formation.

Insulin-like growth factor independent effects of growth hormone on growth plate chondrogenesis and longitudinal bone growth

Wu S, Yang W, De Luca F
Section of Endocrinology and Diabetes, St Christopher's Hospital for Children, Drexel University College of Medicine, Philadelphia, PA, USA
francesco.deluca@drexelmed.edu
Endocrinology 2015;156:2541–2551

Background: Growth hormone (GH) plays a key role in the regulation of growth plate chondrogenesis and longitudinal bone growth. However, it is not clear whether GH effects are mediated by local secretion of IGF-1 and IGF-2. The aim of this study was to test whether GH has IGF-independent effects on growth plate physiology.
Methods: Mice were generated with excision of the Igf1 receptor (Igf1r) gene exclusively in the growth plate inducible on postnatal systemic injection of tamoxifen ^{TamCart}Igf1r$^{flox/flox}$ (KO mice). The control animals were Igf1r$^{flox/flox}$ littermates. Both KO and controls were subdivided into three groups: untreated; daily injection of IGF-1 for four weeks; or daily injection of GH for four weeks.
Results: KO mice receiving GH showed higher body and tibial growth compared with untreated KO and control mice. Increased phosphorylation of Janus kinase 2 as well as signal transducer and activator of transcription 5B in the tibial growth plate was observed in GH-treated control and KO mice. GH increased mRNA expression of bone morphogenetic protein-2 and mRNA expression and protein phosphorylation of nuclear factor-κB p65 in the tibial growth plate both in control and KO mice. GH stimulated Igf2 mRNA expression in growth plate both in control and KO mice. When cultures of chondrocytes transfected with Igf1rsiRNA were exposed to GH, increased thymidine incorporation and collagen X mRNA expression was observed.
Conclusions: GH promotes growth plate chondrogenesis and longitudinal bone growth through IGF-1R-independent mechanisms in the growth plate. The intracellular molecular mechanisms underlying the IGF-independent growth-promoting GH effects have yet to be elucidated.

Bone growth is a complex mechanism, mainly involving chondrogenesis at the growth plate regulated by several autocrine/paracrine factors and finely modulated by endocrine factors. The central role of the GH-IGF-1 axis in regulating longitudinal growth is well established. GH promotes growth mainly by stimulating IGF-1 production both systematically and locally in the growth plate [39]. IGF-2 also exerts some effects on bone growth as suggested by the severely impaired birth size in animal models with *Igf1* or *Igf2* gene deletion [40]. Evidence from knockout (KO) mice also suggests a direct effect of GH on growth [41–43].

Here, the authors elegantly confirm the ability of GH to influence body and tibial growth, independently of IGF-1. Indeed, *Igfr* KO mice exhibited a reduced length of tibial growth plate, which was due to reduced width of all three cartilage zones (germinal, proliferative and hypertrophic). The systemic injection of GH in *Igfr* KO mice for four weeks increased the growth plate width, reflecting increased widths of all three epiphyseal, proliferative and hypertrophic zones. Interestingly, the authors propose that the mechanism responsible for this IGF-independent GH action might involve the transcription factor nuclear factor (NF)-κB p65 which has been previously linked to chondrocyte proliferation and differentiation [44,45]. Indeed, the injection of GH to *Igfr* KO mice increased phosphorylation (that is, activation) of NF-κB p65 in the growth plate. Regarding additional factors involved in the IGF-independent effects of GH, bone morphogenetic protein-2 (BMP-2) is expressed in the growth plate and stimulates longitudinal bone growth by favouring growth plate chondrocyte proliferation and hypertrophy. GH administration induced BMP-2 mRNA expression in the growth plate of *Igfr* KO mice thus suggesting that also the increased expression of BMP-2 in the growth plate may contribute to the IGF-independent, growth-promoting effects of GH. A potential bias is that IGF-1 and IGF-2 might affect growth plate chondrogenesis and bone growth through the insulin receptor. In conclusion, this study provides strong evidence in favour of a direct IGF-independent action of GH on cartilage growth.

New paradigms

Insulin like growth factor 2 overexpression induces beta-cell dysfunction and increases beta-cell susceptibility to damage

Casellas A, Mallol C, Salavert A, Jimenez V, Garcia M, Agudo J, Obach M, Haurigot V, Vilà L, Molas M, Lage R, Morrò M, Casana E, Ruberte J, Bosch F
Universitat Autonoma de Barcelona, Barcelona, Spain
fatima.bosch@uab.es
J Biol Chem 2015;290:16772–16785

Background: Type 1 diabetes mellitus (DM) is characterised by beta-cell failure, whose mechanism is not yet fully understood. Beta-cell dedifferentiation and endoplasmic reticulum stress are involved in beta-cell dysfunction. The INS/IGF2 locus is associated with DM susceptibility but the pathogenic role of IGF-2 in the development of DM has been poorly investigated. This study aimed to assess the role of IGF-2 in the pathogenesis of DM.
Methods: A transgenic mice model overexpressing IGF-2 specifically in beta-cells (Tg-IGF2) was used. Mice expressing human IFNbeta (Tg-IFNbeta) were used as models of high susceptibility to autoimmune diabetes. Both immunohistochemical analysis and beta-cell ultrastructural analysis were performed. qPCR was used to assess the expression of genes involved in beta-cell function. Microarray analysis on islets of Tg-IGF2 and wild type (WT) mice was performed. Pancreatic islets from WT animals underwent in vitro transfection with adenoviral vectors encoding IGF2.
Results: Tg-IGF2 mice showed beta-cell dysfunction and inadequate secretory response as indicated by glucose intolerance, reduced insulin release, downregulation of GLUT2 and increased number of immature insulin secretory granules. Downregulation of several genes characteristic of fully differentiated and functional beta-cells, upregulation of endoplasmic reticulum stress markers and increased autophagy were observed in islets from Tg-IGF2 mice. The same phenotype was obtained after transfection of islets from WT animals with adenoviral vectors encoding IGF2. In Tg-IGF2 islets, a decreased expression of insulin-receptor A (IR-A) was detected whereas no differences were found in IR-B, IGF2R and IGF1R. Both adenoviral-mediated overexpression of IGF2 and treatment of adult wild-type islets with recombinant IGF2 confirmed the direct implication of IGF2 on beta-cell dysfunction. Streptozotocin treatment or crossing the mice with a transgenic model of islet lymphocytic infiltration promoted the development of overt diabetes, thus suggesting that IGF2 makes islets more susceptible to beta-cell damage and immune attack.
Conclusions: In mice, beta-cell overexpression of IGF-2 leads to beta-cell dedifferentiation and dysfunction increasing the susceptibility to damage. These findings suggest that IGF-2 may play a role in the pathophysiology of DM.

Recently, beta-cell dedifferentiation has been proposed as one of the mechanisms underlying type 1 diabetes. The loss of differentiation involves downregulation of many genes that are highly expressed in beta-cells and necessary for function, such as insulin, solute carrier family member 2 (SLC2A2 or GLUT2), glucokinase (GCK) and pancreatic and duodenal homeobox 1 (PDX1) [46]. In animal models, endoplasmic reticulum (ER) stress is a proposed additional mechanism for beta-cell dysfunction and death in type 2 diabetes [47]. IGF-2 is a key regulator of fetal growth. Interestingly, the *IGF2* gene is located on chromosome 11p15.5 close to the insulin gene and the *INS/IGF2* locus is robustly associated with type 1 diabetes susceptibility [48]. Genetic variants in *IGF2* are associated with insulin resistance [49] and circulating IGF-2 seems to regulate insulin sensitivity [50]. Devedjian et al. previously reported that overexpression of IGF-2 in beta-cells causes a pre-diabetic state [51].

Here, the authors describe that IGF-2 overexpression in beta-cells causes cell dedifferentiation and induces ER stress. The exposure to high IGF-2 levels also increases beta-cell susceptibility to damage, thus contributing to the development of diabetes. Interestingly, by means of adenoviral vectors encoding IGF-2, the authors proved that IGF-2 has direct effects on beta-cells, ruling out the possibility that the observed findings might be caused by exposure to IGF-2 overexpression from early embryonic development. This study demonstrates a novel and detrimental effect of IGF-2 on beta-cell function. Local overexpression of IGF-2 in beta-cells causes profound changes that lead to their dedifferentiation, ER stress and beta-cell dysfunction. As a consequence, the islets are more sensitive to immune and non-immune mediated beta-cell damage. These findings contrast with previous studies showing a protective role of IGF-2 on beta-cell survival [52,53]. In conclusion, these findings highlight a novel role for IGF-2 in beta-cell dedifferentiation and ER stress, and suggest that novel preventive and therapeutic strategies may be based on the balance of the IGF system.

New perspective

The optimal postnatal growth trajectory for term small for gestational age babies: a prospective cohort study

Lei X, Chen Y, Ye J, Ouyang F, Jiang F, Zhang J
MOE-Shanghai Key Laboratory of Children's Environmental Health, Xinhua Hospital, Shanghai Jiao Tong University School of Medicine, Shanghai, China
junjimzhang@gmail.com
J Pediatr 2015;166:54–58

Background: Subjects born small for gestational age (SGA) are at higher risk of cardiometabolic disease in adulthood. Without early postnatal catch-up growth, they are also at risk of permanent short stature. However, early rapid postnatal catch-up growth may further increase the cardiometabolic risk. The aim of this study was to identify the optimal growth trajectory in SGA infants from birth to seven years of age.
Methods: A prospective cohort study involved 12 US medical centres from 1959 to 1976. 1,957 full-term SGA (birthweight <10th percentile) were followed for seven years, with five measurements of weight and length/height during the follow-up. Infants born at term with birthweight appropriate for gestational age were the control group. Five different weight growth trajectories were identified using a latent class model: no catch-up growth, regression after four months, slow catch-up growth, appropriate catch-up growth and excessive catch-up growth. At the age of seven years the presence of obesity or overweight, growth restriction, hypertension, infections and IQ were assessed. The optimal growth trajectory was chosen according to the lowest overall risk of childhood diseases.
Results: SGA infants with no catch-up growth (n=439, 22.4%) showed higher risk of infection in infancy (aOR 1.2, 95% CI 1.0–1.6), growth restriction (11.2, 8.6–14.6) and low IQ (2.1, 1.7–2.8) at seven years compared with controls. SGA babies with excessive catch-up growth (n=176, 8.9%) had a higher risk of overweight/obesity (7.5, 5.4–10.5) and increased blood pressure (1.7, 1.1–2.4) at seven years. Infants with a growth characterised by regression at four months (n=285, 14.6%) had higher risk of growth restriction (2.2, 1.5–3.2). SGA children with slow catch-up growth (n=328, 16.8%) showed higher risk of low IQ (1.6, 1.2–2.1). Babies with appropriate catch-up growth (n=729, 37.3%) did not

have increased risk of any adverse outcome. Testing of the same cohort for linear growth trajectories yielded similar findings.
Conclusions: In term SGA infants the best growth trajectory, associated with the lowest overall risk, is represented by a rapid catch-up growth to reach the 30th percentile during the first months of life, thereafter followed by moderate catch-up growth to be around the 50th percentile by the age of seven years. Both rapid and poor early postnatal growth lead to worst outcomes.

Low birthweight as well as SGA have been associated with a higher risk of metabolic alterations such as insulin resistance, glucose intolerance and type 2 diabetes in adult life. SGA babies usually show early catch-up growth that tends to be completed by two years [54]. A rapid postnatal catch-up growth is associated with a higher risk of metabolic diseases [54-56], whereas infants having poor catch-up growth show higher risk of infection, short stature and neurodevelopment anomalies [57,58]. To date, the postnatal growth pattern associated with the best outcome has not yet been ascertained in SGA children.

Here, the authors identify for the first time the optimal growth trajectory in infants born SGA. The lowest risk of disease is associated with a trajectory characterised by an initial rapid catch-up growth leading to the 30th percentile and followed by a growth allowing the maintenance on the 50th percentile track. Both poor and excessive catch-up growth patterns are associated with poor outcomes. In particular, excessive postnatal catch-up growth in term SGA infants increases the risk of overweight/obesity and hypertension. The neurodevelopmental performance at seven years was better in SGA with faster catch-up growth in the first four months of life than in those with poor growth in the same period. The clinical implication is that strategies aimed at optimising early postnatal growth may prevent cardiometabolic disease in adulthood and interventions should be pursued. Although thought provoking, the study has several limitations. First, the definition of SGA used differed from that established by the consensus conference on SGA children [54]. Second, the use of last menstrual period to calculate gestational age may underestimate the duration of pregnancy and over-diagnose SGA. Third, the influence of nutrition was not investigated. Fourth, the follow-up was conducted only up to seven years of age thus not being able to consider the important changes in the main outcomes occurring at puberty. Finally, the study was performed 30–40 years ago and the findings may not be relevant to contemporary populations. Nevertheless, this study indicates for the first time the optimal growth trajectory which SGA infants should follow to reduce the risks of adverse consequences, showing, once again, that 'in medio stat virtus'.

Genetically determined height and coronary artery disease

Nelson CP, Hamby SE, Saleheen D, Hopewell JC, Zeng L, Assimes TL, Kanoni S, Willenborg C, Burgess S, Amouyel P, Anand S, Blankenberg S, Boehm BO, Clarke RJ, Collins R, Dedoussis G, Farrall M, Franks PW, Groop L, Hall AS, Hamsten A, Hengstenberg C, Hovingh GK, Ingelsson E, Kathiresan S, Kee F, König IR, Kooner J, Lehtimäki T, März W, McPherson R, Metspalu A, Nieminen MS, O'Donnell CJ, Palmer CN, Peters A, Perola M, Reilly MP, Ripatti S, Roberts R, Salomaa V, Shah SH, Schreiber S, Siegbahn A, Thorsteinsdottir U, Veronesi G, Wareham N, Willer CJ, Zalloua PA, Erdmann J, Deloukas P, Watkins H, Schunkert H, Danesh J, Thompson JR, Samani NJ; CARDIoGRAM+C4D Consortium
njs@le.ac.uk
N Engl J Med 2015;372:1608-1618

Background: An inverse relationship between stature and risk of coronary artery disease (CAD) has long been recognised but the underlying mechanisms are still unclear. By using a genetic approach, this study aimed to investigate the relationship between adult height and CAD.
Methods: 180 genetic variants, previously associated with height but not implicated in susceptibility to CAD, were used to study the association between adult height and CAD. A cohort of 65,066 cases (65% with a history of myocardial infarction) and 128,383 controls was evaluated to assess the association between a change in genetically determined height of 1 SD (6.5cm) and the risk of CAD. 18,429 subjects (including 8,240 cases) with individual-level genotype data were subdivided into quartiles according to increasing numbers of height-raising alleles. The associations between genetically determined height and 12 established cardiovascular risk factors were analysed and a pathway analysis of the height-associated genes was performed.
Results: Height-increasing variants in combination were inversely associated with CAD (odds ratio, 0.88; 95% CI, 0.82–0.95; P<0.001); there was a relative increase of 13.5% (95% CI, 5.4–22.1, P<0.001) in the risk of CAD for each 1 SD decrease in genetically determined height. The association was still present when

analysing subjects with a history of myocardial infarction. In sex-specific analyses, the association was significant in males and not in females, but in an interaction test this gender difference was not significant. Subjects with higher numbers of height-raising alleles showed lower risks of CAD (odds ratio for quartile 4 versus quartile 1 was 0.74; 95% CI, 0.68 to 0.84; P<0.001). Among the analysed cardiovascular risk factors, a small but significant association was found between height-associated variants and LDL cholesterol and triglyceride levels (accounting for approximately 30% of the association with CAD). Several overlapping pathways involving genes associated with both development and atherosclerosis were detected.
Conclusions: The association between a genetically determined shorter height and higher risk of CAD was identified. This finding may be partially explained by a more adverse lipid profile. Common biological pathways involving both height growth and atherosclerosis might also contribute to this association.

The relationship between short stature and higher risk for cardiovascular diseases has been reported since the 1950s. A recent systematic review, assessing >3,000,000 subjects from 52 studies, concluded that adults in the shortest height category have a 50% higher relative risk of CAD mortality and morbidity than tall subjects [59]. The underlying mechanisms are unclear. Short stature is associated with well-known risk factors for coronary disease such as LDL-cholesterol levels, hypertension and diabetes. However, the association between height and CAD persists even after adjustment for those factors [60]. Short stature might be a consequence of exposure to a poor intrauterine environment and fetal growth restriction which is per se associated with higher risk of CAD in adulthood [61]. Finally, the relationship between short stature and CAD may be confounded by other factors affecting both conditions, such as undernutrition or infections.

By analysis in a huge case-control study of 180 height-associated genetic variants accounting for about 10% of the variation in adult height, the authors describe an association between variants that confer shorter stature and CAD. Similar associations also emerged with lipid profile (specifically LDL-cholesterol and triglyceride levels), thus confirming previous findings [60]. However, statistical analysis showed that lipid profile explains only 30% of the association with CAD, therefore other pathways may be involved. The pathway analysis identified a number of overlapping pathways linking height-associated variants to risk of CAD, including the BMP- and TGF-beta signalling pathways, axon guidance pathways and the STAT3 and IGF-1 pathways, all of which have experimentally documented roles in atherosclerosis. Body size is positively related to the diameter of coronary arteries. Therefore, a potential simple explanation is that shorter adults have proportionally smaller coronary vessels and consequently higher risk of plaque-induced ischaemia. The risk of CAD attributable to any single variant is small, but is significant in the combination of all considered variants [62]. However, the overall effect remains lower than that of other well-known risk factors, such as overweight, smoking or diabetes.

This study is also extremely helpful in interpreting data on the safety of long-term GH therapy, especially in non-GH deficient patients. This innate relationship between shorter height and higher CAD risk must be taken into account in the analysis of cardiovascular morbidity and mortality in subjects with short stature. In conclusion, the recognised association between shorter adult height and higher risk of CAD is partially explained by a worse lipid profile as well as other common biological processes involved in height growth and the development of atherosclerosis.

Vitamin B12-dependent taurine synthesis regulates growth and bone mass

Roman-Garcia P, Quiros-Gonzalez I, Mottram L, Lieben L, Sharan K, Wangwiwatsin A, Tubio J, Lewis K, Wilkinson D, Santhanam B, Sarper N, Clare S, Vassiliou GS, Velagapudi VR, Dougan G, Yadav VK
Systems Biology of Bone Laboratory, Wellcome Trust Sanger Institute, Cambridge, UK
vy1@sanger.ac.uk
J Clin Invest 2014;124:2988–3002

Background: Fetal exposure to maternal environment influences late-life health of the offspring. Vitamin B12 deficiency is associated with growth retardation, reduced serum osteocalcin levels, low bone mineral density and increased bone fracture risk but the underlying mechanism is unclear. The aim of this study was to define the role of maternally derived vitamin B12 on offspring growth and bone mass.
Methods: A mouse genetic model of B12 deficiency obtained by deleting the gene essential for gut absorption of B12 ($Gif^{-/-}$), was generated to study the role of maternally or offspring-derived B12 on growth

and bone mass homeostasis. Both first- ($Gif^{-/-}_{(F1)}$) and second-generation ($Gif^{-/-}_{(F2)}$) mice were evaluated. Pregnant $Gif^{-/-}_{(F1)}$ mothers received a single injection of B12. Primary osteoblasts were cultured in B12-deficient medium and treated with different B12 doses. Metabolomic analysis was performed in liver samples of $Gif^{-/-}_{(F2)}$ and WT mice. HepG2 cells were transfected with transcobalamin 2-oleosin construct (TCOL) in order to obtain B12 chelation. $Gif^{-/-}_{(F2)}$ mice were treated orally with taurine. Children's serum samples with low B12 levels were also analysed.

Results: Growth was similar among $Gif^{-/-}_{(F1)}$, $Gif^{-/-}_{(F2)}$ and wild-type (WT) mice until 21 days after birth (P21). Thereafter, $Gif^{-/-}_{(F2)}$ mice had impaired weight gain and reduced body size. Compared with $Gif^{-/-}_{(F1)}$ and WT mice, $Gif^{-/-}_{(F2)}$ mice showed decreased bone mass both in vertebrae and in long bones. 48-week-old $Gif^{-/-}_{(F1)}$ mice had normal growth but a severe decrease of bone mass suggesting that B12 deficiency during ageing influenced bone mass independently of body growth. Primary osteoblasts of B12-deficient mice exposed to different doses of B12 proliferated and differentiated similarly to WT cells. $Gif^{-/-}_{(F2)}$ mice showed elevated serum GH levels as well as a higher expression of GH-releasing hormone and reduced IGF-1 levels. Decreased STAT5 phosphorylation was shown both in liver and in muscle. A single B12 injection to $Gif^{-/-}_{(F1)}$ mothers prevented bone anomalies in $Gif^{-/-}_{(F2)}$ mice by rescuing growth retardation and bone loss, and normalised GH/IGF-1 levels. A suppression of taurine metabolism was found in the liver of $Gif^{-/-}_{(F2)}$ mice. HepG2 cells transfected with TCOL had no increase in STAT5 phosphorylation and taurine production when exposed to GH treatment. The administration of taurine restored GH responsiveness. $Gif^{-/-}_{(F2)}$ mice treated with taurine showed a rescue of growth retardation associated with a normalisation of IGF-1 and GH levels, as well as of histological and histomorphometry parameters. Taurine treatment increased osteoblast proliferation. In children's serum samples, positive correlations between B12 and taurine, B12 and osteocalcin, taurine and osteocalcin levels were found.

Conclusions: These findings reveal the importance of vitamin B12 in the regulation of growth and bone mass through taurine synthesis.

Vitamin B12 deficiency is associated with anomalies of growth and bone homeostasis [63,64]. In addition, in wasted, underweight and stunted children, B12 supplementation improves both weight and height [65]. Using a B12-deficient animal model, the authors clearly show that maternally derived B12 crucially regulates offspring growth and bone mass. In particular, B12 deficiency reduces liver taurine production which in turn decreases IGF-1 hepatic synthesis. Exogenous taurine restores the GH-dependent synthesis of IGF-1 and osteoblast function with consequent rescue of growth retardation. Taurine was previously associated with growth retardation [66], and this study elucidates the mechanism by which it affects bone growth. These results are consistent with a recent report that taurine increases growth plate thickness by promoting JAK2-STAT phosphorylation and increasing IGF-1 levels [67]. Finally, positive associations between B12 and taurine, B12 and osteocalcin, taurine and osteocalcin were found in children's serum, suggesting the possibility of transferring these results to humans. An important limitation of this study is the lack of information regarding other consequences of long-term vitamin B12 deficiency (for example growth arrest, hypotonia and nerve demyelination), which are deleterious to bone and skeletal muscle function and might explain the findings. Further studies should assess the relative contributions to the bone phenotype of all the potential interfering variables [68]. In conclusion, these in vitro and in vivo results support the concept that B12 regulates growth and bone mass via GH sensitivity by regulating liver taurine production and may be translated into novel B12-based preventive and therapeutic approaches for bone health.

Low circulating levels of IGF-1 in healthy adults are associated with reduced β-cell function, increased intramyocellular lipid, and enhanced fat utilization during fasting

Thankamony A, Capalbo D, Marcovecchio MD, Sleigh A, Jørgensen SW, Hill NR, Mooslehner K, Yeo GSH, Bluck L, Juul A, Vaag A, Dunger DB
Department of Paediatrics and Wolfson Brain Imaging Centre, University of Cambridge, Cambridge, UK
ajaytg@hotmail.com
J Clin Endocrinol Metab 2014;99:2198–2207

Background: An association between low IGF-1 serum levels and a higher risk of developing type 2 diabetes mellitus (T2DM) has been reported, but the effects of IGF-1 on glucose metabolism are unclear. This

study aimed to investigate the consequences of IGF-1 serum variations on glucose and lipid metabolism.
Methods: First, serum IGF-1 levels were measured from a biobank of 275 healthy, non-obese, adult male volunteers (age range 18–50 years). Consequently, 24 men (mean age 34.8 ± 8.9 years) belonging to the lowest quartile (n=12) or the highest quartile (n=12) were selected for further investigations. After a 24-hour fast, glucose and glycerol turnover rates using tracers, intravenous glucose tolerance test to assess peripheral insulin sensitivity and acute insulin and C-peptide responses (indexes of insulin secretion), magnetic resonance spectroscopy to assess intramyocellular lipids (IMCLs), calorimetry and gene expression in muscle biopsy samples, were evaluated.
Results: Men with lowest quartile IGF-1 had lower fasting insulin and C-peptide levels as well as lower endogenous glucose production (estimated using glucose Ra adjusted for insulin levels), suggesting higher hepatic insulin sensitivity compared with high-IGF-1 men. Acute insulin and C-peptide responses were also lower, whereas the whole-body insulin sensitivity was similar between groups. This resulted in a lower disposition index in low-IGF men. Overnight levels of FFA and beta-hydroxybutyrate were higher in low IGF-1 men, as well as higher increase of IMCLs in tibialis anterior muscle. Hepatic fat content and in vivo mitochondrial function did not differ between groups. Low-IGF-1 men showed upregulated expression of genes involved in fatty acid metabolism and a downregulation of GLUT1 in skeletal muscle.
Conclusions: Serum IGF-1 levels might represent a marker of beta-cell function and glucose as well as lipid homeostasis in fasting conditions.

There is increasing evidence that IGF-1 regulates beta-cell mass [69,70], by antagonising apoptosis and stimulating pancreatic islet growth. In animals, *Igf1r* deletion specifically in beta-cell impairs both glucose-stimulated insulin secretion and glucose tolerance [70]. In humans, low IGF-1 levels are associated with impaired glucose tolerance and T2DM [71]. IGF-1 administration improves insulin sensitivity in subjects with and without T2DM [72]. These findings show a crucial role for IGF-1 in glucose metabolism and T2DM pathogenesis. During fasting, GH diverts substrate metabolism from carbohydrate utilisation to lipid mobilisation from adipose tissue and oxidation in skeletal muscle. As IGF-1 is the downstream effector of GH metabolic actions, the authors hypothesised that variations in circulating IGF-1 levels may reflect the changes in glucose and lipid metabolism during fasting. By studying healthy men with IGF-1 at the extreme quartiles of the normal distribution, they found a relationship between low IGF-1 levels and lower insulin secretion, as well as higher hepatic insulin sensitivity during fasting. Low IGF-1 levels were also associated with enhanced lipid metabolism, accumulation of IMCLs and upregulation of genes involved in fat oxidation. Interestingly, although GH is the key hormone driving metabolic responses to fasting, differences in GH secretion were not observed. The authors speculate that the higher hepatic insulin sensitivity in low-IGF men may be a compensatory mechanism for the reduced insulin secretion. The lower *GLUT1* gene expression in low IGF-1 men supports a role for IGF-1 in glucose distribution but functional studies are required to confirm this. Notably, the differences in substrate metabolism observed in low-IGF-1 men during fasting might account for the higher risk for T2DM previously observed in subjects with low IGF-1 levels.

Food for thought

Environmental rather than genetic factors determine the variation in the age of the infancy to childhood transition: a twins study

German A, Livshits G, Peter I, Malkin I, Dubnov J, Akons H, Shmoish M, Hochberg Z
Department of Pediatrics, Bnai Zion Medical Center, Haifa, Israel
alinagerman@gmail.com
J Pediatr 2015;166:731–735

Background: The infancy to childhood transition (ICT) in growth is a time window of the utmost importance to determine adult height but the relative contribution of genetic and environmental factors is not well defined. The aim of this study was to assess the relative impact of genes and environment in regulating timing of the ICT.

Methods: A longitudinal study, based on a retrospective cohort of 536 individuals, included 56 monozygotic (MZ) twin pairs, 106 dizygotic (DZ) twin pairs and the remainder were other (singleton) siblings (SB). Placental examination, haematologic and serologic tests defined twin concordance. Subjects underwent anthropometry at birth and during the following 24 months. ICT-age was determined and a variance component analysis was performed to estimate familial components of the total variance, with adjustment for potential covariates.
Results: ICT occurred earlier in preterm infants and was dependent on gestational age. ICT-age ranged from 7.5 to 13.3 months in boys and 6.1 to 14.1 months in girls. Such differences explained approximately 7cm in adult height (28% of the total variance) with each month of ICT change contributing approximately 0.9cm in adult height. Intrapair correlations were almost identical in MZ and DZ twins (r=0.59 versus r=0.60, both P<0.001), and were higher than in other SB pairs (r=0.29, P=0.003). The common environment shared by all types of SB explained 27.7% of the total variance in ICT, whereas the common twin environment explained 9.2%. Gestational age and birthweight contributed 3.5% and 1.8% of the variance in ICT, respectively. Additionally, 8.7% was attributable to sex differences. No contribution of genetic factors to the inter-individual variation in ICT-age was found.
Conclusions: Environmental factors determine the age of infancy to childhood transition in growth. No detectable genetic influence was found.

Human growth is influenced by both genetic and environmental factors which seem to exert their relative contribution differently according to the life phases [73,74]. Environmental factors, including those acting in early life, deeply influence child growth and development. The transition from infancy to childhood growth, which occurs at age 7–12 months in Western countries, is responsible for up to 50% of the variance in adult height [75]. ICT is indicated by a growth acceleration when the growth hormone (GH) axis takes over from nutrition as the major driver for growth. Delayed ICT has a lifelong impact on stature and is responsible for as many as 44% of children with 'idiopathic' short stature. These same authors had previously suggested that delayed ICT is a 'predictive-adaptive' strategy to withstand environmental cues for low energy availability, resulting in short stature. This study clarifies the relative contributions of genetic and environmental factors in ICT timing, revealing that environmental factors have the predominant influence. MZ and DZ twins alike have high intrapair correlations in ICT timing, indicating that shared household and/or intrauterine environments determine 36.9% of its variation. The finding that ICT timing is associated with gestational age and birthweight supports previous reports of the importance of intrauterine environment on early growth [76]. In conclusion, this study highlights the importance of environmental factors in ICT timing, which is an important determinant of adult height.

Mechanism of the year

Insulin and insulin-like growth factor 1 receptors are required for normal expression of imprinted genes

Boucher J, Charalambous M, Zarse K, Mori MA, Kleinridders A, Ristow M, Ferguson-Smith AC, Kahn CR
Section on Integrative Physiology and Metabolism, Joslin Diabetes Center and Department of Medicine, Brigham and Women's Hospital and Harvard Medical School, Boston, MA, USA
c.ronald.kahn@joslin.harvard.edu
Proc Natl Acad Sci U S A 2014;111:14512–14517

Background: Insulin receptor (IR) and insulin-like growth factor 1 receptor (IGF1R) can emit signals in the unoccupied state, independently of the tyrosine kinase pathway. The aim of this study was to investigate the effects of unoccupied IR and IGF1R on gene expression.
Methods: Brown preadipocyte cell lines were generated with double deletions (DKO) of IR and IGF1R. mRNA and miRNA expression profiles were assessed in control (WT) and DKO cells under normal or proapoptotic conditions. Microarray analysis of WT and DKO cells was performed. Embryonic fibroblasts (MEFs) were obtained from IR-lox/CreERT2 mice with tamoxifen-inducible IR disruption. Mice with fat-specific IR deletion (FIRKO) were also evaluated. Methylation analysis was performed.

Results: 134 miRNAs were differentially expressed between WT and DKO cells: 45 miRNAs were upregulated in DKO cells while 89 miRNAS were downregulated. This downregulation of miRNAs in the DKO cells was observed in both the serum-fed and starved conditions with differences in expression of 100-fold or more. The downregulation occurred without any changes in enzymes or proteins involved in miRNA formation or maturation, indicating decreased expression of the primary miRNA transcripts rather than a change in miRNA processing. 61 of 89 downregulated miRNAs resided in clusters on two imprinted regions of chromosome 12 and chromosome 2. DKO cells displayed decreased expression of multiple maternally and paternally expressed imprinted genes. To test whether the observed changes in imprinted gene expression was related to a loss of insulin or IGF-1 signaling, WT brown pre-adipocytes and differentiated adipocytes were treated with 100nM insulin or IGF1. All imprinted genes that were found decreased in the DKO cells were either unchanged or only modestly decreased by insulin/IGF1 stimulation. Both MEFs cells lacking the IR and FIRKO mice showed changes in the expression of imprinted genes, as observed in DKO mice. The expression of transcription factor Zac1, a well-known regulator of a large imprinted gene network, was decreased by 80% in DKO cells. The induced re-expression of Zac1 only partially restored the expression of some imprinted genes. A different methylation pattern was found between WT and DKO cells. The repression of the imprinted genes in DKO cells was reversed by cell treatment with the DNA methyltransferase inhibitor 5-azacytidine alone or with the histone deacetylase inhibitor trichostatin A, suggesting that repression of the imprinted genes in DKO cells is related to increased DNA methylation.
Conclusions: Unoccupied IR and IGF1R modulate the expression of multiple imprinted genes. This novel pathway is stably maintained by changes in DNA methylation.

Insulin and IGFs act by binding to their specific receptors, IR and IGF1R, activating the intrinsic tyrosine kinase pathway. IR and IGFR may also signal independently of this canonical ligand-dependent pathway. Preadipocytes with deleted IR and IGF1R genes (this lacking insulin and IGF-1 signalling) are resistant to apoptosis [77] due to post-transcriptional modulation of pro-apoptotic and anti-apoptotic protein expression [77,78]. Genomic imprinting is an epigenetic process that silences one parental allele resulting in monoallelic expression. Imprinted gene regulation is strictly controlled by means of different DNA methylation of specific regions (differentially methylated regions and imprinting control regions). They are involved in several physiological processes being particularly important for fetal growth and development. The underlying mechanism by which imprinted genes influence growth is not fully clear. In mice, an imprinted locus on chromosome 12 modulates IGF-1 signalling [78]. In humans, altered imprinted gene dosage is associated with multiple disorders, including Beckwith-Wiedemann, Silver-Russell, Angelman and Prader-Willi syndromes.

Here, the authors describe that somatic cells lacking both IR and IGF1R display a decreased expression of several maternally and paternally imprinted genes. This repression is associated with changes in DNA methylation, particularly with increased DNA methylation and is obtained through a non-classical imprinting control. They discovered a completely new mechanism of IR and IGF1R actions, independent of their ligands (that is, insulin and IGF-1) by which IR and IGF1R may regulate growth and metabolism during early development [79] and thereafter.

References

1. Anckaert E, Schiettecatte J, Vanbesien J, Smitz J, Velkeniers B, De Schepper J. Variability among five different commercial IGF-1 immunoassays in conditions of childhood-onset GH deficiency and GH therapy. Acta Clin Belg 2006;61:335–339.
2. Clemmons DR. Consensus statement on the standardization and evaluation of growth hormone and insulin-like growth factor assays. Clin Chem 2011;57:555–559.
3. Bidlingmaier M, Friedrich N, Emeny RT, Spranger J, Wolthers OD, Roswall J, et al. Reference intervals for insulin-like growth factor-1 (igf-i) from birth to senescence: results from a multicenter study using a new automated chemiluminescence IGF-I immunoassay conforming to recent international recommendations. J Clin Endocrinol Metab 2014;99:1712–1721.
4. Ohlsson C, Mohan S, Sjogren K, Tivesten A, Isgaard J, Isaksson O, et al. The role of liver-derived insulin-like growth factor-I. Endocr Rev 2009;30:494–535.
5. Berneis K, Oehri M, Kraenzlin M, Keller U. Effects of IGF-I combined with GH on glucocorticoid-induced changes of bone and connective tissue turnover in man. J Endocrinol 1999;162:259–264.
6. Mauras N, Doi SQ, Shapiro JR. Recombinant human insulin-like growth factor I, recombinant human growth hormone, and sex steroids: effects on markers of bone turnover in humans. J Clin Endocrinol Metab 1996;81:2222–2226.

7. Rosen HN, Chen V, Cittadini A, Greenspan SL, Douglas PS, Moses AC, et al. Treatment with growth hormone and IGF-I in growing rats increases bone mineral content but not bone mineral density. J Bone Miner Res 1995;10:1352–1358.
8. Midyett LK, Rogol AD, Van Meter QL, Frane J, Bright GM, MS301 Study Group. Recombinant insulin-like growth factor (IGF)-I treatment in short children with low IGF-I levels: first-year results from a randomized clinical trial. J Clin Endocrinol Metab 2010;95:611–619.
9. Carel JC, Ecosse E, Landier F, Meguellati-Hakkas D, Kaguelidou F, Rey G, et al. Long-term mortality after recombinant growth hormone treatment for isolated growth hormone deficiency or childhood short stature: preliminary report of the French SAGhE study. J Clin Endocrinol Metab 2012;97:416–425.
10. Brevetti G, Marzullo P, Silvestro A, Pivonello R, Oliva G, di Somma C, et al. Early vascular alterations in acromegaly. J Clin Endocrinol Metab 2002;87:3174–3179.
11. Li G, Del Rincon JP, Jahn LA, Wu Y, Gaylinn B, Thorner MO, et al. Growth hormone exerts acute vascular effects independent of systemic or muscle insulin-like growth factor I. J Clin Endocrinol Metab 2008;93:1379–1385.
12. Savendahl L, Maes M, Albertsson-Wikland K, Borgstrom B, Carel JC, Henrard S, et al. Long-term mortality and causes of death in isolated GHD, ISS, and SGA patients treated with recombinant growth hormone during childhood in Belgium, The Netherlands, and Sweden: preliminary report of 3 countries participating in the EU SAGhE study. J Clin Endocrinol Metab 2012;97:E213–E217.
13. Ichord RN. Adult stroke risk after growth hormone treatment in childhood: first do no harm. Neurology 2014;83:776–777.
14. Hindmarsh PC, Peters CJ. Growth hormone treatment and stroke: should we be concerned? A case for cohort studies. Clin Endocrinol 2015;82:178–179.
15. Geffner ME, Santen R, Kopchick J. Growth hormone treatment for childhood short stature and risk of stroke in early adulthood. Neurology 2015;84:1062–1063.
16. Coste J, Touze E, Carel JC. Growth hormone treatment for childhood short stature and risk of stroke in early adulthood: author's response. Neurology 2015;84:1063.
17. Roberts AE, Allanson JE, Tartaglia M, Gelb BD. Noonan syndrome. Lancet 2013;381:333–342.
18. Romano AA, Allanson JE, Dahlgren J, Gelb BD, Hall B, Pierpont ME, et al. Noonan syndrome: clinical features, diagnosis, and management guidelines. Pediatrics 2010;126:746–759.
19. Regelmann MO, Rapaport R. Growth hormone treatment in patients with hypochondroplasia. Horm Res Paediatr 2014;82:353–354.
20. Key LL Jr, Gross AJ. Response to growth hormone in children with chondrodysplasia. J Pediatr 1996;128(5 Pt 2):S14–S17.
21. Burren CP, Werther GA. Skeletal dysplasias: response to growth hormone therapy. J Pediatr Endocrinol Metab 1996;9(1):31–40.
22. Rothenbuhler A, Linglart A, Piquard C, Bougneres P. A pilot study of discontinuous, insulin-like growth factor 1-dosing growth hormone treatment in young children with FGFR3 N540K-mutated hypochondroplasia. J Pediatr 2012;160:849–853.
23. Whitman B, Carrel A, Bekx T, Weber C, Allen D, Myers S. Growth hormone improves body composition and motor development in infants with Prader-Willi syndrome after six months. J Pediatr Endocrinol Metab 2004;17:591–600.
24. Eiholzer U, L'allemand D, Schlumpf M, Rousson V, Gasser T, Fusch C. Growth hormone and body composition in children younger than 2 years with Prader-Willi syndrome. J Pediatr 2004;144:753–758.
25. Carrel AL, Myers SE, Whitman BY, Eickhoff J, Allen DB. Long-term growth hormone therapy changes the natural history of body composition and motor function in children with Prader-Willi syndrome. J Clin Endocrinol Metab 2010;95:1131–1136.
26. Deal CL, Tony M, Hoybye C, Allen DB, Tauber M, Christiansen JS, et al. Growth Hormone Research Society workshop summary: consensus guidelines for recombinant human growth hormone therapy in Prader-Willi syndrome. J Clin Endocrinol Metab 2013;98:E1072–E1087.
27. Kershaw EE, Flier JS. Adipose tissue as an endocrine organ. J Clin Endocrinol Metab 2004;89:2548–2556.
28. Cohen CA, Shea AA, Heffron CL, Schmelz EM, Roberts PC. Intra-abdominal fat depots represent distinct immunomodulatory microenvironments: a murine model. PLoS One 2013;8:e66477.
29. Tateya S, Kim F, Tamori Y. Recent advances in obesity-induced inflammation and insulin resistance. Front Endocrinol 2013;4:93.
30. Ip BC, Hogan AE, Nikolajczyk BS. Lymphocyte roles in metabolic dysfunction: of men and mice. Trends Endocrinol Metab 2015;26:91–100.
31. Berryman DE, Glad CA, List EO, Johannsson G. The GH/IGF-1 axis in obesity: pathophysiology and therapeutic considerations. Nat Rev Endocrinol 2013;9:346–356.
32. Ukropec J, Penesova A, Skopkova M, Pura M, Vlcek M, Radikova Z, et al. Adipokine protein expression pattern in growth hormone deficiency predisposes to the increased fat cell size and the whole body metabolic derangements. J Clin Endocrinol Metab 2008;93:2255–2262.
33. Odle AK, Drew PD, Childs GV. Giant mice reveal new roles for GH in regulating the adipose immune microenvironment. Endocrinology 2015;156:1613–1615.

34. Kintscher U, Hartge M, Hess K, Foryst-Ludwig A, Clemenz M, Wabitsch M, et al. T-lymphocyte infiltration in visceral adipose tissue: a primary event in adipose tissue inflammation and the development of obesity-mediated insulin resistance. Arterioscler Thromb Vasc Biol 2008;28:1304–1310.
35. Bach LA. Endothelial cells and the IGF system. J Mol Endocrinol 2015;54(1):R1–R13.
36. Grant M, Jerdan J, Merimee TJ. Insulin-like growth factor-I modulates endothelial cell chemotaxis. J Clin Endocrinol Metab 1987;65:370–371.
37. Nicosia RF, Nicosia SV, Smith M. Vascular endothelial growth factor, platelet-derived growth factor, and insulin-like growth factor-1 promote rat aortic angiogenesis in vitro. Am J Pathol 1994;145:1023–1029.
38. Liu W, Liu Y, Lowe Jr WL Jr. The role of phosphatidylinositol 3-kinase and the mitogen-activated protein kinases in insulin-like growth factor-I-mediated effects in vascular endothelial cells. Endocrinology 2001;142:1710–1719.
39. Yakar S, Rosen CJ, Beamer WG, Ackert-Bicknell CL, Wu Y, Liu JL, et al. Circulating levels of IGF-1 directly regulate bone growth and density. J Clin Invest 2002;110:771–781.
40. DeChiara TM, Efstratiadis A, Robertson EJ. A growth-deficiency phenotype in heterozygous mice carrying an insulin-like growth factor II gene disrupted by targeting. Nature 1990;345:78–80.
41. Wang J, Zhou J, Cheng CM, Kopchick JJ, Bondy CA. Evidence supporting dual, IGF-I-independent and IGF-I-dependent, roles for GH in promoting longitudinal bone growth. J Endocrinol 2004;180:247–255.
42. Lupu F, Terwilliger JD, Lee K, Segre GV, Efstratiadis A. Roles of growth hormone and insulin-like growth factor 1 in mouse postnatal growth. Dev Biol 2001;229:141–162.
43. Dobie R, Ahmed SF, Staines KA, Pass C, Jasim S, MacRae VE, et al. Increased Linear Bone Growth by GH in the Absence of SOCS2 is Independent of IGF-1. J Cell Physiol 2015;230(11):2796–2805.
44. Wu S, Flint JK, Rezvani G, De Luca F. Nuclear factor-kappaB p65 facilitates longitudinal bone growth by inducing growth plate chondrocyte proliferation and differentiation and by preventing apoptosis. J Biol Chem 2007;282:33698–33706.
45. Wu S, Morrison A, Sun H, De Luca F. Nuclear factor-kappaB (NF-kappaB) p65 interacts with Stat5b in growth plate chondrocytes and mediates the effects of growth hormone on chondrogenesis and on the expression of insulin-like growth factor-1 and bone morphogenetic protein-2. J Biol Chem 2011;286:24726–24734.
46. Wang Z, York NW, Nichols CG, Remedi MS. Pancreatic beta cell dedifferentiation in diabetes and redifferentiation following insulin therapy. Cell Metab 2014;19:872–882.
47. Hotamisligil GS. Endoplasmic reticulum stress and the inflammatory basis of metabolic disease. Cell 2010;140:900–917.
48. Pugliese A, Miceli D. The insulin gene in diabetes. Diabetes Metab Res Rev 2002;18(1):13–25.
49. Ukkola O, Sun G, Bouchard C. Insulin-like growth factor 2 (IGF2) and IGF-binding protein 1 (IGFBP1) gene variants are associated with overfeeding-induced metabolic changes. Diabetologia 2001;44:2231–2236.
50. Rossetti L, Barzilai N, Chen W, Harris T, Yang D, Rogler CE. Hepatic overexpression of insulin-like growth factor-II in adulthood increases basal and insulin-stimulated glucose disposal in conscious mice. J Biol Chem 1996;271:203–208.
51. Devedjian JC, George M, Casellas A, Pujol A, Visa J, Pelegrin M, et al. Transgenic mice overexpressing insulin-like growth factor-II in beta cells develop type 2 diabetes. J Clin Invest 2000;105:731–740.
52. Cornu M, Yang JY, Jaccard E, Poussin C, Widmann C, Thorens B. Glucagon-like peptide-1 protects beta-cells against apoptosis by increasing the activity of an IGF-2/IGF-1 receptor autocrine loop. Diabetes 2009;58:1816–1825.
53. Estil les E, Tellez N, Soler J, Montanya E. High sensitivity of beta-cell replication to the inhibitory effects of interleukin-1beta: modulation by adenoviral overexpression of IGF2 in rat islets. J Endocrinol 2009;203:55–63.
54. Clayton PE, Cianfarani S, Czernichow P, Johannsson G, Rapaport R, Rogol A. Management of the child born small for gestational age through to adulthood: a consensus statement of the International Societies of Pediatric Endocrinology and the Growth Hormone Research Society. J Clin Endocrinol Metab 2007;92:804–810.
55. Barker DJ, Osmond C, Forsen TJ, Kajantie E, Eriksson JG. Trajectories of growth among children who have coronary events as adults. N Engl J Med 2005;353:1802–1809.
56. Cianfarani S, Germani D, Branca F. Low birthweight and adult insulin resistance: the "catch-up growth" hypothesis. Arch Dis Child Fetal Neonatal Ed 1999;81:F71–F73.
57. Han TY, Wang XL, Cui YP, Ye HM, Tong XM, Piao MH. No weight catch-up growth of SGA infants is associated with impaired insulin sensitivity during the early postnatal period. Int J Pediatr 2010;2010:704642.
58. Adair LS, Fall CH, Osmond C, Stein AD, Martorell R, Ramirez-Zea M, et al. Associations of linear growth and relative weight gain during early life with adult health and human capital in countries of low and middle income: findings from five birth cohort studies. Lancet 2013;382:525–534.
59. Paajanen TA, Oksala NK, Kuukasjarvi P, Karhunen PJ. Short stature is associated with coronary heart disease: a systematic review of the literature and a meta-analysis. Eur Heart J 2010;31:1802–1809.
60. Emerging Risk Factors Collaboration. Adult height and the risk of cause-specific death and vascular morbidity in 1 million people: individual participant meta-analysis. Int J Epidemiol 2012;41:1419–1433.
61. Barker DJ, Gluckman PD, Godfrey KM, Harding JE, Owens JA, Robinson JS. Fetal nutrition and cardiovascular disease in adult life. Lancet 1993;341:938–941.
62. Karhunen PJ, Meinander T. Coronary artery disease: complex association between height and CHD-size matters. Nat Rev Cardiol 2015;12:385–386.

63. Muthayya S, Kurpad AV, Duggan CP, Bosch RJ, Dwarkanath P, Mhaskar A, et al. Low maternal vitamin B12 status is associated with intrauterine growth retardation in urban South Indians. Eur J Clin Nutr 2006;60:791–801.
64. Merriman NA, Putt ME, Metz DC, Yang YX. Hip fracture risk in patients with a diagnosis of pernicious anemia. Gastroenterology 2010;138:1330–1337.
65. Strand TA, Taneja S, Kumar T, Manger MS, Refsum H, Yajnik CS, et al. Vitamin B-12, folic acid, and growth in 6- to 30-month-old children: a randomized controlled trial. Pediatrics 2015;135:e918–e926.
66. Verner A, Craig S, McGuire W. Effect of taurine supplementation on growth and development in preterm or low birth weight infants. Cochrane Database Syst Rev 2007;(4):CD006072.
67. Moon PD, Kim MH, Lim HS, Oh HA, Nam SY, Han NR, et al. Taurine, a major amino acid of oyster, enhances linear bone growth in a mouse model of protein malnutrition. Biofactors 2015;41:190–197.
68. Clemens TL. Vitamin B12 deficiency and bone health. N Engl J Med 2014;371:963–964.
69. Clemmons DR. Role of insulin-like growth factor iin maintaining normal glucose homeostasis. Horm Res 2004;62 Suppl 1:77–82.
70. Kulkarni RN, Holzenberger M, Shih DQ, Ozcan U, Stoffel M, Magnuson MA, et al. Beta-cell-specific deletion of the Igf1 receptor leads to hyperinsulinemia and glucose intolerance but does not alter beta-cell mass. Nat Genet 2002;31:111–115.
71. Rajpathak SN, He M, Sun Q, Kaplan RC, Muzumdar R, Rohan TE, et al. Insulin-like growth factor axis and risk of type 2 diabetes in women. Diabetes 2012;61:2248–2254.
72. Moses AC, Young SC, Morrow LA, O'Brien M, Clemmons DR. Recombinant human insulin-like growth factor I increases insulin sensitivity and improves glycemic control in type II diabetes. Diabetes 1996;45:91–100.
73. Dubois L, Ohm Kyvik K, Girard M, Tatone-Tokuda F, Perusse D, Hjelmborg J, et al. Genetic and environmental contributions to weight, height, and BMI from birth to 19 years of age: an international study of over 12,000 twin pairs. PLoS One 2012;7:e30153.
74. Silventoinen K, Kaprio J, Yokoyama Y. Genetics of pre-pubertal growth: a longitudinal study of Japanese twins. Ann Hum Biol 2011;38:608–614.
75. Hochberg Z. Evo-devo of child growth II: human life history and transition between its phases. Eur J Endocrinol 2009;160:135–141.
76. Livshits G, Peter I, Vainder M, Hauspie R. Genetic analysis of growth curve parameters of body weight, height and head circumference. Ann Hum Biol 2000;27:299–312.
77. Boucher J, Macotela Y, Bezy O, Mori MA, Kriauciunas K, Kahn CR. A kinase-independent role for unoccupied insulin and IGF-1 receptors in the control of apoptosis. Sci Signal 2010;3(151):ra87.
78. Mehlen P. Dependence receptors: the trophic theory revisited. Sci Signal 2010;3(151):pe47.
79. Radford EJ, Ferron SR, Ferguson-Smith AC. Genomic imprinting as an adaptative model of developmental plasticity. FEBS Lett 2011;585:2059–2066.

Bone, Growth Plate and Mineral Metabolism

Outi Mäkitie[a,b], Agnès Linglart[c], Adalbert Raimann[d] and Gabriele Häusler[d]

[a] Children's Hospital, University of Helsinki and Helsinki University Hospital, Helsinki, Finland

[b] Department of Molecular Medicine and Surgery, Karolinska Institutet, and Department of Clinical Genetics, Karolinska University Hospital, Stockholm, Sweden

[c] Department of Endocrinology and Diabetes for Children, Center of Reference for Rare Disorders of Calcium and Phosphorus Metabolism, APHP, Hôpital Bicêtre Paris Sud, Le Kremlin-Bicêtre, France

[d] Department of Pediatrics and Adolescent Medicine, Medical University of Vienna, Vienna, Austria

While research during the past years has elucidated the multitude of signalling molecules and pathways involved in skeletal homeostasis, a few researchers have now focused on the fundamental questions: where do the bone cells come from, what is their origin and fate? The identification of the skeletal stem cell and the presented evidence for versatility between the chondrocyte and osteoblast lineages have great scientific importance but also hold the potential for new therapeutic approaches to combat skeletal disorders. While these are awaited, ongoing attempts to apply novel treatments for conditions such as hypophosphataemic rickets, hypoparathyroidism, hyperparathyroidism and achondroplasia give promising results. Further, the selected papers describe some novel techniques, such as HR-pQCT, that allow *in vivo* detailed characterisation of bone pathology on the tissue level, and dynamic 4D imaging of cellular functions, for example in the growth plate. And to the readers who stay awake until the last page of this chapter, we disclose how bones suffer from disturbed sleep.

Important for clinical practice: dissecting bone problems in coeliac disease

Abnormal skeletal strength and microarchitecture in women with celiac disease

Stein EM, Rogers H, Leib A, McMahon DJ, Young P, Nishiyama K, Guo XE, Lewis S, Green P, Shane E
Divisions of Endocrinology and Gastroenterology, Department of Medicine, Columbia University College of Physicians and Surgeons, NY, USA
es2029@columbia.edu
J Clin Endocrinol Metab 2015;100:2347–2353

Background: Osteoporosis may be the presenting sign of coeliac disease (CD) but the skeletal characteristics on the tissue level remain unknown. This study evaluated bone microarchitecture and biomechanical properties in CD.
Methods: The authors recruited from a university hospital out-patient facility premenopausal women with newly diagnosed CD (n=33) and healthy controls (n=33) to this case-control study. Areal BMD was determined by DXA. Trabecular and cortical volumetric BMD and microarchitecture were assessed by high resolution peripheral computed tomography (HR-pQCT) of the distal radius and tibia; whole bone stiffness was estimated by finite element analysis. Peripheral blood PTH, 25-hydroxyvitamin D and bone turnover markers were measured.
Results: Groups had similar age, race and BMI and all subjects were vitamin D sufficient and had normal calcium and PTH. Areal BMD was lower in CD. By HR-pQCT, CD had lower trabecular volumetric BMD, and fewer, more widely and irregularly spaced trabeculae at both radius and tibia (8–33%). At the tibia, they also had lower total density and thinner cortices. Whole bone stiffness and failure load were lower in CD at both sites. Biomechanical deficits were associated with trabecular abnormalities.
Conclusions: Women with CD had abnormal volumetric BMD and microarchitecture at both radius and tibia. Trabecular bone was preferentially affected. These deficits were associated with reduced estimated skeletal strength. The authors conclude that the findings suggest a potential structural mechanism for skeletal fragility in CD.

Significant bone microarchitecture impairment in premenopausal women with active celiac disease

Zanchetta MB, Costa F, Longobardi V, Longarini G, Mazure RM, Moreno ML, Vazquez H, Silveira F, Niveloni S, Smecuol E, Temprano Mde L, Hwang HJ, Gonzalez A, Maurino EC, Bogado C, Zanchetta JR, Bai JC
IDIM, Instituto de Diagnostico e Investigaciones Metabolicas, Buenos Aires, Argentina; Catedra de Osteologia y Metabolismo Mineral, Universidad del Salvador, Buenos Aires, Argentina; Seccion Intestino Delgado, Departamento de Medicina, Hospital de Gastroenterologia 'Dr. C. Bonorino Udaondo', Buenos Aires, Argentina
mbzanchetta@idim.com.ar
Bone 2015;76:149–157

Background: Patients with active coeliac disease (CD) are more likely to have osteoporosis and increased risk of fractures. The authors aimed to determine the volumetric and microarchitectural characteristics of peripheral skeletal sites at diagnosis in adult premenopausal women with active CD to gain insight into mechanisms leading to skeletal pathology.
Methods: The authors enrolled 31 consecutive premenopausal women with newly diagnosed CD (median age 29 years, range 18–49 years) and 22 healthy women of similar age (median age 30 years, range 21–41 years) and BMI. High-resolution peripheral quantitative computed tomography (HR-pQCT), which permits three-dimensional assessment of bone microarchitectural characteristics, was used to measure cortical and trabecular compartments.
Results: Compared with controls, peripheral bones – distal radius and tibia – of CD patients were lower in terms of total volumetric density mg/cm^3 (P=0.0006 at the radius; P=0.002 at the tibia), trabecular density mg/cm^3 (P<0.0001 at the radius; P<0.0001 at the tibia); bone volume/trabecular volume ratio percentage (P<0.0001 at the radius; P<0.0001 at the tibia); trabecular spacing (P=0.009 at the radius; P=0.002 at the tibia); and trabecular thickness (P<0.0001 at the radius; P=ns at the tibia). Cortical density was lower in both radius and tibia. Patients with symptomatic CD (n=22) had a greater bone microarchitectural deficit than those with subclinical CD.
Conclusions: The authors were able to detect by HR-pQCT a significant deterioration in the microarchitecture of trabecular and cortical compartments of peripheral bones in patients with CD. Impairment was characterised by lower trabecular number and thickness, and lower cortical density and thickness. Prospective follow-up of the cohort will show whether bone microarchitecture recovers during gluten-free diet.

Coeliac disease (CD) is a chronic intestinal disorder that affects ~1% of the population in Europe and North America. Osteomalacia and osteoporosis are potential extraintestinal manifestations of CD. Several studies have reported low bone mineral density (BMD) in patients with CD. According to a recent meta-analysis [1], CD associates with an increased risk of fractures; fractures can also be the presenting feature of CD. Malabsorption of calcium, magnesium and vitamin D and inflammation contribute to low BMD. Lactose intolerance, often present in CD, may be an additional risk factor for calcium and vitamin D insufficiency. Inflammatory cytokines increase osteoclast activity, decrease osteoblast activity, resulting in uncoupled bone turnover. Other potential risk factors for skeletal fragility include zinc deficiency and low IGF-1, low BMI, malnutrition and hypogonadism. High-resolution peripheral quantitative computed tomography (HR-pQCT) is a fairly novel tool for assessment of bone characteristics at peripheral sites. It has the ability to measure true volumetric BMD and to separately assess cortical and trabecular bone. Data can be computationally modelled to assess bone stiffness and failure load, surrogate measures of strength.

These two studies are the first to evaluate volumetric BMD, microarchitecture and strength in patients with CD. Both studies applied almost an identical approach: assessment of distal radius and tibia by HR-pQCT in a cohort of premenopausal women with CD and a matched healthy control group. The findings indicated that premenopausal women with CD had lower volumetric BMD, abnormal bone microarchitecture and lower strength compared with normal premenopausal women. There were pronounced deficits in trabecular bone, associated with impaired biomechanical properties. Biomechanical deficits were directly related to abnormalities in trabecular bone volumetric BMD and microarchitecture, and existed despite sufficient calcium and 25-OH-vitamin D and normal PTH at the time of evaluation. Whether similar skeletal deficits are present in children and adolescents with CD remains unknown but is very likely. In the paediatric population such changes may have even greater implications than in adults. Active, undiagnosed or inadequately treated CD may result in suboptimal peak bone mass attainment and thereby increase future risk of osteoporosis. While similar paediatric studies are awaited, it is important to keep in mind that skeletal effects of CD extend beyond compromised growth and require surveillance.

Important for clinical practice: BMD deficits conquered in Crohn's disease?

Improvements in bone density and structure during anti-TNF-alpha therapy in pediatric Crohn's disease

Griffin LM, Thayu M, Baldassano RN, DeBoer MD, Zemel BS, Denburg MR, Denson LA, Shults J, Herskovitz R, Long J, Leonard MB

Department of Radiology, NY University School of Medicine, New York, NY, USA

J Clin Endocrinol Metab 2015;100:2630–2639

Background: Paediatric Crohn's disease (CD) is associated with deficits in trabecular bone mineral density (BMD) and cortical structure, potentially related to tumour necrosis factor alpha (TNF-alpha) which decreases bone formation and promotes bone resorption. The authors examined changes in bone density and structure in children and adolescents with CD following initiation of anti-TNF-alpha therapy.

Methods: Altogether 74 participants (age five to 21 years) with CD completed the 12-month prospective study. Tibia peripheral quantitative CT scans were obtained at initiation of anti-TNF-alpha therapy and 12 months later. Musculoskeletal outcomes were compared with age-, sex- and race-specific reference values and expressed as Z-scores.

Results: At baseline, CD participants had lower Z-scores for height, trabecular BMD, bone cortical area and muscle area (all $P<0.01$). Paediatric CD activity index decreased during the 10-week induction ($P<0.001$), with subsequent gains in height, trabecular BMD, cortical area and muscle area Z-scores over 12 months (height $P<0.05$; others $P<0.001$). The bone formation marker bone-specific alkaline phosphatase increased a median of 75% ($P<0.001$) during induction with associated 12-month improvements in trabecular BMD and cortical area Z-scores (both $P<0.001$). Younger age was associated with greater increases in trabecular BMD Z-scores ($P<0.001$) and greater linear growth with greater recovery of cortical area ($P<0.001$).

Conclusions: The improvements in trabecular BMD and cortical structure during anti-TNF-alpha therapy were greater in younger and growing participants, suggesting a window of opportunity for treatment of bone deficits.

Children with Crohn's disease (CD) have multiple risk factors for impaired bone health, including malnutrition, decreased physical activity, inflammation and glucocorticoid therapy. These may result in fractures, suboptimal peak bone mass and increased risk of osteoporosis in adulthood. Studies have documented significant trabecular and cortical bone deficits and increased fracture rates in CD. Increased tumour necrosis factor alpha (TNF-alpha) may have a causative role as it has direct adverse effects on bone and is increased in CD. TNF-alpha inhibits osteoblast differentiation, maturation and activity, and promotes bone resorption by activation of osteoclasts. Glucocorticoids used in treatment have similar effects and further aggravate imbalance in bone cell function.

The authors have previously described reductions in trabecular volumetric BMD, cortical dimensions and muscle area, as measured by tibia peripheral quantitative computed tomography (pQCT), in newly diagnosed children with CD [2]. After treatment onset these bone deficits improved only partly and persisted even three to four years later, despite low disease activity. In the present study they evaluated whether anti-TNF-alpha therapy, used to treat CD, has the ability to more completely restore the bone defects. Infliximab, a monoclonal antibody against TNF-alpha, is the first-line biologic agent in refractory paediatric CD. Studies have documented that infliximab induces and maintains clinical remission in moderate to severe CD and improves linear growth but its impact on bone homeostasis has not been evaluated. This prospective cohort study on tibial pQCT parameters over a 12-month interval from initiation of infliximab therapy showed a rapid improvement in disease activity and an increase in bone turnover. Rapid improvements in trabecular BMD and cortical structure were seen. Future studies are needed to examine whether these changes result in reduced fracture risk over time. Biological therapies are widely used in also other paediatric inflammatory conditions. The results of this study give a reason for optimism - the modern therapies of childhood chronic diseases may be able to not only cure the disease itself but to alleviate the harmful skeletal effects induced by the disease and its treatment.

Concepts revised: the challenging parathyroid

Hypoparathyroidism or pseudohypoparathyroidism, what is your diagnosis?

A homozygous [Cys25]PTH(1-84) mutation that impairs PTH/PTHrP receptor activation defines a novel form of hypoparathyroidism

Lee S, Mannstadt M, Guo J, Kim SM, Yi HS, Khatri A, Dean T, Okazaki M, Gardella TJ, Juppner H
Department of Internal Medicine and Laboratory of Molecular Endocrinology, Gachon University School of Medicine, Incheon, South Korea
J Bone Miner Res 2015 (Epub ahead of print) doi:10.1002/jbmr.2532

Background: Hypoparathyroidism results from the insufficient secretion or action of the parathyroid hormone (PTH) leading to hypocalcaemia, hyperphosphataemia and low or undetectable PTH levels. In contrast, resistance to the biologically active PTH is due to genetic or epigenetic defects downstream of the PTH receptor that cause a similar biochemical phenotype.
Methods: This study describes a family in which three siblings were affected by idiopathic hypoparathyroidism while the parents were healthy. The affected patients presented with hypocalcaemia and hyperphosphataemia but PTH was elevated or low depending on the bioassay and suggested either hypoparathryoidism or pseudohypoparathryoidism type 1B as the diagnosis. Whole-exome sequencing and Sanger sequencing were used to determine the underlying cause.
Results: The authors identified a homozygous arginine-to-cysteine mutation at position 25 of the mature PTH(1-84) polypeptide in the PTH gene in the three affected siblings. In vitro and in vivo studies showed that 1) the mutated PTH molecule is secreted, 2) the mutant PTH has a lower binding affinity for the PTH receptor than the wild-type PTH and 3) the mutant PTH failed to induce a significant calcaemic and phosphataemic response in mice.
Conclusions: The association of hypocalcaemia, hyperphosphataemia and elevated PTH may be due to biologically inactive PTH due to an underlying PTH gene mutation.

Idiopathic isolated hypoparathyroidism is a rare disorder most likely due to gene defects in factors involved in parathyroid development, PTH secretion or action. The causative gene defects are identified in about 30% of the cases when the disease is familial (more than one affected case), and in only 5% of sporadic cases, which is by far the more frequent situation. Among the involved genes, mutations in the PTH gene itself have been identified thus far in only six families, including this report. The identified mutation in this family was exceptional in that it is the first germline PTH mutation that changes an amino acid residue in the bioactive portion of PTH(1-84) rather than the prepro leader sequence, as in the five other cases. In this respect this is similar to other endocrine disorders where loss-of-function mutations in ligands are also exceptionally identified while mutations in other parts of the involved pathways are more common [3]. Here, the authors challenge the differential diagnosis between PTH resistance in the context of pseudohypoparathyroidism type 1B (PHP1B) (the association of hypocalcaemia, hyperphosphataemia and elevated PTH) and hypoparathyroidism (low PTH levels associated with hypocalcaemia and hyperphosphataemia). Several elements may contribute to the final diagnosis. Patients with PHP1B usually present with other hormone resistances, especially TSH and calcitonin resistance. In addition, as nicely demonstrated here, the PTH infusion test will discriminate between these disorders by the presence or absence of cAMP and phosphaturic response to PTH. In exceptional cases of 'pseudohypoparathyroidism' without any epigenetic or genetic defect at the *GNAS* locus, investigations should include after vitamin D repletion, multiple PTH measurements with different bioassays, a PTH infusion test and PTH gene sequencing. Differentiating between idiopathic hypoparathyroidism and PHP1B has considerable implications for genetic counselling, therapy and long-term outcome, since treatment of patients with idiopathic hypoparathyroidism with inappropriately high doses of active vitamin D and calcium can contribute to the development of nephrocalcinosis and chronic kidney disease.

Thyroid or parathyroid problems – which come first?

TSH elevations as the first laboratory evidence for pseudohypoparathyroidism type Ib (PHP-Ib)

Molinaro A, Tiosano D, Takatani R, Chrysis D, Russell W, Koscielniak N, Kottler ML, Agretti P, De Marco G, Ahtiainen P, Christov M, Mäkitie O, Tonacchera M, Juppner H

Endocrine Unit, Massachusetts General Hospital and Harvard Medical School, Boston, MA, USA

J Bone Miner Res 2015;30:906–912

Background: PHP1B is caused by methylation defects at the *GNAS* locus that alter the expression of Gsa, the alpha subunit of the stimulatory G protein. Gsa mediates the signals of hormones, which binds to 7-transmembrane receptors, including PTH and TSH. Patients affected with PHP1B present resistance towards these hormones, PTH resistance being the most pre-eminent.

Methods: The authors characterised patients who had been diagnosed first with hypothyroidism and only later with PTH resistance. *GNAS* locus was evaluated for genetic changes. Further, they evaluated patients with hypothyroidism for methylation changes at the *GNAS* locus.

Results: Four patients were initially diagnosed with hypothyroidism and later were found to also have PTH resistance. Diagnosis of PHP1B was confirmed by identifying epigenetic defects at the *GNAS* locus in each of the four patients. These included broad methylation changes in three patients, and loss of methylation restricted to the A/B promoter associated to the *STX16* deletion in one patient. In contrast, no methylation defects at the *GNAS* locus were identified in a cohort of 23 children and 39 adults with subclinical hypothyroidism.

Conclusions: TSH elevation as evidence for subclinical or overt hypothyroidism can occur in some PHP1B patients with methylation changes at the *GNAS* locus before PTH-resistant hypocalcaemia becomes apparent.

PHP1B was defined through the discovery of the imprinting defects at the *GNAS* locus, responsible for a decreased expression of Gsa in imprinted tissues. For years, PHP1B was described as a 'pure PTH resistance' and, consequently, several research groups have locked for mutations in the PTH receptor. This dogma was later challenged when patients affected with PHP1B and some features of Albright osteodystrophy were reported. Eventually, TSH resistance was also associated with PHP1B, although the level of TSH was only slightly elevated and most patients did not require any treatment. The four patients described in this article presented with symptomatic hypothyroidism in infancy (three out of four) requiring L-thyroxine to compensate for their TSH resistance. Romanet et al. recently described another patient who was diagnosed with congenital hypothyroidism in the neonatal screening, based on a TSH level of 50mIU/L [4]. These observations indicate that 1) in contrast to the PTH resistance that develops overtime, the TSH resistance in PHP1B may be present since birth, 2) although rare, PHP1B may be a cause of subclinical hypothyroidism and congenital hypothyroidism in children. Furthermore, these findings imply that significant silencing of Gsa expression from the paternal *GNAS* allele may occur in tissues other than the proximal renal tubules, including the thyroid. In line with this, the authors speculate that other disorders such as isolated obesity, intrauterine growth retardation or short stature, may in some patients be caused by *GNAS* methylation changes without obvious changes in PTH and/or TSH levels.

Treatment trials: How to restore PTH signalling, by injecting PTH or by modifying PTH release?

Calcilytic ameliorates abnormalities of mutant calcium-sensing receptor (CaSR) knock-in mice mimicking autosomal dominant hypocalcemia (ADH)

Dong B, Endo I, Ohnishi Y, Kondo T, Hasegawa T, Amizuka N, Kiyonari H, Shioi G, Abe M, Fukumoto S, Matsumoto T
Department of Medicine and Bioregulatory Sciences, University of Tokushima Graduate School of Medical Sciences, Tokushima, Japan
J Bone Miner Res 2015 (Epub ahead of print) doi:10.1002/jbmr.2551

Background: Autosomal dominant hypocalcaemia (ADH) is caused by activating mutations in the calcium sensing receptor (CaSR) gene. Current treatment of ADH with vitamin D analogues and/or recombinant PTH does not prevent hypercalciuria and renal calcifications. Calcilytics, the allosteric antagonists of the CaSR, are expected to reverse the disease phenotype.
Methods: In order to evaluate the potential effect of the calcilytic JTT-305/MK-5442, the authors generated two mouse strains, each of them bearing a different knock-in activating mutation of the *CaSR*.
Results: Animals bearing the activating mutation of the *CaSR* recapitulate the phenotype of ADH, that is, hypocalcaemia, hyperphosphataemia, low PTH, low bone turnover, hypercalciuria, renal calcifications and growth retardation. The acute oral administration of the calcilytic restored calcium, phosphate and PTH levels. In addition, long-term oral administration restored urinary calcium reabsorption in the nephron, an effect that was not observed with the long-term administration of PTH. Both the calcilytic and PTH ameliorated bone turnover.
Conclusions: Calcilytics restore mineral metabolism in mice with ADH and counteract the bone defect induced by the *CaSR* activating mutation.

ADH is a rare, yet devastating disorder, caused by activated signalling of the CaSR. The *CaSR* is mainly expressed in the parathyroid glands and in the kidneys, where its activation leads to a suppressed PTH excretion and prevents the urinary calcium paracellular reabsorption. Therefore, consequences of the enhanced CaSR activity are numerous, including hypocalcaemia, hyperphosphataemia, hypercalciuria, hypomagnesaemia and, in some cases, growth retardation and neurocognitive impairment. The hypercalciuria results from the lack of PTH signalling in the distal tubule and from the activation of the CaSR in the Henle's loop. CaSR antagonists modify the receptor's allostery, facilitate PTH release by the parathyroid cells and may restore reabsorption of calcium in the kidney. CaSR antagonists represent an attractive therapeutic approach for the ADH patients. Calcilytics have first been developed for the treatment of osteoporosis, because of their anabolic action on the bone, likely due to increased PTH [5].

In the present study, the authors successfully used the calcilytics to reverse the activation of the CaSR in transfected cells and in ADH mice. Upon increasing doses of JTT-305/MK-5442, ADH mice showed increased calcium, decreased phosphate, increased PTH and urinary cAMP excretion and decreased urinary calcium excretion. It is remarkable that this effect was sustained overtime, demonstrating its potential for therapeutic use. The experimental design allowed dissecting the respective roles of calcilytics and PTH on the renal reabsorption of calcium. Interestingly, in ADH mice, only calcilytics prevented hypercalciuria, whereas they did not observe an anticalciuric effect with PTH. While we eagerly await clinical trials of calcilytics in ADH patients, different calcilytics are currently tested on various ADH mice with similarly promising results [6]. Safety profiles of these drugs need to be carefully addressed.

Effects of pump versus twice-daily injection delivery of synthetic parathyroid hormone 1-34 in children with severe congenital hypoparathyroidism

Winer KK, Fulton KA, Albert PS, Cutler GB Jr
Eunice Kennedy Shriver National Institute of Child Health and Human Development, National Institutes of Health, Bethesda, MD, USA
karenwiner@gmail.com
J Pediatr 2014;165:556-63.e1

Background: Recombinant PTH 1-34 may be used for the treatment of congenital hypoparathyroidism but optimal dosing in children remains unknown.

Methods: The authors recruited to this treatment study 12 children affected with hypoparathyroidism due to autoimmune polyglandular syndrome type 1 or *CasR* activating mutations. They were randomly assigned to receive PTH 1-34 for 13 weeks, either with twice-daily subcutaneous injections or by insulin pump, followed by crossover to the opposite delivery method. The objective was to compare the effects of these two treatment regimens on mineral metabolism and bone turnover.
Results: Continuous injection of PTH through pump delivery resulted in a stable near normalisation of serum calcium, a better reduction in urinary calcium excretion and reduced markers of bone turnover. In addition, the dosage of PTH was lower when given by pump compared with twice-daily injections.
Conclusions: Recombinant PTH 1-34 provides an effective and safe way to improve calcium homeostasis in children with hypoparathyroidism. In this study, pump delivery was superior to twice-daily injections in the ability to restore biochemical parameters of calcium and bone homeostasis.

Hypoparathyroidism is often severe and refractory to conventional treatment with vitamin D analogues and calcium supplements. In children, most cases are due to *CaSR* mutation-related autosomal dominant hypoparathyroidism or autoimmune polyglandular syndrome type 1. Several reports and studies have established the efficacy of recombinant PTH (recPTH) as a substitutive treatment of hypoparathyroidism also in children, with near-normalisation of serum calcium during therapy. However, several issues remain unclear especially regarding the effect of recPTH on urinary calcium excretion, phosphate response and bone turnover. The accumulating data suggested that the route of hormone administration could explain some of the unsolved issues.

The authors here clearly demonstrate that continuous administration of recPTH allows a sustained near-normal calcium level throughout the day as compared with the biphasic calcium response during treatment with twice daily injections of recPTH 1-34. This result could at first glance appear contradictory as both modes of administration lead to identical levels of 1,25-OH_2D, which is important for intestinal absorption of calcium. In addition, this study shows for the first time that recPTH reduces urinary calcium excretion upon continuous infusion. In adults the REPLACE study, designed to test the efficacy of once daily recPTH 1-84 for the treatment of hypoparathyroidism, failed in this particular aspect [7]. In the current study, serum phosphate and urinary calcium levels were at the upper level of the normal range in both groups of patients (even if the urinary calcium level was lower in the pump group). Using recPTH as replacement therapy, the target should be to normalise serum calcium and give enough PTH to stimulate the reabsorption of calcium in the renal distal tubule. The authors may not have obtained the optimal response to PTH, because their patients still presented with features of hypoparathyroidism, that is, hypocalcaemia, hyperphosphataemia and high urinary calcium. As for today, the use of recPTh in children is off-label and should be used only in children with severe hypoparathyroidism or under trial protocols.

Clinical trials: X-linked hypophosphatemia: 20 years after the discovery of the gene, how far are we from the 'ideal' therapy?

Prolonged correction of serum phosphorus in adults with X-linked hypophosphatemia using monthly doses of KRN23

Imel EA, Zhang X, Ruppe MD, Weber TJ, Klausner MA, Ito T, Vergeire M, Humphrey JS, Glorieux FH, Portale AA, Insogna KL, Peacock M, Carpenter TO
Indiana University School of Medicine, Indianapolis, IN, USA
J Clin Endocrinol Metab 2015;100:2565–2573

Background: In patients with X-linked hypophosphataemia (XLH), excessive FGF23 secretion by osteocytes leads to hypophosphataemia secondary to renal phosphate wasting and impaired vitamin D hydroxylation. Hypophosphataemia results in rickets in children and osteomalacia in adults.
Methods: In this multi-centre open-label phase 1/2 study with escalating doses (from 0.05 to 0.6mg/kg), KRN23, a recombinant human FGF23 antibody, was administered subcutaneously to 28 XLH adults

every four weeks for four months. A 12-month extension study with 22 participants followed, with doses ranging from 0.1 to 1.0mg/kg.

Results: During the dose-escalation study, after each dose of KNR23 mean serum Pi peaked by day seven, decreasing to a trough on day 28. On the highest dose, serum phosphate was normal in 88% of patients one week after each drug injection. During the 12-month extension, peak Pi was in the normal range in 58–85% of patients and ≥25% maintained trough Pi levels within the normal range. TmP/GFR, 1,25-$(OH)_2D$ and bone biomarkers increased. Serum calcium, urinary calcium excretion and PTH values remained unchanged throughout the study.

Conclusions: Monthly KRN23 has a beneficial effect on the biochemical profile of XLH adult patients.

XLH is a rare metabolic bone disease due to mutations in the *PHEX* gene that lead to an uncontrolled secretion of FGF23, lack of tubular reabsorption of phosphate in the kidney proximal tubule and impaired production of 1,25-OH_2-vitamin D. In children, the disease manifests primarily as rickets and dental complications; in adults, the clinical picture is variable, depending on the care provided during childhood, yet, bone pain, pseudofractures, enthesopathies (inflammation of the attachment of tendon or ligament to bone), altered quality of life and limited mobility seem to be frequent in these patients, even when treated. The authors clearly demonstrate here, and in their previous report [8], that KRN23 – an antibody targeted against FGF23 – is an attractive therapeutic option for XLH, as it reverses most of the biochemical abnormalities. Both single and repeated subcutaneous injections maintain phosphate concentrations within the normal range (low normal range) through the increase in tubular reabsorption of phosphate and, maybe, increased intestinal absorption of phosphate. It is reassuring to observe normalisation of 1,25-OH_2-vitamin D levels upon long-term administration of KRN23, as this is likely to prevent calcification. Based on these findings, KRN23 rescues phosphate wasting and vitamin D hydroxylation, thereby diminishing signs of osteomalacia in adults. Further trials in XLH adults with also functional and symptomatic endpoints, are needed to establish the use of the therapy and to determine optimal dosing and target population. Undeniably, children would most likely benefit from KRN23, as restoring the phosphate balance will prevent rickets and improve bone and tooth mineralisation.

Effect of paricalcitol on circulating parathyroid hormone in X-linked hypophosphatemia: a randomised, double-blind, placebo-controlled study

Carpenter TO, Olear EA, Zhang JH, Ellis BK, Simpson CA, Cheng D, Gundberg CM, Insogna KL
Departments of Pediatrics, Internal Medicine, Orthopaedics and Rehabilitation, and Diagnostic Radiology, Yale University School of Medicine, New Haven, CT, USA
J Clin Endocrinol Metab 2014;99:3103–3111

Background: Patients affected with X-linked hypophosphataemia (XLH) often develop hyperparathyroidism and this may exacerbate phosphaturia, potentially affecting skeletal abnormalities.

Methods: This prospective double-blind, one-year randomised placebo-controlled trial investigated whether paricalcitol, a vitamin D analogue, could control PTH secretion in XLH patients without inducing hypercalcaemia.

Results: Thirty adults and three children were included; all had XLH and modest to moderate hyperparathyroidism. Paricalcitol diminished the PTH area under the curve in treated patients and increased phosphate reabsorption in the kidney. Hypercalciuria developed in six subjects.

Conclusions: Paricalcitol might be an adjuvant therapy for patients with XLH and increased PTH. Careful monitoring of serum and urine calcium levels is indicated.

Patients with X-linked hypophosphataemic rickets (XLH) usually have at diagnosis PTH levels within the normal range or higher. It is still unclear why some patients have slightly elevated PTH. On one hand, it is expected because of their low 1,25-OH_2-vitamin D levels inducing a PTH response. On the other hand, elevated FGF23 should suppress PTH secretion. The relative importance of the two mechanisms might change overtime and influence the natural history of the disease as well as the response to therapies. However, as mentioned by the authors, and unanimously experienced by physicians caring for XLH patients, PTH levels rise during treatment with phosphate supplements leading sometimes to symptomatic hyperparathyroidism. Increased PTH also has adverse effects on bone homeostasis and may contribute to development of nephrocalcinosis and enthesopathies. It is in such cases important to consider adjuvant drugs with a potential effect on PTH secretion. Careful control of phosphate supplementation is a prerequisite for any patient with XLH and elevated PTH level. There is no published data on the potential role of vitamin D supplementation. Administration of CaSR agonists - calcimimetics - leads to decreased PTH secretion and increased serum Pi [9].

Here, the authors show that paricalcitol, a vitamin D analogue, could be an additional adjuvant therapy for XLH. Despite the relatively small numbers studied, they found that paricalcitol suppressed elevated PTH levels and increased tubular phosphate reabsorption despite increases in FGF23 level. Further, serum alkaline phosphatase activity, a measure of skeletal disease severity, was decreased in paricalcitol-treated adults. Twenty years after the disease-causing gene defect was discovered, and 15 years after the identification of the disease-causing hormone, we are still searching for optimal treatment for XLH! Even today, the complicated links between FGF23, PTH, mineral homeostasis and bone tissue in XLH remain inadequately understood. Interventional studies like this are needed to elucidate the potential benefits of various new and old treatment options.

New hope: statins to stabilise overactive FGFR3

Statin treatment rescues FGFR3 skeletal dysplasia phenotypes

Yamashita A, Morioka M, Kishi H, Kimura T, Yahara Y, Okada M, Fujita K, Sawai H, Ikegawa S, Tsumaki N
Cell Induction and Regulation Field, Department of Cell Growth and Differentiation, Center for iPS Cell Research and Application, Kyoto University, Kyoto, Japan
ntsumaki@cira.kyoto-u.ac.jp
Nature 2014;513:507–511

Background: The severe bone and growth disorders, thanatophoric dysplasia and achondroplasia (ACH), arise when fibroblast growth factor receptor 3 is constitutively activated by gain-of-function mutations. The lack of disease models using human cells has hampered the identification of a clinically effective treatment for these diseases.
Methods: The authors transdifferentiated fibroblasts from patients with thanatophoric dysplasia type I (TD1) or ACH into induced pluripotent stem cells (iPSCs). Chondrogenic differentiation of these cells and those in a mouse model of FGFR3 skeletal dysplasia resulted in the formation of degraded cartilage. Statins were applied.
Results: Statins corrected the degraded cartilage in chondrogenically differentiated iPSCs from patients with TD1 or ACH. Further, statin treatment of ACH model mice led to recovery of bone growth.
Conclusions: These findings suggest that statins could potentially be used to treat infants and children with TD1 and ACH.

Achondroplasia (ACH) and thanatophoric dysplasia (TD) are caused by gain-of-function mutations in the fibroblast growth factor receptor 3 gene (*FGFR3*). Specific therapeutic options are lacking but some new pharmacological approaches have been developed, as reviewed in previous Yearbook chapters [10]. While data only from animal studies have confirmed effects of the specific FGFR3-binding peptide P3 [11], the efficacy and safety of C-type natriuretic peptide analogoues [12] is currently being tested in phase 2 clinical trials.

Here, the authors aimed to overcome excessive FGFR3 activity with yet another novel approach with a not-so-novel drug. They screened drugs for their ability to rescue chondrocytic cartilage production. They found that statins led the cells to produce less degraded cartilage, although the exact mechanism remains unclear. The researchers found that FGFR3 protein levels—but not FGFR3 mRNA levels—were decreased in statin-treated cells, indicating that the drug increased degradation of the protein. As FGFR3 is a signalling molecule that resides in chondrocyte membranes, statins may increase cartilage production by suppressing overexpressed mutant *FGFR3*. They then showed in mice with ACH mutations in *FGFR3* that statins increased longitudinal bone growth.

Statins are among the most thoroughly investigated therapeutics, but it is still unclear whether they are safe for use in young children. Since the symptoms of TD1 and ACH begin to manifest prenatally, statin treatment in these conditions should start as early as possible, preferably even prenatally. Before moving to clinical tests, safety and efficacy of statins for FGFR3 chondrodysplasia need to be tested more extensively in animal models. The precise working mechanism of statins in this group of skeletal disorders, and optimal dosing and treatment regimens, remain to be established. However, the wide use of statins and the large number of adult and paediatric patients receiving statin treatment for other conditions gives hope for expeditious development of well-tolerated and specific treatments for FGFR3-associated skeletal dysplasias.

Important for clinical practice: anti-angiogens disturb growth plate function

Growth plate abnormalities in pediatric cancer patients undergoing phase 1 anti-angiogenic therapy: a report from the Children's Oncology Group Phase I Consortium

Voss SD, Glade-Bender J, Spunt SL, DuBois SG, Widemann BC, Park JR, Leary SE, Nelson MD, Adamson PC, Blaney SM, Weigel B
Department of Radiology, Boston Children's Hospital Dana-Farber Cancer Institute, Boston, MA, USA
stephan.voss@childrens.harvard.edu
Pediatr Blood Cancer 2015;62:45-51

Background: Pre-clinical studies suggest that anti-angiogenic agents may be toxic to the developing growth plate. This study investigated potential toxic effects of anti-angiogenic therapy on growth plates in children with refractory cancer.
Methods: The authors reviewed targeted radiographic studies from 53 children enrolled on six separate Children's Oncology Group Phase 1 and Pilot Consortium clinical trials evaluating new anti-cancer agents that interfere with angiogenesis. Altogether 35 children received tyrosine kinase inhibitors with anti-angiogenic effects, 13 monoclonal antibodies targeting vascular endothelial growth factor (VEGF) and five antibodies against angiopoietin. Radiographs of the distal femur / proximal tibia were obtained at baseline. Follow-up radiographs were obtained in patients with open growth plates.
Results: Baseline and follow-up radiographs were available for 90% of the children. Growth plate abnormalities were found in five patients (9.4%) who were all then treated with VEGF/VEGFR antibodies (one with sunitinib and four with pazopanib). Four of them had growth plate widening in radiographs; one child had progressive growth plate widening and physeal cartilage hypertrophy on MRI. Reversibility of the abnormalities was observed after discontinuation of treatment.
Conclusions: Abnormalities of the growth plate were seen in a sufficient proportion of patients receiving anti-angiogenic therapy to warrant further studies and careful monitoring of children with open growth plates. Further, improved methods to evaluate toxic skeletal effects of anti-angiogenic agents are needed.

Anti-angiogenic therapies have increasingly become established in paediatric oncological treatment protocols in recent years. They are reasonably well-tolerated and result in objective and sustained tumour responses in a variety of paediatric cancers. Therefore it is likely that treatment regimens will increasingly include prolonged use of anti-angiogenic agents. Concerns about the effects of anti-angiogenic agents on the developing skeleton have been vindicated by animal studies. Longitudinal bone growth and growth plate maturation depend on recruitment of new blood vessels, and various angiogenic growth factors and their receptors are expressed in the growth plate. Due to the essential role of angiogenesis in bone growth and adverse effects in preclinical animal studies using anti-angiogenic agents, there have been concerns that anti-angiogenic therapies used to treat paediatric cancer would result in toxic skeletal effects. Previous clinical data are limited by small patient numbers.

Here, the authors describe in data from 53 patients that among the anti-angiogenic agents VEGF inhibition in particular impedes the growing skeleton and results in growth plate toxicity in a small but significant proportion of patients. Further, radiographs revealed reversibility of the changes when treatment was discontinued. Although the long-term effects on fracture risk and final patient height remain unclear, the study underscores the need for careful monitoring of patients receiving anti-angiogenic therapies, especially VEGF inhibition.

Gremlin 1 identifies a skeletal stem cell with bone, cartilage, and reticular stromal potential

Worthley DL, Churchill M, Compton JT, Tailor Y, Rao M, Si Y, Levin D, Schwartz MG, Uygur A, Hayakawa Y, Gross S, Renz BW, Setlik W, Martinez AN, Chen X, Nizami S, Lee HG, Kang HP, Caldwell JM, Asfaha S, Westphalen CB, Graham T, Jin G, Nagar K, Wang H, Kheirbek MA, Kolhe A, Carpenter J, Glaire M, Nair A, Renders S, Manieri N, Muthupalani S, Fox JG, Reichert M, Giraud AS, Schwabe RF, Pradere JP, Walton K, Prakash A, Gumucio D, Rustgi AK, Stappenbeck TS, Friedman RA, Gershon MD, Sims P, Grikscheit T, Lee FY, Karsenty G, Mukherjee S, Wang TC
Department of Medicine and Irving Cancer Research Center, Columbia University, New York, NY, USA
sm3252@columbia.edu; tcw21@columbia.edu
Cell 2015;160:269–284

Background: The stem cells responsible for maintenance and renewal of the postnatal skeleton remain uncharacterised. Peri-sinusoidal mesenchymal stem cells (MSCs) have been suggested to give rise to osteoblasts, chondrocytes, marrow stromal cells and adipocytes. However the existence and fate of these cells has not been proven.
Methods: Various animal models and cell-based assays were used.
Results: The authors demonstrate here that expression of the bone morphogenetic protein antagonist gremlin 1 defines a population of osteochondroreticular (OCR) stem cells in the bone marrow. OCR stem cells self-renew and generate osteoblasts, chondrocytes and reticular marrow stromal cells, but not adipocytes. OCR stem cells are concentrated within the metaphysis of long bones and are needed for bone development, bone remodelling and fracture repair. Grem1 expression also identifies intestinal reticular stem cells (iRSCs) that are cells of origin for the periepithelial intestinal mesenchymal sheath.
Conclusions: These findings confirm the existence and relevance of bone, cartilage and reticular stromal stem cells. These observations present a paradigm shift in our understanding of the diverse origins of connective tissues in health, ageing and disease.

Identification and specification of the mouse skeletal stem cell

Chan CK, Seo EY, Chen JY, Lo D, McArdle A, Sinha R, Tevlin R, Seita J, Vincent-Tompkins J, Wearda T, Lu WJ, Senarath-Yapa K, Chung MT, Marecic O, Tran M, Yan KS, Upton R, Walmsley GG, Lee AS, Sahoo D, Kuo CJ, Weissman IL, Longaker MT
Department of Surgery, Stanford University, Palo Alto, CA, USA
chazchan@stanford.edu; longaker@stanford.edu
Cell 2015;160:285–298

Background: The skeletal stem cells and how skeletal tissues are derived from them remain unknown. The authors hypothesised that skeletogenesis may proceed through a developmental hierarchy of lineage-restricted progenitors as occurs in haematopoiesis.
Methods: The authors mapped bone, cartilage and stromal development from a population of pure, postnatal mouse skeletal stem cells (mSSCs) to their downstream progenitors of bone, cartilage and stromal tissue. They then investigated the transcriptome of the stem/progenitor cells for unique gene-expression patterns that would indicate potential regulators of mSSC lineage commitment.
Results: The results indicate that mSSC niche factors can be potent inducers of osteogenesis and several specific combinations of recombinant mSSC niche factors can activate mSSC genetic programs in situ. This activation can take place even in nonskeletal tissues, resulting in de novo formation of cartilage or bone and bone marrow stroma.
Conclusions: These results imply that inducing mSSC formation with soluble factors and subsequently regulating the mSSC niche to specify its differentiation toward bone, cartilage or stromal cells could provide new means for therapeutic regeneration of skeletal tissues.

The existence, true nature and function of skeletal stem cells have been incompletely evaluated. The existing model for the development and growth of long bones proposes two phases. First, cartilage cells lay down a matrix that forms a scaffold for bone formation. Osteoblasts then invade this matrix and lay down the mineralised parts of bone. Although this process of endochondral ossification has been known for decades, it has remained unclear whether these postnatal processes are performed by osteoblasts and chondrocytes already committed to their respective lineages or whether specialised multipotent cells are involved.

Two independent studies published concurrently now identify mouse stem cells that give rise to various skeletal tissues — bone, cartilage and bone marrow stroma — but not to adipose, haematopoietic or muscle tissue. The authors identify in mice a stem cell for skeletal tissues, along with downstream progenitors, that have a role in skeletal tissue maintenance and regeneration. In the first study, the authors applied a transgenic mouse model to identify cells that express the BMP antagonist gremlin 1. They traced a novel population of stem cells, osteochondroreticular stem cells, which have the capacity to self-renew and generate osteoblasts, chondrocytes and reticular marrow stromal cells. In the second study, the authors searched for the parental cell type of all skeletal progenitor cells. Investigation of clonal relationships and lineage development in mice led to the isolation of a population of postnatal mouse skeletal stem cells (mSSCs) and to the characterisation of downstream progenitors giving rise to bone, cartilage and stromal cells. Transcriptome analysis of these cell populations clarified the pathways involved in mSSC self-renewal and specification of progenitor lineages. By modulating niche signalling the researchers were able to stimulate skeletal stem cell proliferation and tissue growth. Furthermore, administration of specific morphogenetic factors led to reprogramming of non-skeletal mesenchymal tissue into cartilage.

The findings of both studies may have important therapeutic applications for various skeletal diseases that involve tissues arising from the particular stem cell. Possible applications could include osteoporosis and osteoarthritis, maybe even short stature. While these observations in mice are extremely exciting, no data from human skeletal stem cells are available. Identification and characterisation of such a stem cell is the next step towards development of new therapeutic approaches. Much work is still to be done, but the potential is great.

Mechanism of the year: the multi-tasking chondrocytes

Hypertrophic chondrocytes can become osteoblasts and osteocytes in endochondral bone formation

Yang L, Tsang KY, Tang HC, Chan D, Cheah KS
Department of Biochemistry and Centre for Reproduction, Development and Growth, LKS Faculty of Medicine, The University of Hong Kong, Pokfulam, Hong Kong
kathycheah@hku.hk
Proc Natl Acad Sci U S A 2014;111:12097–12102

Background: The lineage of osteoblasts has attracted intense interest, as maintenance of bone throughout life requires their continual renewal. The idea that hypertrophic chondrocytes (HCs) are an alternative source of osteoblasts is controversial.
Methods: The authors developed a Col10a1-Cre:RLacZ mice with specific gene expression in HCs to determine in vivo whether HCs contribute to the osteoblast lineage. X-Gal staining, immunohistochemistry and in situ hybridisation were used to follow the fate of HCs.
Results: HC-derived cells were found in the endosteum of Col10a1-cre:RLacZ mice. They expressed Col1a1 (marker of osteoblasts) but not Col10a1 (marker of HCs), suggesting lineage progression of HCs to osteoblasts and osteocytes in vivo. The presence of HC-derived cells at the chondro-osseous junction and in cortical bone of three-month-old mice suggests that HCs continue to commit to the osteogenic fate in adulthood and may thrive as osteocytes.
Conclusions: HCs can survive the cartilage-to-bone transition. They become osteogenic cells in fetal and postnatal endochondral bones and persist into adulthood.

Chondrocytes transdifferentiate into osteoblasts in endochondral bone during development, postnatal growth and fracture healing in mice

Zhou X, von der Mark K, Henry S, Norton W, Adams H, de Crombrugghe B
Department of Genetics, The University of Texas MD Anderson Cancer Center, Houston, TX, USA
xiinzhou@mdanderson.org
PLoS Genet 2014;10:e1004820

Background: Endochondral bone formation requires replacement of a chondrocyte-derived cartilage matrix with bone trabeculae made by osteoblasts. However, the sources of osteoblasts responsible for trabecular bone formation have remained unclear. The authors investigated whether cells derived from hypertrophic chondrocytes contribute to the osteoblast pool in trabecular bones.
Methods: The authors genetically labelled either hypertrophic chondrocytes with *Col10a1-Cre* or chondrocytes with tamoxifen-induced *Agc1-Cre ERT2* using *EGFP*, *LacZ* or *Tomato* expression to establish specific expression in chondrocytic cells.
Results: Labelled non-chondrocytic cells were abundant in the primary spongiosa. They were distributed throughout trabeculae surfaces and later in the endosteum, and were embedded within the bone matrix. About 60% of all mature osteoblasts in the endochondral bones of one-month-old mice derived from *Col10a1*-expressing hypertrophic chondrocytes. Chondrocytes also transdifferentiated to osteoblasts during bone fracture healing in adult mice.
Conclusions: Chondrocytes are a major source of osteoblasts and contribute to endochondral bone formation.

According to current dogma, chondrocytes and osteoblasts are considered independent lineages derived from a common osteochondroprogenitor. Lineage determination towards the chondrocyte or osteoblast fate is controlled by the relative expression of *Sox9* and *Runx2*. Programmed death has been generally accepted as the ultimate fate of terminally differentiated hypertrophic chondrocytes (HCs). However, it has also been debated whether a HC could become an osteoblast and contribute to the full osteogenic lineage.

These two recent studies now provide evidence that some HCs survive the cartilage-to-bone transition and that descendants of HCs may become *Col1a1*-expressing osteoblasts and sclerostin-expressing osteocytes. Both groups show independently that there is a chondrocyte-to-osteoblast lineage continuum and that HCs and perichondrial/periosteal osteoblast progenitors contribute to the osteogenic pool during endochondral bone formation and growth. The differential origin of osteoblasts may assure a steady supply of osteoblasts for building bone and provide diverse sources of progenitors for fracture repair. These findings have implications for our understanding of the mechanisms controlling bone homeostasis and interpretation of the underlying pathology in bone disorders. Knowing that HCs are a source of osteoblasts in bone, we should re-examine the bone phenotypes arising from mutations in genes that are expressed in cartilage. These important findings indicate a need to reconsider current concepts of bone formation and regeneration, and to re-evaluate the theories of pathogenetic mechanisms underlying skeletal disorders.

New methods: chondrocytes in live show

Dynamic imaging of the growth plate cartilage reveals multiple contributors to skeletal morphogenesis

Li Y, Trivedi V, Truong TV, Koos DS, Lansford R, Chuong CM, Warburton D, Moats RA, Fraser SE
Division of Biology and Biological Engineering, California Institute of Technology, Pasadena, CA, USA
Nat Commun 2015;6:6798

Background: The complex orchestration of skeletal formation in vertebrates is only partly understood. In this study, cell behaviour in the growth plate cartilage during growth was quantitatively analysed to gain insight into cellular regulation and physiology.

Methods: Behaviours of proliferative cells in avian embryonic organ culture during linear growth were monitored using a time-lapse two-photon laser scanning microscopy, which revealed cellular trajectories with a spreading displacement mainly along the tissue elongation axis. The authors developed software to quantify the extent to which various cellular processes contributed to tissue elongation.
Results: Extracellular matrix deposition and cell volume enlargement were the main contributors to tissue elongation in avian embryonic cartilage. By contrast, other contributors such as mitotic cell division and daughter cell rearrangement only had minor effects on cartilage growth.
Conclusions: Extracellular matrix deposition and cell volume enlargement are major contributors to cartilage elongation in the avian embryo. The applied methodology provides means to systematically dissect cell behaviour during skeletal shaping using quantitative approaches.

This study uses 21st century technology to perform quantitative imaging on a living tissue and to generate models to understand cellular dynamics during tissue maturation. The growth plate cartilage of long bones is ideal for 4D analyses of cell behaviours - assessment of 3D growth in time - due to its largely unidirectional growth and cylindrical shape. Long bone growth is accompanied by progressive differentiation of chondrocytes along the proximo-distal axis from resting chondrocytes to proliferative, prehypertrophic and hypertrophic chondrocytes. During the process various extracellular matrix proteins are deposited. Hypertrophic chondrocytes produce type X collagen, which then serves as a scaffold for the invasion of osteoblasts and subsequent formation of calcified bony matrix for long bone maturation. The process is controlled by multiple signalling pathways. Static imaging has limitations and has not provided us with a complete understanding of this dynamic, complex and yet so orderly process. The applied quantitative live optical imaging allows longitudinal visualisation of individual cells and quantitative description of their behaviours in 4D. The study findings beautifully confirm reports from pioneers of growth plate research. However, the dynamic analyses also offer several novel insights into cell behaviours during embryonic cartilage elongation. Among other things, the authors show that cells in the proliferating zone show progressive anisotropic spreading mainly along the proximo-distal axis; the relative speed between individual cells is constant and this homogenous behaviour additively contributes to the orderly cell motions at a global level; cell spreading is largely due to the expansion of the extracellular matrix, with a secondary contribution from increases in cell volume. The authors conclude that a central task of modern biology is to understand how cells build a tissue in a 4D context. Live imaging provides a unique approach due to its noninvasive ability to collect longitudinal data from cells in their normal context of the live tissues. In this way cell behaviour during skeletal shaping can be systematically dissected using quantitative approaches.

Novel therapeutic approach: targeting drug targets

Human monoclonal antibody fragments targeting matrilin-3 in growth plate cartilage

Cheung CS, Zhu Z, Lui JC, Dimitrov D, Baron J
Section on Growth and Development, National Institute of Child Health and Development, National Institutes of Health, Bethesda, MD, USA
luichunk@mail.nih.gov
Pharm Res 2015;32:439–449

Background: Growth plate abnormalities and impaired bone elongation are features of many genetic disorders such as chondrodysplasias. Signalling factors and molecules potentially correcting or improving these phenotypes cannot be directly applied into growth plate cartilage to reach optimal therapeutic levels locally. The authors aimed to find an antibody target in the growth plate for specific delivery of therapeutic agents into the physeal cartilage, with minimum effects on non-target tissues.
Methods: The cartilage-specific extracellular matrix protein matrilin-3 was chosen as a target candidate. Single-chain variable antibody fragments that bound to human and murine matrilin-3 were selected by yeast display technology. Matrilin-3 binding of the selected antibody fragments was investigated in vivo and in vitro and the data analysed by ELISA and immunohistochemistry.

Results: The authors were able to develop high-affinity matrilin-3 antibody fragments with high tissue specificity in vitro and in vivo. When injected intravenously in mice, the antibody fragments specifically homed to cartilage.
Conclusions: High-affinity antibody fragments for targeting cartilage tissue can be successfully selected using yeast display technology. Targeted drug delivery for patients with disorders of the growing skeleton could potentially be achieved by developing factors coupled to matrilin-3 antibody fragments.

Longitudinal bone growth is a complex process and requires normal function of multiple intracellular, endocrine and paracrine pathways. Mutations in the several genes involved in growth plate function give rise to disorders of growth, including the skeletal dysplasias. In addition to genetic disorders, acquired endocrine, nutritional or inflammatory disorders can impair growth plate function and result in severe short stature. Treatment options in several such disorders are severely limited.

To develop novel cartilage-targeting therapies, the authors aimed to identify polypeptides that specifically home onto growth plate cartilage. They selected matrilin-3, an extracellular matrix protein expressed with high tissue specificity in the growth plate cartilage, as their target and used a yeast display human antibody library to select specific binders to matrilin-3. Three antibody fragments showed high-affinity binding *in vitro* to homogenates of cartilage tissue and cartilage sections of mouse embryos. Most importantly, after intravenous injection to mice, the antibody fragments were specifically localised in cartilage and were not detectable in other tissues. The targeting antibody fragment would thus be preferentially taken up by the growth plate cartilage, resulting in high local concentrations of molecules and thereby improving efficacy at the growth plate and decreasing potential adverse effects on other tissues. Tissue-specific drug development, for example recombinant alkaline phosphatase, has already proved to be a successful therapeutic concept in skeletal disorders [13]. Extending this concept to cartilage-specific protein targets may open further possibilities for local drug delivery in conditions affecting the growth plate, including many skeletal dysplasias that lack specific therapies. This study gives a new perspective for drug development for several growth disorders. It remains to be shown whether the described approach is applicable in human therapies.

New genes: another communicator between osteoblast and osteoclast

Osteoblast-derived WNT16 represses osteoclastogenesis and prevents cortical bone fragility fractures

Moverare-Skrtic S, Henning P, Liu X, Nagano K, Saito H, Borjesson AE, Sjogren K, Windahl SH, Farman H, Kindlund B, Engdahl C, Koskela A, Zhang FP, Eriksson EE, Zaman F, Hammarstedt A, Isaksson H, Bally M, Kassem A, Lindholm C, Sandberg O, Aspenberg P, Sävendahl L, Feng JQ, Tuckermann J, Tuukkanen J, Poutanen M, Baron R, Lerner UH, Gori F, Ohlsson C
Centre for Bone and Arthritis Research at Institute of Medicine, Sahlgrenska Academy at University of Gothenburg, Gothenburg, Sweden
claes.ohlsson@medic.gu.se; roland_baron@hsdm.harvard.edu
Nat Med 2014;20:1279–1288

Background: The disability, mortality and costs caused by osteoporosis-related non-vertebral fractures are enormous. Based on previous genetic studies, the *WNT16* locus is a major determinant of cortical bone thickness and nonvertebral fracture risk in humans.
Methods: This study explored the mechanisms by which *WNT16* regulates both general bone homeostasis and specifically the cortical bone compartment. The authors generated and analysed several mouse strains with global as well as cell-specific Wnt16 inactivation.
Results: Wnt16-deficient mice developed spontaneous fractures as a result of low cortical thickness and high cortical porosity. In contrast, trabecular bone volume was not altered. Mechanistic studies showed that *WNT16* is osteoblast-derived and inhibits human and mouse osteoclastogenesis both directly, by acting on osteoclast progenitors, and indirectly by increasing expression of osteoprotegerin (Opg) in osteoblasts. In osteoclast progenitors *WNT16* activates the noncanonical signalling pathway, whereas

in osteoblasts both canonical and noncanonical signalling pathways are activated. Conditional Wnt16 inactivation revealed that osteoblast-lineage cells are the principal source of *WNT16*, and its targeted deletion in osteoblasts increases fracture susceptibility.
Conclusions: The osteoblast-derived *WNT16* is a new key regulator of osteoclastogenesis and influences fracture susceptibility. This discovery opens new avenues for the specific prevention or treatment of non-vertebral fractures.

Evidence from multiple sources confirms the key role of the WNT-signalling pathway in skeletal homeostasis. WNT proteins are secreted cysteine-rich glycoproteins that signal through both the canonical and non-canonical WNT pathway. Activation of canonical beta-catenin signalling increases bone mass, while impaired signalling results in reduced bone mass. This is evidenced also in human conditions were mutations in the genes coding for WNT pathway proteins, for example, LRP5 and WNT1, result in variable low bone mass phenotypes [14]. Genome-wide association studies have suggested the *WNT16* locus to be a major determinant of cortical bone thickness and non-vertebral fracture risk in humans.

To explore the mechanisms by which *WNT16* regulates bone homeostasis, and especially in the cortical bone compartment, the authors analysed several mouse strains with global or cell-specific Wnt16 inactivation. Absence of Wnt16 resulted in lower cortical bone thickness and higher porosity and increased fracture susceptibility. In fact, the Wnt16-/- mice had spontaneous fractures which otherwise are rare events in mouse models. The cortical bone defects were primarily caused by increased cortical bone resorption. Importantly, the skeletal defects seemed to be restricted to cortical bone while trabecular bone was unaffected, contrasting the findings in *LRP5* and *WNT1* osteoporosis where mainly the trabecular bone is affected. Further, based on study findings, *WNT16* is derived from osteoblast-lineage cells and activates both canonical and non-canonical WNT signalling to inhibit human and mouse osteoclastogenesis through direct effects on osteoclast progenitors and indirect effects that increase *Opg* expression in osteoblasts. This study also evaluated the possible beneficial effect of *WNT16* treatment in a mouse model, showing that *WNT16* improves bone mass in pathological bone loss. Local *WNT16* treatment in rat tibiae increased bone mineral density. These exciting findings provide important new insights to the role of WNT signalling in the cortical bone. New treatment strategies targeting regulators of *WNT16* might provide means to reduce fracture risk at cortical bone sites.

Food for thought – strong bones require a good night's sleep

Obstructive sleep apnea and metabolic bone disease: insights into the relationship between bone and sleep

Swanson CM, Shea SA, Stone KL, Cauley JA, Rosen CJ, Redline S, Karsenty G, Orwoll ES
Division of Endocrinology, Oregon Health and Science University, Portland, OR, USA
J Bone Miner Res 2015;30:199–211

Background: Obstructive sleep apnoea (OSA) and low bone mass are both common conditions, particularly among older adults. OSA, the most common form of sleep-disordered breathing, has been linked to multiple cardiovascular, metabolic, hormonal and inflammatory derangements and may have adverse effects on bone. However, little is known about the mechanisms through which OSA and the associated hypoxia and sleep loss affect bone metabolism.
Methods: In order to gain insight into the relationship between sleep and bone, the authors reviewed the current literature on OSA and metabolic bone disease.
Results: Several pathophysiological mechanisms are recognised by which OSA may affect bone metabolism and architecture. These include: metabolic disturbances, inflammation, hypoxia, hypogonadism, vitamin D deficiency, depression and use of medications. Some of these are causes for OSA, some represent features commonly seen in patients with OSA. Skeletal effects include abnormal bone turnover, low BMD and strength and increased risk for falls – all risk factors for fractures.

Conclusions: OSA may be an unrecognised cause of secondary osteoporosis. The rising prevalence of obesity may increase the numbers of patients at risk for both osteoporosis and OSA. It is therefore important to determine the relationship between these, understand the biological processes that drive the relationship and establish appropriate screening and interventions to decrease morbidity associated with OSA/osteoporosis.

This interesting review summarises a surprising amount of evidence to support the idea that obstructive sleep apnoea (OSA) is bad for bones. Nocturnal hypoxia is a cardinal feature of OSA. Hypoxia is harmful to bone by inducing acidosis and inflammation. The episodic nocturnal hypoxia in OSA (throughout the night and over years if untreated) can cause recurrent ischaemic injury, creating inflammation and a hypoxic, acidotic microenvironment for bone cells. In animal studies acidosis activates osteoclasts and inhibits mineral deposition by osteoblasts. The effects of hypoxia on human bone cells remain poorly understood but may depend on the duration, severity, frequency and chronicity of the hypoxia. OSA disturbs also normal circadian rhythm which is important for several biological processes. Many hormones have day-night rhythms of secretion and pulsatility that can be disturbed in sleep disturbance. Even bone turnover markers have a clear day-night pattern. Bone resorption and, to a lesser degree, bone formation markers, increase overnight, with a peak in the early morning and a nadir in the late afternoon. Concentration patterns of the osteocyte-derived proteins FGF23 and sclerostin have suggested the presence of a circadian rhythm also in osteocytes. The implications of disturbed circadian pattern in bone homeostasis *per se* remain unknown. The authors speculate that OSA during adolescence is likely to be of increasing importance due to the growing prevalence of childhood obesity; up to 45% of adolescents with moderate to severe obesity have polysomnographic evidence of OSA. These adolescents may be especially susceptible to OSA-mediated insults to bone. If left untreated, peak bone mass attainment may be compromised, predisposing to low bone mass later in life. A wake-up call for clinicians treating obese adolescents...

References

1. Heikkilä K, Pearce J, Maki M, Kaukinen K. Celiac disease and bone fractures: a systematic review and meta-analysis. J Clin Endocrinol Metab 2015;100:25–34.
2. Tsampalieros A, Lam CK, Spencer JC, Thayu M, Shults J, Zemel BS, et al. Long-term inflammation and glucocorticoid therapy impair skeletal modeling during growth in childhood Crohn disease. J Clin Endocrinol Metab 2013;98:3438–3445.
3. Bouligand J, Ghervan C, Tello JA, Brailly-Tabard S, Salenave S, Chanson P, et al. Isolated familial hypogonadotropic hypogonadism and a GNRH1 mutation. N Engl J Med 2009;360:2742–2748.
4. Romanet P, Osei L, Netchine I, Pertuit M, Enjalbert A, Reynaud R, et al. Case report of GNAS epigenetic defect revealed by a congenital hypothyroidism. Pediatrics 2015;135:e1079–1083.
5. Filopanti M, Corbetta S, Barbieri AM, Spada A. Pharmacology of the calcium sensing receptor. Clin Cases Miner Bone Metab 2013;10:162–165.
6. Hannan FM, Walls GV, Babinsky VN, Nesbit MA, Kallay E, Hough TA, et al. The calcilytic agent NPS 2143 rectifies hypocalcemia in a mouse model with an activating calcium-sensing-receptor (CaSR) mutation: relevance to autosomal dominant hypocalcemia type 1 (ADH1). Endocrinology 2015:en20151269.
7. Mannstadt M, Clarke BL, Vokes T, Brandi ML, Ranganath L, Fraser WD, et al. Efficacy and safety of recombinant human parathyroid hormone (1–84) in hypoparathyroidism (REPLACE): a double-blind, placebo-controlled, randomised, phase 3 study. Lancet Diabetes Endocrinol 2013;1:275–283.
8. Carpenter TO, Imel EA, Ruppe MD, Weber TJ, Klausner MA, Wooddell MM, et al. Randomised trial of the anti-FGF23 antibody KRN23 in X-linked hypophosphatemia. J Clin Invest 2014;124:1587–1597.
9. Alon US, Levy-Olomucki R, Moore WV, Stubbs J, Liu S, Quarles LD. Calcimimetics as an adjuvant treatment for familial hypophosphatemic rickets. Clin J Am Soc Nephrol 2008;3:658–664.
10. Mäkitie O, Linglart A, Heino TJ. Growth plate, bone and mineral metabolism; in Ong K, Hochberg Z (eds). Yearbook of Pediatric Endocrinology 2013. Basel, Karger, 2013.
11. Jin M, Yu Y, Qi H, Xie Y, Su N, Wang X, et al. A novel FGFR3-binding peptide inhibits FGFR3 signalling and reverses the lethal phenotype of mice mimicking human thanatophoric dysplasia. Hum Mol Genet 2012;21:5443–5455.
12. Lorget F, Kaci N, Peng J, Benoist-Lasselin C, Mugniery E, Oppeneer T, et al. Evaluation of the therapeutic potential of a CNP analog in a Fgfr3 mouse model recapitulating achondroplasia. Am J Hum Genet 2012;91:1108–1114.
13. Whyte MP, Greenberg CR, Salman NJ, Bober MB, McAlister WH, Wenkert D, et al. Enzyme-replacement therapy in life-threatening hypophosphatasia. N Engl J Med 2012;366:904–913.
14. Baron R, Kneissel M. WNT signalling in bone homeostasis and disease: from human mutations to treatments. Nat Med 2013;19:179–192.

Reproductive Endocrinology

Lena Sahlin and Olle Söder

Pediatric Endocrinology Unit, Q2:08, Department of Women's and Children's Health, Karolinska Institutet and University Hospital, Solna, SE-171 76 Stockholm, Sweden

Reproductive endocrinology constitutes a busy research area covering the whole developmental journey from fertilisation through pregnancy, childhood, puberty, fertile life and finally ending in senescence, with obvious gender differences. This chapter focuses on the paediatric angle of this journey, including aspects of fetal development and fertility. A survey with relevant search terms for articles published during the past year resulted in more than 1,200 hits which were screened and sorted into different topics for final selection. A total of 21 articles were chosen covering epidemiological, molecular, experimental animal and human aspects of the theme. The selected articles are sorted under headings such as new genes, important for clinical practice, clinical trials, new mechanisms and new paradigms. As in previous Yearbooks, other chapters of this volume also describe papers dealing with reproduction. We realise that there are also many other excellent papers within the field published during the past year that we probably have missed and yet others which we could not include due to space limitation. Our aim was to present a mix of experimental and clinical publications advancing the knowledge within the field of reproductive endocrinology. A few articles may not seem to be in the mainstream of the topic but they are selected to inspire you to think along new lines. The selection obviously represents our own bias but we hope you find it interesting and useful for your work in the clinic or at the lab bench.

New mechanisms

Loss of BMAL1 in ovarian steroidogenic cells results in implantation failure in female mice

Liu Y, Johnson BP, Shen AL, Wallisser JA, Krentz KJ, Moran SM, Sullivan R, Glover E, Parlow AF, Drinkwater NR, Schuler LA, Bradfield CA

McArdle Laboratory for Cancer Research, and Carbone Cancer Center, School of Medicine and Public Health University of Wisconsin-Madison, Madison, WI, USA

bradfield@oncology.wisc.edu

Proc Natl Acad Sci U S A 2014;111:14295–14300

Background: Many aspects of female reproductive biology, such as estrous cycling, ovulation, embryonic implantation, onset of puberty and parturition, are influenced by the circadian clock.
Methods: A promoter that controls expression of Steroidogenic Factor-1 (SF1) was inserted to drive Cre-recombinase-mediated deletion of the brain muscle arnt-like 1 (Bmal1) gene, which is known to encode an essential component of the circadian clock.
Results: SF1-Bmal1(-/-) females exhibited embryonic implantation failure, which could be rescued by addition of progesterone, or transplantation of wild-type (wt) ovaries into SF1-Bmal1(-/-) dams. The central clock, and many of the peripheral, were fully functional in this model which makes an assignment of the implantation phenotype to the clock in ovarian steroidogenic cells. This phenotype is different from the more general circadian related systemic pathology (such as early onset arthropathy, premature ageing, anovulation, late onset puberty and abnormal estrous cycle).
Conclusions: This ovarian transcriptome analysis identifies a deletion of ovarian Bmal1 expression disrupting transcripts associated with the circadian machinery and also genes critical for regulation of progesterone production, for example, steroidogenic acute regulatory factor (StAR). This study provides a model to probe the interlocking and synergistic network of the circadian clock and reproductive system.

The authors created a mouse model to determine if cellular circadian clocks in peripheral tissues influence reproductive biology. They provide evidence that promoter-driven deletions, induced to knock out the circadian clock in ovarian steroidogenic cells, results in a total implantation failure in homozygotic dams. The female mice showed characteristics of an early pregnancy loss. When transplanted either uni- or bi-laterally with wild type ovaries, or supplemented with progesterone, the fertility of the knock-out animals was rescued. The results support that the Bmal1 gene has a role in the intrinsic clock of ovarian steroidogenic cells and also in regulation of progesterone production. Hence, there is evidence that the circadian clock is of direct importance for implantation, and thus female reproduction. The results add to the list of mechanisms behind female infertility. Further phenotyping of this disruption in humans is warranted. The article was highlighted by Claire Greenhill in *Nature Endocrinology Reviews* [1].

New paradigms in sperm competition

Sexual selection and the evolution of sperm quality

Fitzpatrick JL, Lupold S
Computational and Evolutionary Biology, Faculty of Life Sciences, University of Manchester, Manchester, UK
john.fitzpatrick@manchester.ac.uk
Mol Hum Reprod 2014;20:1180–1189

Background: Sperm experience intense and varied selection that impacts the evolution of sperm quality. Selection acts to ensure that sperm are fertilisation-competent and able to overcome the many challenges experienced on their journey to the oocyte. However, simply being able to fertilise an egg is not enough to ensure male fertility in most species. Female multiple mating is common throughout the animal kingdom, therefore successful fertilisation requires sperm to outcompete rival sperm. In addition, females can actively affect sperm quality, storage or utilisation to influence male fertility.
Methods: This paper reviews how selection forces influence the evolution of sperm quality.
Results: After exploring the link between sperm traits and male fertility, the authors examined how post-mating competition between rival ejaculates influences the evolution of sperm quality. They further described how complex genetic, social and sexual interactions influence the quality of sperm, focusing on the importance of seminal fluid and interactions between sperm and the female's reproductive tract. In light of the complexities of selection on sperm traits, it is envisaged that use of multivariate approaches incorporating male-male, sperm-sperm and sperm-female interactions to study sperm quality will enhance the understanding of how selection acts on sperm traits and factors influencing male fertility.
Conclusions: Because the metric of male reproductive success, fertilisation, is the same across the animal kingdom, the authors argue that information about sperm evolution gained from animals has great potential to inform the understanding of the factors that impact human fertility.

Sperm competition and the evolution of spermatogenesis

Ramm SA, Scharer L, Ehmcke J, Wistuba J
Evolutionary Biology, Bielefeld University, Bielefeld, Germany
steven.ramm@uni-bielefeld.de
Mol Hum Reprod 2014;20:1169–1179

Background: Spermatogenesis is a long and complex process that, despite the shared overall goal of producing the male gamete, displays striking interspecies diversity. In this review, the authors argue that sperm competition has been an important selection pressure acting on multiple aspects of spermatogenesis, causing variation in the number and morphology of sperm produced and in the underlying molecular and cellular processes.
Methods: The authors review the basic biology of spermatogenesis in some of the main animal model systems to illustrate this diversity and then describe the extent to which this variation arises from the evolutionary forces acting on spermatogenesis, most notably sperm competition.
Results: Five specific aspects of spermatogenesis from an evolutionary perspective were explored, namely: (i) interspecific diversity in the number and morphology of sperm produced; (ii) the testicular organisations and stem cell systems used to produce them; (iii) the large number and high evolutionary rate of genes underpinning spermatogenesis; (iv) the repression of transcription during spermiogenesis and its link to

the potential for haploid selection; and (v) the phenomenon of selection acting at the level of the germline.
Conclusions: The authors conclude that adopting an evolutionary perspective can shed light on many otherwise opaque features of spermatogenesis, and helps to explain the diversity of ways in which males of different species perform this fundamentally important process.

These two papers were published in a special issue of *Molecular Human Reproduction*, focusing on sperm competition, and introduced by Ramm [2].

Sperm competition occurs when sperm from several males compete to fertilise one or more ova in a single female. Males who win the sperm competition, or find ways to avoid it, produce more offspring in the long run. In evolution this leads to higher frequency of the features that are important for such successful outcome in sperm competition. If this assumption is correct, such fitness should have been selected for and be enriched in the reproductive biology observed today. Fitzpatrick and Lüpold describe how to define a 'successful' sperm. They show how selection by sperm competition strongly affects sperm phenotypes including clinical parameters such as morphology, speed of movement and longevity. They also discuss the role of the seminal fluid and the female reproductive tract where sperm have to perform. Humans are no exception in the array of different species covered. Ramm et al. consider how male gametes should be produced in order to succeed in fertilising eggs. They describe and discuss the evolutionary forces acting on the process and the machinery of spermatogenesis. Features such as the amount and proportion of spermatogenic tissue the testes contain, the number and morphology of sperm that must be produced there and the spermatogonial stem cell systems that support this process are considered. One notion is that the relative testis size as a measure of sperm production capacity is just one of the multiple ways spermatogenesis has been affected by the selection pressure. Taken together these two papers give interesting new insights into the phenomenon of sperm competition and its evolutionary perspective including that of humans.

New mechanisms

In utero effects. In utero undernourishment perturbs the adult sperm methylome and intergenerational metabolism

Radford EJ, Ito M, Shi H, Corish JA, Yamazawa K, Isganaitis E, Seisenberger S, Hore TA, Reik W, Erkek S, Peters AH, Patti ME, Ferguson-Smith AC
Department of Physiology, Development and Neuroscience, University of Cambridge, Cambridge, UK
afsmith@mole.bio.cam.ac.uk
Science 2014;345:1255903

Background: Adverse prenatal environments can promote metabolic disease in offspring and subsequent generations. Animal models and epidemiological data implicate epigenetic inheritance, but the mechanisms remain unknown.
Methods: In an intergenerational developmental programming model affecting 2nd (F2) generation mouse metabolism, the authors demonstrate that the in utero nutritional environment of 1st (F1) generation embryos alters the germline DNA methylome of F1 adult males in a locus-specific manner.
Results: Differentially methylated regions are hypomethylated and enriched in nucleosome-retaining regions. A substantial fraction is resistant to early embryo methylation reprogramming, which may have an impact on F2 development. Differential methylation is not maintained in F2 tissues, yet locus-specific expression is perturbed.
Conclusions: In utero nutritional exposures during critical windows of germ cell development can impact the male germline methylome, associated with metabolic disease in offspring.

Undernutrition in utero may result in low birthweight and compromised energy metabolism and health in adulthood. Accumulating research indicate that such environmentally induced effects are memorised and last for generations. The mechanisms behind such long lasting perturbations are not well understood but epigenetic changes have been implicated.

The authors employed a mouse model of low birthweight induced by calorie restriction to investigate the effects of the undernourishment and altered in utero environment on the DNA methylation profile of adult germ cells. The first generation offspring in these mice were small for gestational age (SGA) at term birth and shows signs of metabolic syndrome. SGA was induced by maternal undernutrition in the final week of pregnancy, which is estimated to parallel the late second trimester and third trimester of human pregnancy. This developmental period coincides with the maturational stage in which male primordial germ cells are reprogrammed by DNA methylation. Male mice from the first generation were crossed with healthy control mice under normal nutritional conditions and the offspring was analysed for metabolic perturbations. The resulting pups were SGA and demonstrated a compromised adult metabolic phenotype very similar to the one displayed by the SGA fathers. In utero examination of fetal mice of the same origin in the last trimester revealed metabolic perturbations already at this early stage when compared with controls. To study possible mechanisms the authors compared the DNA methylation patterns in sperm from male first generation mice and control mice. They observed 166 differentially methylated regions (DMRs) of which 111 were hypomethylated and 55 hypermethylated. Loss of methylation in hypomethylated DMRs was confirmed in 90% of the unique regions in an independent set of sperm samples whereas none of the hypermethylated changes were confirmed. The genomic distribution of the hypomethylated DMRs in primordial germ cells of affected male first generation mice revealed a unique temporal pattern of reprogramming. This indicates that in utero undernutrition interferes with the DNA remethylation process that normally starts at mid gestation. There were also indications that these effects are transmitted via altered chromatin structures. The differential methylation pattern did not persist in fetal brain and liver demonstrating that the metabolic phenotypes seen in this generation do not result from long-term heritable memory from previous generations. In summary the results show that paternal exposure in fetal life may affect the health of his offspring. Questions that remain to be addressed include whether these observed changes are reversible and if maternal contribution may also add to these effects via the first generation offspring. This article is highlighted by Schubert in *Biology of Reproduction* [3] and by Sarget in *Nature Reviews* [4].

Estrogens and their genotoxic metabolites are increased in obese prepubertal girls

Mauras N, Santen RJ, Colon-Otero G, Hossain J, Wang Q, Mesaros C, Blair IA
Division of Endocrinology, Diabetes and Metabolism, Nemours Children's Health System, Jacksonville, FL, USA
J Clin Endocrinol Metab 2015;100:2322–2328

Background: Levels of estrogen and their metabolites are higher in obese as compared with lean postmenopausal women and obesity increases breast cancer risk. Quinone derivatives of 4-hydroxylated estrogen metabolites, independently of the estrogen receptor, cause depurination and impaired DNA repair and thus denoted to be 'genotoxic'. As an example, 16alpha-OH-E1 promotes tumour proliferation while 2-methoxy (MeO)-E2 may be chemoprotective. Obesity in childhood is known to increase breast cancer death risk in adulthood, but the levels of estrogen derivatives have not been assessed in young girls.
Methods: Serum samples from 12 lean and 23 obese prepubertal girls (breast and pubic hair Tanner stage I) were assayed for estrone (E1), estradiol (E2) and their multiple metabolites (in total 12) by LC/MS-MS.
Results: Estradiol and 16alpha-OH-E1 levels were higher in obese than in lean girls. 2-MeO-E2 concentrations were lower in the obese group as compared with the lean group. The 16alpha-OH-E1 concentrations were positively correlated with BMI, percentage fat mass and interleukin-6.
Conclusions: Estradiol and genotoxic metabolites were higher in obese than lean prepubertal girls. Thus, obesity seems to be associated with increased extraglandular estrogen production and metabolism also before the onset of puberty in girls.

Highly sensitive estrogen analysis was employed to detect the relatively low hormone levels in prepubertal girls accurately. In addition to the steroid hormone levels also a great number of their genotoxic metabolites were assessed. The results indicate that obesity might be associated with increased extraglandular estrogen production and metabolism already before the onset of puberty. The study indicates that prepubertal obesity may affect breast cancer risk in adulthood by the increased levels of the genotoxic metabolites. The possibility that girls may differ in their production capacity of genotoxic metabolites and that this may affect breast cancer risk in adulthood remains to be investigated. Such possibility opens up for personalised prevention regimes based on monitoring of the genotoxic metabolites.

Gender development in Indonesian children, adolescents, and adults with disorders of sex development

Ediati A, Juniarto AZ, Birnie E, Drop SL, Faradz SM, Dessens AB
Department of Clinical Psychology, Faculty of Psychology, Diponegoro University, Tembalang, Semarang, Indonesia
aediati@gmail.com
Arch Sex Behav 2015;44:1339-1361

Background: Clinical management of disorders of sex development (DSD) begins in most high-income countries at diagnosis, soon after birth. In the low-income country Indonesia, DSD patients often have limited access to medical treatment. Therefore, affected individuals are often raised with ambiguous genitalia and atypical secondary sex characteristics.
Methods: Gender identity and gender role behaviour were investigated for gender, age and residential setting (rural, suburban, urban), in 118 Indonesian subjects (77 males, 41 females) with different types of DSD in comparison with 118 healthy matched controls.
Results: The majority of participants with DSD had never received any medical or surgical treatment prior to this study. A gender change was observed in all age groups, with the greatest incidence in adults. Among patients who changed, most switched from female to male, possessed a 46,XY karyotype and had experienced significant masculinisation during life. Confusion in gender identity and a cross-gender behaviour were more frequently observed in children with DSD raised as girls compared with boys.
Conclusions: In this setting an integrated clinical and psychological follow-up on gender outcome is necessary prior to puberty and adulthood.

The resources available for management of DSD patients differ between high-income countries and other settings without universal access to qualified medical care. Individuals affected by DSD in Indonesia are often raised with ambiguous genitalia and atypical sex characteristics. The authors uniquely describe gender development in a large sample of DSD individuals who did not receive any medical or surgical treatment at birth or early childhood. The authors found that the highest incidence of gender change was in the adult group (44%, as compared with 7% and 8% in children and adolescents, respectively). They also show that adolescent girls and women, who never received any medical treatment for their DSD condition reported more dissatisfaction with their gender identities and more frequent cross-gender behaviour, than those who had received some treatment. Consequently, it is important to perform appropriate investigation of DSD early and to provide medical and surgical treatments prior to puberty where necessary, in order to improve quality of life. The patients reported here may be the tip of the iceberg as we do not know how many patients with DSD in this setting remain undisclosed and do not present to healthcare professionals even as adults.

Changes over time in sex assignment for disorders of sex development

Kolesinska Z, Ahmed SF, Niedziela M, Bryce J, Molinska-Glura M, Rodie M, Jiang J, Sinnott RO, Hughes IA, Darendeliler F, Hiort O, van der Zwan Y, Cools M, Guran T, Holterhus PM, Bertelloni S, Lisa L, Arlt W, Krone N, Ellaithi M, Balsamo A, Mazen I, Nordenström A, Lachlan K, Alkhawari M, Chatelain P, Weintrob N
Developmental Endocrinology Research Group, School of Medicine, University of Glasgow, Yorkhill, Glasgow, UK
faisal.ahmed@glasgow.ac.uk
Pediatrics 2014;134:e710-715

Background: The International Disorder of Sex Development (I-DSD) Registry was used to determine if the proportion of infants with DSD who are raised as males or females has changed over time.
Methods: DSD cases reported as partial androgen insensitivity syndrome (PAIS; n=118), disorder of gonadal development (DGD; n=232) and disorder of androgen synthesis (DAS; n=104) were divided into three birth cohort periods: those born before 1990, those born 1990–1999 and those born after 1999. The appearance of the external genitalia was described by the external masculinisation score.

Results: The median external masculinisation score of the infants with PAIS, DGD or DAS who were raised as boys were all 6, and were higher than in those raised as girls (2, 2 and 0, respectively). This difference in external severity was maintained in all three birth cohorts. In contrast, 35% of the pre-1990 cohort, 41% of the 1990–1999 cohort and 68% of the post-1999 cohort were raised as boys.
Conclusions: Expectedly, there was an association between the external appearance of the genitalia and the choice of sex assignment. However, there was a clear temporal trend towards an increased likelihood of affected infants being raised as boys.

The international web-based I-DSD Registry was created in 2008. The authors used this registry to assess evidence for a change in the practice of sex assignment over the past few decades, when important changes in the field of DSD occurred. The post-1999 period can be regarded as the start of a new era with increased awareness of gender assignment and with less emphasis on the appearance of the external genitalia at birth. This changed view may have been influenced by the John versus Joan case [5], which challenged the tradition not to choose a male gender if the external genitalia of a Y chromosome-carrying individual was judged to predict poor future male sexual function. That landmark case centred on an XY infant, whose penis was accidentally ablated and who was subsequently raised as a female. This seemed at first to work out well, but later gender dysphoria developed and the gender was reassigned to male after puberty. The present results show that a growing proportion of severely affected infants are being raised as boys. Close monitoring and long-term follow-up into adulthood of these children are highly warranted and will reveal if this approach is successful.

New genes

Genome-wide association analyses identify variants in developmental genes associated with hypospadias

Geller F, Feenstra B, Carstensen L, Pers TH, van Rooij IA, Korberg IB, Choudhry S, Karjalainen JM, Schnack TH, Hollegaard MV, Feitz WF, Roeleveld N, Hougaard DM, Hirschhorn JN, Franke L, Baskin LS, Nordenskjöld A, van der Zanden LF, Melbye M
Department of Epidemiology Research, Statens Serum Institut, Copenhagen, Denmark
fge@ssi.dk
Nature Genetics 2014;46:957–963

Background: Hypospadias is a common congenital condition in boys in which the urethra opens towards the ventral side of the penis. Deficiency or poor action of androgens may be one cause but in most cases the aetiology is obscure.
Methods: A genome-wide association study on 1,006 surgery-confirmed hypospadias cases and 5,486 controls from Denmark was performed.
Results: After replication genotyping of an additional 1,972 cases and 1,812 controls from Denmark, the Netherlands and Sweden, 18 genomic regions were detected to show independent association.
Conclusions: The discovered loci explain 9% of the probability of developing hypospadias. Several of the identified regions contain well known genes with key roles in embryonic development, for example, HOXA4, IRX5, IRX6 and EYA1.

The authors included a large number of patients with hypospadias in a genome-wide association study and detected 18 independent associated genomic regions. Many of these regions hosted genes crucial for embryonic development, the disruption of which would result in much more serious consequences than just hypospadias. Despite this and other extensive studies, a clear majority of cases with hypospadias still remain unexplained. There are recent reports indicating an increasing prevalence of hypospadias, at least in certain geographical regions. Such rapid and ongoing changes are not consistent with genetic causes but more so with environmental influences. Hypothetically, exposure to endocrine-disrupting chemicals with anti-androgenic actions may be one such mechanism.

Increased gene copy number of VAMP7 disrupts human male urogenital development through altered estrogen action

Tannour-Louet M, Han S, Louet JF, Zhang B, Romero K, Addai J, Sahin A, Cheung SW, Lamb DJ
Scott Department of Urology, Baylor College of Medicine, Houston, TX, USA
mounia.louet@gmail.com and dlamb@bcm.edu
Nature Medicine 2014;20:715-724

Background: Although genitourinary defects are among the most common birth defects in newborns, still little is known about their aetiology.
Methods: Samples from children born with congenital genitourinary tract masculinisation disorders were analysed by array-comparative genomic hybridisation.
Results: In 1.35% of cases the presence of de novo copy number gains at Xq28 encompassing the *VAMP7* gene, were found. The *VAMP7* gene encodes a vesicle-trafficking protein that is part of the SNARE complex. Transgenic mice carrying an artificial chromosome encoding human *VAMP7* mimicked the defective urogenital traits observed in boys with masculinisation disorders such as cryptorchidism, urethral defects and hypospadias. The mice were also found to have reduced penile length, focal spermatogenic anomalies, diminished sperm motility and subfertility. VAMP7 co-localises with estrogen receptor alpha (ESR1) in the presence of its cognate ligand, 17beta-estradiol. Increased levels of VAMP7 strengthened ESR1-potentiated transcriptional activity by raising the cellular content of ESR1 protein upon ligand stimulation. The expression of estrogen-responsive genes such as ATF3, CYR61 and CTGF were upregulated, all being genes previously known to be associated with hypospadias.
Conclusions: An increased gene dosage of *VAMP7*, and its protein product, enhances estrogen receptor action in male genitourinary tissues, with subsequent undermasculinisation of the reproductive tract and genitourinary birth defects in humans.

The authors identified extra copies of *VAMP7* in a small proportion of children born with congenital genitourinary tract masculinisation disorders. The protein encoded by *VAMP7* enhances estrogen receptor ESR1 transcriptional activity. ESR1 is known to be involved in some genitourinary birth defects in newborn boys, for example, hypospadias. *VAMP7* also exerts a partial inhibitory effect on androgen receptor action. To examine which phenotypes the gene could give rise to, a transgenic mouse model was generated. Interestingly, these mice exhibited defects similar to those observed in the affected boys. The mice also displayed sperm production deficiencies and subfertility with ageing. Additional studies on the mice revealed that high levels of *VAMP7* resulted in elevated levels of ESR1. The exact mechanism of how *VAMP7* affects ESR1 activity is not clear, but one hypothesis is that this could be by stabilisation of the ESR1 complex in membrane fusion or intracellular transport. Nevertheless, this study opens up novel means by which environmental estrogen may influence the masculinisation process in male prenatal development. This study was highlighted in *Biology of Reproduction* [6].

Genome-wide association study of sexual maturation in males and females highlights a role for body mass and menarche loci in male puberty

Cousminer DL, Stergiakouli E, Berry DJ, Ang W, Groen-Blokhuis MM, Körner A, Siitonen N, Ntalla I, Marinelli M, Perry JR, Kettunen J, Jansen R, Surakka I, Timpson NJ, Ring S, McMahon G, Power C, Wang C, Kahonen M, Viikari J, Lehtimäki T, Middeldorp CM, Hulshoff Pol HE, Neef M, Weise S, Pahkala K, Niinikoski H, Zeggini E, Panoutsopoulou K, Bustamante M, Penninx BW, Murabito JM, Torrent M, Dedoussis GV, Kiess W, Boomsma DI, Pennell CE, Raitakari OT, Hypponen E, Davey Smith G, Ripatti S, McCarthy MI, Widen E
Institute for Molecular Medicine, Finland
elisabeth.widen@helsinki.fi
Hum Mol Genet 2014;23:4452-4464

Background: Little is known about the genes that regulate male puberty. Many identified pubertal timing gene variants are associated with age at menarche and body mass in females. However, their relationships to pubertal initiation or tempo is not known.
Methods: A genome-wide association meta-analysis was performed on more than 11,000 European samples with data on early pubertal traits, male genital and female breast development, measured as Tanner scores.

Results: The authors identified a locus for male puberty timing upstream of myocardin-like 2 (*MKL2*), a known menarche locus tagging a developmental pathway linking earlier puberty with reduced pubertal growth and short adult stature in both males and females. Some menarche loci are thus important for pubertal initiation in both sexes. Epidemiological correlations between increased prepubertal body mass and earlier pubertal timing in girls have been described. In accordance, body mass index (BMI)-increasing alleles correlated with earlier breast development. In boys, some BMI-increasing alleles associated with earlier but others with later sexual development. This mimics the directionally discordant epidemiological associations reported between prepubertal BMI and the timing of male puberty.
Conclusions: The results give novel insights into the puberty initiation program in both boys and girls, and indicate that mechanisms regulating pubertal onset in males and females to a large extent seem to be shared. However, the relationship between body mass and pubertal timing may be more complex in boys than in girls.

Many attempts have been made to find the genes that regulate puberty. Many gene variants are associated with age at menarche, but that is a late manifestation of puberty in girls. Here, the authors performed a genome-wide association study to find genes linked with early puberty. The authors report the first locus for male pubertal timing near the gene *MKL2* on chromosome 16. This locus also associates with both the timing of pubertal development and the pubertal growth spurt. No novel genetic associations for female breast development were found but markers of early puberty in both genders were investigated. The authors conclude that previously reported menarche loci also appear to be important for pubertal timing in both sexes. These markers are likely tagging biological effects upstream of sex-specific mechanisms, as demonstrated by the high correlation between menarche-advancing effects and earlier pubertal development in both boys and girls. This study increases our understanding of the similarities and differences of pubertal regulation between the sexes.

Parent-of-origin-specific allelic associations among 106 genomic loci for age at menarche

Perry JR, Day F, Elks CE, Sulem P, Thompson DJ, Ferreira T, He C, Chasman DI, Esko T, Thorleifsson G, Albrecht E, Ang WQ, Corre T, Cousminer DL, Feenstra B, Franceschini N, Ganna A, Johnson AD, Kjellqvist S, Lunetta KL, McMahon G, Nolte IM, Paternoster L, Porcu E, Smith AV, Stolk L, Teumer A, Tsernikova N, Tikkanen E, Ulivi S, Wagner EK, Amin N, Bierut LJ, Byrne EM, Hottenga JJ, Koller DL, Mangino M, Pers TH, Yerges-Armstrong LM, Hua Zhao J, Andrulis IL, Anton-Culver H, Atsma F, Bandinelli S, Beckmann MW, Benitez J, Blomqvist C, Bojesen SE, Bolla MK, Bonanni B, Brauch H, Brenner H, Buring JE, Chang-Claude J, Chanock S, Chen J, Chenevix-Trench G, Collee JM, Couch FJ, Couper D, Coviello AD, Cox A, Czene K, D'Adamo A P, Davey Smith G, De Vivo I, Demerath EW, Dennis J, Devilee P, Dieffenbach AK, Dunning AM, Eiriksdottir G, Eriksson JG, Fasching PA, Ferrucci L, Flesch-Janys D, Flyger H, Foroud T, Franke L, Garcia ME, Garcia-Closas M, Geller F, de Geus EE, Giles GG, Gudbjartsson DF, Gudnason V, Guenel P, Guo S, Hall P, Hamann U, Haring R, Hartman CA, Heath AC, Hofman A, Hooning MJ, Hopper JL, Hu FB, Hunter DJ, Karasik D, Kiel DP, Knight JA, Kosma VM, Kutalik Z, Lai S, Lambrechts D, Lindblom A, Magi R, Magnusson PK, Mannermaa A, Martin NG, Masson G, McArdle PF, McArdle WL, Melbye M, Michailidou K, Mihailov E, Milani L, Milne RL, Nevanlinna H, Neven P, Nohr EA, Oldehinkel AJ, Oostra BA, Palotie A, Peacock M, Pedersen NL, Peterlongo P, Peto J, Pharoah PD, Postma DS, Pouta A, Pylkas K, Radice P, Ring S, Rivadeneira F, Robino A, Rose LM, Rudolph A, Salomaa V, Sanna S, Schlessinger D, Schmidt MK, Southey MC, Sovio U, Stampfer MJ, Stockl D, Storniolo AM, Timpson NJ, Tyrer J, Visser JA, Vollenweider P, Volzke H, Waeber G, Waldenberger M, Wallaschofski H, Wang Q, Willemsen G, Winqvist R, Wolffenbuttel BH, Wright MJ, Boomsma DI, Econs MJ, Khaw KT, Loos RJ, McCarthy MI, Montgomery GW, Rice JP, Streeten EA, Thorsteinsdottir U, van Duijn CM, Alizadeh BZ, Bergmann S, Boerwinkle E, Boyd HA, Crisponi L, Gasparini P, Gieger C, Harris TB, Ingelsson E, Jarvelin MR, Kraft P, Lawlor D, Metspalu A, Pennell CE, Ridker PM, Snieder H, Sorensen TI, Spector TD, Strachan DP, Uitterlinden AG, Wareham NJ, Widen E, Zygmunt M, Murray A, Easton DF, Stefansson K, Murabito JM, Ong K
MRC Epidemiology Unit, University of Cambridge School of Clinical Medicine, Institute of Metabolic Science, Cambridge, UK
Nature 2014;514:92-97

Background: Age at menarche is a marker of timing of puberty in females that varies widely between individuals. It is an inheritable trait and is associated with risks for obesity, type 2 diabetes, cardiovascular disease, breast cancer and all-cause mortality. Studies of rare human disorders of puberty, as well as animal models, point to a complex hypothalamic-pituitary-hormonal regulation. The mechanisms that determine pubertal timing and underlie its links to disease risk still remain unclear.

Methods: Genome-wide and custom-genotyping arrays were analysed in up to 182,416 women of European descent from 57 studies.
Results: Robust evidence was found for 123 signals at 106 genomic loci associated with age at menarche. Many loci were associated with other pubertal traits in both sexes. There was a substantial overlap with genes implicated in body mass index and various diseases. Menarche signals were enriched in imprinted regions. Pathway analyses implicated nuclear hormone receptors, particularly retinoic acid and gamma-aminobutyric acid-B2 receptor signalling, among novel mechanisms regulating pubertal timing in humans.
Conclusions: The results indicate a genetic architecture involving at least hundreds of common variants in the coordinated timing of pubertal transition.

These authors also used genome-wide analysis to detect genes important for the timing of puberty. They could confirm the overlap between loci associated with menarche and adult BMI; at all nine loci found to be in common, the age at menarche-raising allele was also associated with lower adult BMI. In addition, three menarche signals overlapped known loci for adult height. These results also indicate both BMI-related and BMI-independent mechanisms that could underlie the epidemiological associations between early menarche and higher risks of adult disease, such as actions of *LIN28B* on insulin sensitivity through the mTOR pathway, $GABA_B$ receptor signalling on inhibition of oxidative stress-related beta-cell apoptosis and *SIRT3* (mitochondrial sirtuin 3), which could link early life nutrition to metabolism and ageing. Thus, there are many genes involved in the timing of puberty with associations also relevant to adult health.

Clinical trial

Effects of low-dose estrogen replacement during childhood on pubertal development and gonadotropin concentrations in patients with Turner syndrome: results of a randomised, double-blind, placebo-controlled clinical trial

Quigley CA, Wan X, Garg S, Kowal K, Cutler GB Jr, Ross JL
Indiana University School of Medicine, Indianapolis, IN, USA
charmianq@gmail.com
J Clin Metabol Metab 2014;99:E1754–E1764

Background: The optimal approach to estrogen replacement in girls with Turner syndrome has not been determined. This study aimed to assess the effects of an individualised regimen of low-dose ethinyl estradiol (EE2) during childhood, followed by a pubertal induction regimen and escalating to full replacement over four years.
Methods: This was a prospective, randomised, double-blind, placebo-controlled clinical trial. Girls with Turner syndrome (n=149), aged 5.0–12.5 years, were enrolled; data from 123 girls were analysable for pubertal onset. Interventions comprised placebo or recombinant GH injections three times a week, with daily oral placebo or oral EE2 during childhood (25ng/kg/d, ages 5–8 years; 50ng/kg/d, ages >8–12 years); after age 12, all patients received escalating EE2 starting at a nominal dosage of 100ng/kg/d. A reduction by 50% of placebo/EE2 dosages was done if there was breast development before age 12 years, vaginal bleeding before age 14 years or undue advance in bone age. The main outcome measures were median ages at Tanner breast stage 2 or higher, median age at menarche and tempo of puberty. Patterns of gonadotropin secretion and impact of childhood EE2 on gonadotropins were also assessed.
Results: Girls who received childhood low-dose EE2 (n=61) had earlier thelarche (median, 11.6 versus 12.6 years) and slower tempo of puberty (median, 3.3 versus 2.2 years,) than the control group (n=62). Both controls and EE2 treated groups had delayed menarche (median, 15.0 years). Girls in the control group who had spontaneous breast development before estrogen exposure (29%) had lower median FSH values than girls who did not.

Conclusions: Childhood estrogen replacement normalised the onset and tempo of puberty. Childhood low-dose estrogen replacement should be considered for girls with Turner syndrome.

Several long-term follow-up studies in young adult Turner syndrome patients have clearly demonstrated that their main concern during childhood and adolescence is their late puberty timing and not short stature. This study is therefore very important for clinical practice as it offers help with the clinical management to reach the goal to start puberty at normal age. The results clearly show a beneficial outcome from EE2 treatment starting already as early as at five years of age, in relation to timing and tempo of puberty in girls with Turner syndrome. The girls had a more physiological onset of puberty as compared with those who began pubertal induction in their teens, as evidenced by optimisation of GH-stimulated height gain and benefits for cognitive development and memory. Baseline bone age was delayed compared with chronological age by a median of 1.3 years in both placebo and treatment groups. Unfortunately final height was not an outcome measure. Use of transdermal estradiol might be a more physiological way of administration, avoiding supraphysiological estrogen doses to the liver. Additionally, an individualisation of the estrogen dosage should be the goal for treatment. The lack of commercially available low-dose (childhood) preparations makes this goal still not fully accessible, although cutting adult estrogen patches into lower dose pieces seems functional. Nevertheless, this study presents promising data for a treatment regimen improving the quality of life for girls growing up with Turner syndrome.

Important for clinical practice

'How should I tell my child?' Disclosing the diagnosis of sex chromosome aneuploidies

Dennis A, Howell S, Cordeiro L, Tartaglia N
Graduate Program in Genetic Counseling, University of Colorado Denver, Aurora, CO, USA
J Genet Couns 2015;24:88–103

Background: The consequences of the disclosure of a sex chromosome aneuploidy (SCA) diagnosis to an affected individual have not been evaluated.
Methods: The best timing and content revealed to an affected child by his or her parent(s), resources accessed in preparation, parental feelings of preparedness, common parental concerns and recommendations for disclosure approaches are not well investigated. To assess this two online surveys were created including one for parents of a child with a diagnosis and another for individuals with a diagnosis. 139 parent surveys (XXY, n=68; XXX, n=21; XYY, n=9; other SCAs, n=41) and 67 individual surveys (XXY, n=58; XXX, n=9) were analysed.
Results: Parents most frequently discussed the topics of learning disabilities (47%) and genetics (45%) with their child during the initial disclosure. A higher proportion of parents reported feeling prepared versus unprepared for disclosure, regardless of their child's diagnosis. Websites, support groups and discussion with the child's physician prior to disclosure were accessed by both prepared and unprepared parents, but with unprepared parents accessing fewer resources than prepared parents. Parental concerns included often making the conversation age-appropriate, discussing infertility and possible impact on the child's self-esteem. Both parents and individual respondents endorsed being honest with the child, disclosing the diagnosis early and before puberty and discussing the diagnosis gradually over time.
Conclusions: These results suggest benefits to parents from additional resources and supports to alleviate concerns when approaching diagnosis disclosure.

Counselling of children/parents/families with chronic medical conditions that affect future health and daily life functions is an everyday activity of paediatricians and paediatric endocrinologists. The authors address this important topic from the view of the medical geneticist for patients with sex chromosome aneuploidies who are frequent visitors also to the paediatric practice. The results from surveys directed separately to patients and parents are presented and give valuable advice on the best approaches disclosing the diagnosis. This information is most certainly of value also in the clinical practice of the paediatric endocrinologist.

Use of propranolol for hypersexual behavior in an adolescent with autism

Deepmala, Agrawal M
University of Arkansas for Medical Sciences, Little Rock, AR, USA
Ann Pharmacother 2014;48:1385–1388

Background: Hypersexual behaviour exhibited by adolescent patients with autism is often a challenge to manage. The pharmacological options are scarce to manage these behaviours in children and adolescents with autism.
Methods: This case report describes a 13-year-old autistic boy who presented to the outpatient psychiatric clinic for hypersexual behaviours starting at the onset of puberty. The behaviours affected his functioning both at school and home. A trial of low-dose propranolol, 0.3mg/kg/d (10mg twice a day) was given.
Results: The treatment led to remarkable clinical improvement. The behaviours remained stable on this dose of propranolol for one year. Clinical data of propranolol use are novel.
Conclusions: This case report shows that a low-dose propranolol treatment lead to clinically significant improvement of hypersexual behaviours in an adolescent with autism. Propranolol use may expand the choice of treatment options to help this patient population.

Hypersexual behaviour in children with neuropsychiatric disorders is unfortunately not rare, is distressing to caregivers and is difficult to treat. This problem is not an infrequent cause of consultation with the paediatric endocrinologist. Studies on institutionalised young adults with autism spectrum disorders indicate that approximately one-third show severe sexual behavioural problems. Similar reports from parents of non-institutionalised children reveal many unwanted public sexual behaviours. Treatment with GnRH analogues and sex steroid blockers has been tried most often but with poor results. Sexual dysfunction in men is a side-effect associated with treatment with beta blockers. The mechanism is unclear, but both decreased levels of testosterone and antagonistic effects on serotonin receptors in the brain have been reported. In this case report a low dose of propranolol improved the hypersexual behaviour after two weeks of treatment in a 13-year-old boy. The public manifestations disappeared after three months and there were no side effects noted after a year. Despite this report describing only a single patient, the approach may be worth trying in patients with this problematic condition. Hopefully, the report will also give inspiration to set up a controlled clinical trial to robustly address this question by a paediatric endocrinologist amongst the readership of this chapter.

Testicular function, semen quality, and fertility in young men after renal transplantation during childhood or adolescence

Tainio J, Jahnukainen K, Nurmio M, Pakarinen M, Jalanko H, Jahnukainen T
Children's Hospital, University of Helsinki and Helsinki University Central Hospital, Helsinki, Finland
juuso.tainio@helsinki.fi
Transplantation 2014;98:987–993

Background: Reproductive function in adult male patients after renal transplantation (RTx) during childhood and adolescence is not well documented.
Methods: Twenty-four RTx recipients were examined as young adults (median chronological age 28.1 years and 18.6 years after transplantation). Reproductive hormone levels and semen samples were studied and compared with those of 56 age-matched controls. Eight RTx men (33%) had been treated with cyclophosphamide. Medical records were retrospectively reviewed and data on puberty, dialysis and immunosuppressive medication were analysed to evaluate the prospects of fertility and sexual health.
Results: Testicular volumes and total sperm counts of the RTx patients were reduced when compared with the controls (median 11.4 versus 33.9mL and 1.3 versus 135.5million, respectively). Only four (22%) of the RTx men had normospermia in the semen sample. The reproductive hormone levels were normal in most of the RTx recipients, with only two patients showing androgen deficiency. Those without history of cyclophosphamide treatment had smaller testes and total sperm counts compared with their healthy peers, whereas those with previous cyclophosphamide treatment showed further worse outcome.
Conclusions: Testicular function is often impaired many years after renal transplantation in the paediatric age group. Poor semen quality decreases the prospect of fertility after paediatric RTx.

This important study evaluated fertility in 24 patients many years after RTx in childhood (at mean age 9.3 years) and clearly shows an impaired testicular function and decreased fertility prospects. In addition, the RTx patients were shorter and lighter than age-matched controls, but their BMIs did not differ. The authors conclude that the effects of lifelong immunosuppressive medication may be of more importance for the endocrine function of the testis and sperm production, than the time with end-stage renal disease or a deteriorating graft function. Thus, long-term surveillance of gonadal function is needed for these patients.

Evaluation of 451 Danish boys with delayed puberty: diagnostic use of a new puberty nomogram and effects of oral testosterone therapy

Lawaetz JG, Hagen CP, Mieritz MG, Blomberg Jensen M, Petersen JH, Juul A
Department of Growth and Reproduction and EDMaRC, Rigshospitalet, University of Copenhagen, Denmark
J Clin Endocrinol Metab 2015;100:1376-1385

Background: There are few data on the diagnostic criteria and effects of puberty induction, in boys with constitutional delay of growth and puberty (CDGP). The authors developed puberty nomograms based on boys with normal pubertal development.
Methods: A retrospective study of 451 boys evaluated for delayed puberty between 1990–2013 was performed and compared with cross-sectional and longitudinal data on Danish boys with normal pubertal development. 36% (164) of the boys evaluated for CDGP were excluded due to missing data, reclassification or associated co-morbidities. The number of patients with CDGP as defined by the current puberty nomogram (genital stage <-2 SD for age) was compared with those defined by classical criteria (Tanner genital stage 1 at ≥14 years). The effect of one year of oral testosterone undecanoate (TU) on pubertal progression, circulating hormones, height and predicted adult height (PAH) was also evaluated.
Results: 27% (78) of the included 287 boys were categorised as having delayed pubertal onset according to the classical criteria, compared with 60% (173) with impaired pubertal progression according to the puberty nomogram. 56% (96) of these 173 boys were treated with oral TU for a median of 0.8 years, with beneficial effects on pubertal progression: height increased from -1.9 to -1.5 SD and median PAH increased from 172.3 to 178.1cm following one year of treatment.
Conclusions: The puberty nomogram evaluated both delayed pubertal onset and delayed pubertal progression, allowing separation of normal versus abnormal pubertal development. Oral TU treatment was followed by pubertal onset and progression, as well as short-term increased growth without compromising final height potential.

This well-performed study describes the application of nomograms for puberty development to discriminate delayed pubertal onset from delayed pubertal progression (CDGP) in boys. The nomograms are built from data of 287 boys finally included in the study. This is, according to the authors, the largest evaluation of CDGP boys before and during treatment with oral testosterone undecanoate (TU). The TU treatment was considered safe, and was followed by pubertal induction and progression, without signs of compromising final height when compared with standard curves. This treatment with TU thus seems to be equally safe and efficient as low-dose treatment with non-aromatisable anabolic steroids that has been practiced by some authors. As delayed puberty and CDGP in boys are very common in paediatric endocrinology practice this paper has important clinical implications.

Benign vaginal bleeding in 24 prepubertal patients: clinical, biochemical and imaging features

Nella AA, Kaplowitz PB, Ramnitz MS, Nandagopal R
Pediatric Endocrinology, National Institute of Child Health and Human Development, Bethesda, MD, USA
J Pediatr Endocrinol Metab 2014;27:821-825

Background: Premature menarche is an uncommon condition characterised by isolated or recurrent menstrual bleeding in the absence of secondary sexual characteristics.
Methods: The authors conducted an observational retrospective study to characterise clinical, biochemical and imaging features of benign prepubertal vaginal bleeding (BPVB). Out of 1,037 girls evaluated for precocious puberty over a five-year period, 24 (2.3%) girls with BPVB were identified based on one or

more episodes of vaginal bleeding, Tanner I or non-progressive Tanner II breast development and lack of physical findings suggesting genital infection, trauma or foreign body.
Results: Age at vaginal bleeding ranged from three years two months to nine years 11 months. Out of the girls with BPVB, ten patients (42%) had one episode of vaginal bleeding, six (25%) had two episodes and eight patients (33%) had three or more. The first bleeding episode lasted three days (range; 1–30 days) and six girls had intermittent spotting for up to one year. Minimal breast was present in five girls, early pubic hair was present in two and no breast development in 19 (79%) of the BPVB patients. LH and FSH levels were prepubertal. Pelvic ultrasound was performed in 11 patients and showed prepubertal uterus and ovaries without adnexal masses.
Conclusions: Without signs of sexual precocity or other vaginal pathology, isolated prepubertal vaginal bleeding is typically benign and self-limiting.

Isolated vaginal bleeding is a rare presentation to the paediatric endocrinology clinic. However, for the parents and the girl such a symptom may seem alarming and requiring immediate attention. The authors here present results that are reassuring, demonstrating that the vaginal bleeding most probably is benign if no other signs of puberty or pathology are present. This and other reports have shown that these girls could experience additional vaginal bleedings but without other sexual precocity manifestations. Some have reported normal ages at the onset of puberty and age at menarche and that these girls have regular menses and normal fertility (see references cited within the paper). The authors conclude that the aetiology of BVBP remains elusive although there are theories of increased endometrial sensitivity. Still, the important message to the clinician is that prepubertal vaginal bleeding without concomitant additional signs of puberty or other pathology should be regarded as a 'benign' condition.

Changing aetiological trends in male precocious puberty: evaluation of 100 cases with central precocious puberty over the last decade

Alikasifoglu A, Vuralli D, Gonc EN, Ozon A, Kandemir N
Department of Pediatric Endocrinology, Hacettepe University, Ankara, Turkey
ayfera@hacettepe.edu.tr
Horm Res Paediatr 2015;83:340–344

Background: Few studies have evaluated the aetiological factors in boys with central precocious puberty (CPP) and those reports are limited in terms of sample size as this condition is much less frequent in boys than in girls.
Methods: Aetiological factors were evaluated in 100 CPP boys, aged between nine months and 10.5 years. Medical records were screened for age at diagnosis, bone age, body weight, height, pubertal stage, imaging findings of the pituitary gland, testosterone and basal and stimulated gonadotropin levels.
Results: No underlying cause was found in 74% of the cases and an organic cause in only 26%. Most of the organic cases were diagnosed in CPP boys aged less than seven years, whereas most idiopathic cases were diagnosed after age seven years.
Conclusions: This proportion of 26% organic cases is among the lowest reported and may indicate the increase over time in the number of idiopathic male CPP cases. Boys who present with CPP older than age seven years are seldom detected with an underlying pathology.

Central precocious puberty (CPP) is defined as the onset of gonadotropin-driven puberty before age eight years in girls and nine years in boys. CPP is much more common in girls than boys and an organic cause is reportedly much more common in boys. In girls there are reports on secular trends towards increasing numbers of idiopathic CPP cases. The situation in boys is less well documented. The authors here report that, in the present Turkish context, the number of CPP boys with organic causes remained constant throughout the study years, whereas the number of idiopathic cases increased until 2009 and was maintained at the higher rate since. One possible explanation for this observation, discussed by the authors, may be greater awareness of parents for signs of precocious puberty and willingness to seek medical help for this condition. This may have been boosted by greater media attention to the issue. However, an increasing rate of idiopathic CPP also in boys, could represent a sign of increasing impact of environmental influences including effects of endocrine-disrupting chemicals.

New methodology

Detection of intra-abdominal testicles with 16β-[^{18}F]-fluoro-5α-dihydrotestosterone positron emission tomography/computed tomography in a pubertal boy

Glaudemans AW, de Vries EF, Luurtsema G, Cornelissen EA, Feitz WF, Farinha Antunes I, Slart RH, Bongaerts AH, Komhoff M
Department of Nuclear Medicine and Molecular Imaging, University of Groningen, University Medical Center Groningen, Groningen, The Netherlands
J Pediatr 2015;166:774.e1

Background: To localise impalpable undescended testicles can be a difficult quest. Unsuccessful efforts had earlier been made to detect gonadal tissue in a 16-year-old pubertal boy diagnosed with confirmed genetically Denys-Drash syndrome. He presented as a neonate with cryptorchidism, penoscrotal hypospadia, renal failure and proteinuria. At six years old he received a kidney transplant in the right iliac fossa. Progression to puberty, including a normal pubertal growth spurt and increasing levels of sex hormones, confirmed the presence of hormonally active gonads.
Methods: A novel imaging approach was used to detect the undescended testes. As androgen receptors are known to be expressed in testicles from pre puberty onward, the authors aimed to localise testicular tissue by positron emission tomography imaging with the androgen receptor tracer 16-beta-[^{18}F]-fluoro-5-alpha-dihydrotestosterone (^{18}F-FDHT).
Results: ^{18}F-FDHT-positron emission tomography/computed tomography revealed two testicles; one at the right side just below the transplanted kidney and the other at the left ventral side of the pelvic area. The ^{18}F-FDHT uptake in the testicles was low, probably due to competition with high levels of testosterone in serum.
Conclusions: This case-report shows that positron emission tomography could help to localise abdominal testes.

Undescended testes are sometimes difficult to localise despite intensive efforts by laparoscopy. Since such testes may show an increased risk of malignant transformation, it is important to find them for surgical removal or for control purposes if orchiectomy is not performed. In this case report the authors developed a novel imaging approach to find testes that were hormonally functional but impossible to localise anatomically. ^{18}F-FDHT-positron emission tomography/computed tomography was used to find the impalpable abdominal testes that the paediatricians knew must be present due to the boy's normal pubertal development. This method may be found useful in similar cases, but of course needs access to technical facilities with the ability to produce the molecular tracer used in the present study.

Food for thought

Sexual attractiveness in male rats is associated with greater concentration of major urinary proteins

Kumar V, Vasudevan A, Soh LJ, Le Min C, Vyas A, Zewail-Foote M, Guarraci FA
Department of Psychology, Southwestern University, Georgetown, TX, USA
guarracf@southwestern.edu
Biol Reprod 2014;91:150

Background: Female rats show a distinct attraction for males. This attraction remains consistent without the necessity for the physical presence of the male. However, the identity of the olfactory cues contributing to sexual attraction in rats remains unknown.
Methods: The authors tested the hypothesis that the high amounts of major urinary proteins (MUPs) present in rat urine may mediate sexual attractiveness in rats.

Results: The member of a male group that received greater copulatory opportunities in competitive mate choice tests was found to excrete higher amounts of MUPs. In addition, the amount of male MUPs positively correlated with both copulatory opportunities received and female exploration of the urine. Females given a two-choice olfactory attraction test, showed that urinary fractions containing MUPs were sufficient to induce attraction. In addition, male MUPs activated neurons in the posterodorsal medial amygdala in female rats.
Conclusions: These results indicate that olfactory signals associated with MUPs act as an attractant to female rats in estrus.

Many studies have been performed on the promiscuous male rats and their mating strategies. Less is known about female rats and their mate choice. Several recent articles have presented results demonstrating that the female rats exhibit definite and consistent mate choice (see references cited in the paper). Female rats show a consistent preference for a particular male in a dyad of male rats, rather than a random choice. The authors tested if it is the MUPs that give males this attribute of attractiveness. Indeed, they found that in males the amounts of MUPs correlated positively to copulatory opportunities and the female exploration of the urine. To what extent these results could be extrapolated to other species, and in particular to humans, remain uncertain. In this study the male MUPs activated neurons in the posterodorsal medial amygdala of female rats, an area known to be involved in pheromonal communication and sexual behaviour in rodents. Rats possess a vomeronasal organ (VNO), which is reactive to volatile pheromones signalling sexual attractiveness. It is up to the reader to imagine how these results might be exploited commercially if translation into humans is possible. Nevertheless, the following paper indicates that a VNO is present also in humans, and opens up the possibility of olfactory chemosensory signalling also in humans.

New hope (?)

Anatomical evidence for an endocrine activity of the vomeronasal organ in humans

Wessels Q, Hoogland PV, Vorster W
Lancaster Medical School, Faculty of Health and Medicine, Lancaster University, Lancaster, UK
Clin Anat 2014;27:856–860

Background: The vomeronasal organ (VNO) in mammals is a well-adjusted chemosensory structure facilitating social and reproductive behaviour. The existence, locality and function of a VNO in human adults remain controversial. Nowadays most authors agree that a neuroreceptive function of the adult human VNO can be excluded, since the absence of both neural receptive cells associated with the VNO in other mammals despite reports on the effects of pheromones on human behaviour.
Methods: Adult human Caucasian cadavers were studied. Parasagittal dissection of the heads allowed access to the nasal septa, which were grossly examined for VNO openings. Tissue samples were collected and processed for histology. Nissl staining was performed as well as immunohistochemical staining with an antibody against calcium-binding protein.
Results: The findings confirm the bilateral presence of the VNO in adult human cadavers and demonstrate morphological connections of VNO receptor cells with the underlying capillaries. In addition, possible endocrine activity associated with the epithelium of this chemosensory structure was demonstrated by the expression of calcium-binding protein in a part of these receptor cells.
Conclusions: The results point to the presence of an anatomically distinct VNO in humans. However, it remains to be shown whether this VNO is functional.

Discoveries in the area of macro-anatomy in higher species is rare these days. The authors describe an anatomical structure in humans that may serve as a homologue to the well-established VNO in rodents, a chemosensory organ important for reproductive behaviour. This subject is controversial and these observations need to be confirmed by independent investigators. Furthermore, the functionality of this human VNO candidate remains to be demonstrated. Nevertheless, taken together with the paper by Kumar et al. described above, the present findings indicate a potential to affect human sexual behaviour by means of nasally transmitted signals.

References

1. Greenhill C. Reproductive endocrinology: circadian clock involved in embryo implantation. Nat Rev Endocrinol [Comment] 2014;10(12):701.
2. Ramm SA. Sperm competition and the evolution of reproductive systems. Mol Hum Reprod 2014;20(12):1159–1160.
3. Schubert C. World of reproductive biology: methylation keeps it in the family. Biol Reprod 2014 July 16, 2014.
4. Sargent J. Reproductive endocrinology: you are what your grandmother ate: inherited effects of in utero undernourishment. Nat Rev Endocrinol 2014;10(9):509.
5. Diamond M, Sigmundson HK. Sex reassignment at birth. Long-term review and clinical implications. Arch Pediatr Adolesc Med 1997;151(3):298–304.
6. Schubert C. World of reproductive biology: messing with masculinisation. Biol Reprod 2014 June 11, 2014.

Adrenals

Erica L T van den Akker[a] and Evangelia Charmandari[b]

[a]Department of Pediatric Endocrinology, Erasmus Medical Center, 3015 GJ Rotterdam, The Netherlands

[b]Department of Endocrinology, Metabolism and Diabetes, University of Athens Medical School, 'Aghia Sophia' Children's Hospital; and Division of Endocrinology and Metabolism, Clinical Research Center, Biomedical Research Foundation of the Academy of Athens, Athens, 11527, Greece

For this year's chapter, we have searched PubMed for articles on 'adrenal' and 'steroidogenesis' published in English between June 1, 2014 and May 31, 2015. Our search yielded more than 5,500 citations. We have examined all citations individually and selected the following collection of basic research and clinical articles. Whenever possible, we have avoided topics that have been discussed in the Yearbook 2014, unless there was significant progress in the field. Emerging themes this year include: 1) the effect of chronic variable stress on haematopoietic stem cells; 2) the role of somatic mutations in *PRKACA* gene, encoding the catalytic subunit of protein kinase A, in cortisol-producing adrenal tumours; 3) the role of thioredoxin reductase 2 (TXNRD2) in familial glucocorticoid deficiency; 4) insights in the management of patients with congenital adrenal hyperplasia and primary aldosteronism; and 5) new therapeutic modalities for the management of patients with classic congenital adrenal hyperplasia.

Mechanism of the year

Chronic variable stress activates hematopoietic stem cells

Heidt T, Sager HB, Courties G, Dutta P, Iwamoto Y, Zaltsman A, von Zur Muhlen C, Bode C, Fricchione GL, Denninger J, Lin CP, Vinegoni C, Libby P, Swirski FK, Weissleder R, Nahrendorf M

Center for Systems Biology, Massachusetts General Hospital and Harvard Medical School, Boston, MA, USA

Nat Med 2014;20(7):754–758

Background: Psychosocial stress represents a risk factor for many diseases, including atherosclerosis. Cross-talk between the brain and immune system includes the hypothalamic-pituitary-adrenal axis and the sympathetic-adrenal-medullary axis. The aim of the present study was to investigate whether chronic stress alters haematopoietic stem cell activity.
Methods and Results: Chronic stress induced monocytosis and neutrophilia in humans, and activated upstream haematopoietic stem cells. Under conditions of chronic variable stress in mice, sympathetic nerve fibres released surplus noradrenaline, which signalled bone marrow niche cells to decrease CXCL12 levels through the beta-3-adrenergic receptor. Consequently, haematopoietic stem cell proliferation was elevated, leading to an increased output of neutrophils and inflammatory monocytes. When atherosclerosis-prone Apoe(-/-) mice were subjected to chronic stress, accelerated haematopoiesis promoted plaque features associated with vulnerable lesions that cause myocardial infarction and stroke in humans.
Conclusions: Stress increases proliferation of the most primitive haematopoietic progenitors, resulting in higher levels of disease-promoting inflammatory leukocytes. The interaction between the psyche and the immune system provides one potential mechanism linking stress and disease inception and progression.

Psychosocial stress is a risk factor for many diseases, including atherosclerosis. These authors report how chronic stress interferes with haematopoiesis, and describe the interactions between the central nervous system, immunity and atherosclerosis. To explore the impact of stress on the human immune system, they analysed blood samples from 29 medical residents working on a tertiary hospital intensive care unit (ICU), a challenging, fast-paced work environment. Compared with when off duty, residents working on the ICU had increased stress perception, and higher stress intensity and frequency. When comparing samples taken during work to samples taken off duty, they observed an increase in blood leukocytes, with higher numbers of neutrophils, monocytes and lymphocytes, after one week of intensive care rotation. To test the hypothesis that stress-induced leukocytosis results from increased leukocyte production, they exposed wild-type mice to chronic variable stressors. In mice exposed to stress, increased sympathetic nervous system activity decreased the expression of chemokine (C-X-C motif) ligand 12 (CXCL12) in the haematopoietic stem cell (HSC) niche, accelerated HSC proliferation and enhanced neutrophil and monocyte production. These events caused extensive release of inflammatory leukocytes into the circulation and promoted plaque inflammation and atherosclerosis. On the other hand, administration of a beta-3-adrenergic receptor blocker limited the progression of atherosclerosis, indicating that sympathetic nervous system targeting the interaction between CXCL12 and its receptor (CXCR4) in the bone marrow should be explored as potential therapeutic avenues. These data provide further evidence of the haematopoietic system's role in cardiovascular disease [1,2] and elucidate a direct biological link between chronic variable stress and chronic inflammation.

New mechanisms

An epithelial circadian clock controls pulmonary inflammation and glucocorticoid action

Gibbs J, Ince L, Matthews L, Mei J, Bell T, Yang N, Saer B, Begley N, Poolman T, Pariollaud M, Farrow S, DeMayo F, Hussell T, Worthen GS, Ray D, Loudon A
Faculty of Medical and Human Sciences, University of Manchester, Manchester Academic Health Sciences Centre, Manchester, UK
Nat Med 2014;20(8):919–926

Background: The circadian system is an important regulator of immune function. In humans, inflammatory lung diseases frequently show time-of-day variation in symptom severity and lung function, however, the underlying mechanisms remain unclear.
Methods and Results: Pulmonary antibacterial responses are modulated by a circadian clock within epithelial club (Clara) cells, which drive circadian neutrophil recruitment to the lung via the chemokine CXCL5. Genetic ablation of the clock gene Bmal1 in bronchiolar cells disrupts rhythmic Cxcl5 expression and results in exaggerated inflammatory responses to lipopolysaccharide and an impaired host response to *Streptococcus pneumoniae* infection. Furthermore, adrenalectomy blocks rhythmic inflammatory responses and the circadian regulation of CXCL5. Glucocorticoid receptor occupancy at the Cxcl5 locus shows circadian oscillations, however, this is disrupted in mice with bronchiole-specific ablation of Bmal1, leading to enhanced CXCL5 expression despite normal corticosteroid secretion. The therapeutic effects of the synthetic glucocorticoid dexamethasone depend on intact clock function in the airway.
Conclusions: This study defines a regulatory mechanism that links the circadian clock and glucocorticoid hormones to control both time-of-day variation and the magnitude of pulmonary inflammation and responses to bacterial infection.

Inflammatory lung diseases, including chronic obstructive pulmonary disease (COPD) and asthma, are responsible for 25% of premature deaths. These conditions frequently show time-of-day variation in symptom severity and lung function, however, the underlying mechanisms have not been elucidated. The recruitment of immune cells to tissues is under circadian control and several immune cells, including macrophages and mast cells, exhibit robust oscillations of circadian clock genes and proinflammatory cytokines. Furthermore, the magnitude of response to pathogenic bacterial challenge varies with time of day. The immune response to bacterial infection is partly mediated by neutrophil recruitment to the affected site, which can also cause tissue damage and must therefore be tightly regulated. The inflammatory responses are inhibited by glucocorticoids, which exert their actions through their ubiquitously expressed receptor, the glucocorticoid receptor (GR). Secretion of glucocorticoids is clock controlled and acts as a potent circadian-entrained stimulus in many peripheral tissues. In addition, the function of the GR is determined by physical interactions with clock component proteins [3,4].

These authors identify resonance between an oscillating circadian systemic glucocorticoid signal and locally operating circadian control of GR function to confer clock control of pulmonary innate immunity. They describe a mechanism that associates the circadian clockwork within pulmonary epithelial cells to the action of glucocorticoids in the control of the chemokine CXCL5, which drives circadian inflammatory responses within the lung. The bronchiolar club cells (nonciliated epithelial cells found mainly in bronchioles as well as basal cells found in large airways), acting through a single neutrophil chemokine, represent the final effector pathway and the efficacy of glucocorticoid treatment depends on intact clock function in the airway. Therefore, conditions characterised by persisting pulmonary neutrophilic inflammation, which are resistant to glucocorticoid therapy, may share a common underlying mechanism of clock disruption, either *de novo* or in response to particular inflammatory signals.

Thioredoxin reductase 2 (TXNRD2) mutations associated with familial glucocorticoid deficiency (FGD)

Prasad R, Chan LF, Hughes CR, Kaski JP, Kowalcyk JC, Savage MO, Peters CJ, Nathwani N, Clark AJL, Storr HL, Metherell LA
Centre for Endocrinology, Queen Mary University of London, William Harvey Research Institute, Barts and the London School of Medicine and Dentistry, London, UK
J Clin Endocrinol Metab 2014;99(8): E1556–E1563

Background: Familial glucocorticoid deficiency (FGD) is characterised by ACTH resistance owing to disruption of ACTH signalling. Recent reports of FGD cases caused by mutations in the mitochondrial antioxidant, nicotinamide nucleotide transhydrogenase, have highlighted the importance of redox regulation in steroidogenesis. The authors hypothesised that other components of mitochondrial antioxidant systems would be good candidates in the aetiology of FGD.
Methods: Seven individuals from a consanguineous Kashmiri kindred, six of whom presented with FGD between 0.1 and 10.8 years, were studied. Whole-exome sequencing was performed in three related patients with FGD, and segregation of putative causal variants was confirmed by Sanger sequencing of all family members. In addition, a TXNRD2-knockdown H295R cell line was created to investigate redox homeostasis.
Results: A stop gain mutation (p.Y447X) in *TXNRD2*, encoding the mitochondrial selenoprotein thioredoxin reductase 2 (TXNRD2) was identified and segregated with disease in this extended kindred. In patients homozygous for the mutation, the complete absence of *TXNRD2* was confirmed by RT-PCR and Western blotting. In human adrenocortical cells, *TXNRD2* deficiency led to impaired redox homeostasis.
Conclusions: *TXNRD2* deficiency in humans leads to glucocorticoid deficiency. This is the first report of a homozygous mutation in a component of the thioredoxin antioxidant system leading to inherited disease in humans.

TXNRD2 is one of 25 human selenoproteins, which require insertion of a highly reactive selenocysteine residue for enzymatic activity. Several selenoproteins, including the thioredoxin reductases and glutathione peroxidases, contribute to redox regulation. TXNRD2, one of three thioredoxin reductases, is mitochondria specific. The N- and C-terminal redox active centres of the two subunits functionally interact and transfer electrons from NADPH/H to thioredoxin 2 (TXN2). Within the mitochondria, the thioredoxin and glutathione systems contribute to the maintenance of redox homeostasis. Individuals with TXNRD2 and NNT mutations primarily develop glucocorticoid deficiency. Oxidative stress impedes steroidogenesis, and steroidogenesis itself induces oxidative stress as a result of electron leak throughout the steroidogenic pathway. This may explain the particular susceptibility of the zona fasciculata to oxidative stress, and hence, why individuals with *TXNRD2* and *NNT* mutations primarily develop glucocorticoid deficiency. The wide variability in age at diagnosis (0.1–10.8years) in the family studied here suggests other disease modifiers, such as genetic or environmental factors that could influence the development of the disease. As *TXNRD2* is widely expressed in humans, individuals with this genetic defect are potentially at risk of extra-adrenal (such as cardiac and haematopoietic) manifestations. In mice, *Txnrd2* deletion is embryonically lethal as a consequence of cardiac (dilated cardiomyopathy) and haematopoietic defects. In humans, dilated cardiomyopathy was diagnosed in three of 227 patients. In addition, one affected family member presented with truncus arteriosus. This study reports the first mutation in *TXNRD2* associated with adrenal insufficiency in humans, which signifies the importance of the thioredoxin system in maintaining redox homeostasis in the adrenocortical environment. Other components of this complex network of mitochondrial antioxidants make good candidates for undiagnosed causes of adrenal insufficiency.

Important for clinical practice – a need for better management of patients with congenital adrenal hyperplasia and primary aldosteronism

Increased mortality in patients with congenital adrenal hyperplasia due to 21-hydroxylase deficiency

Falhammar H, Frisén L, Norrby C, Hirschberg AL, Almqvist C, Nordenskjöld A, Nordenström A
Department of Endocrinology, Metabolism and Diabetes, Karolinska University Hospital, Stockholm, Sweden
J Clin Endocrinol Metab 2014;99(12):E2715–E2721

Background: The prevalence of mortality in patients with Congenital Adrenal Hyperplasia (CAH) is unknown. The authors aimed to describe mortality rates and causes of death in patients with CAH.
Patients and Methods: Information on mortality and causes of death was obtained from patients with CAH (n=588) and normal controls (n=58,800) from a Swedish national population-based register.
Results: In patients with CAH, the mean age of death (41.2 ± 26.9 years) was lower than in control subjects (47.7 ± 27.7 years, $P<0.001$). In males with CAH, the hazard ratio of death was 2.3 (95% CI 1.2–4.3) and in females 3.5 (95% CI 2.0–6.0). The causes of death in patients with CAH included adrenal crisis (42%), cardiovascular disease (32%), cancer (16%) and suicide (10%).
Conclusions: CAH is a potentially lethal condition and is associated with increased mortality due to adrenal crises.

Prior to availability of replacement therapy with glucocorticoids and mineralocorticoids, patients with classic congenital adrenal hyperplasia (CAH) could not survive due to adrenal crises. Now, when CAH is treatable, survival has been presumed to be normal. However, fatal adrenal crises still occur. The introduction of neonatal screening for CAH gave hope that mortality in CAH would be decreased by avoiding fatal adrenal crises in undiagnosed boys with classic CAH. Only one previous study has reported on mortality rates in young patients with the various forms of CAH. Increased mortality was noted at one to four years of age in girls from the Indian subcontinent [5].

Here, the authors raise awareness about the long-term risks and mortality rates in patients with CAH. They found an increased mortality with 6.5 years earlier mean age of death in patients with CAH compared with matched controls. The increased mortality was due to adrenal crises and was noted not only during the first year of life but also during childhood and adulthood. These findings indicate that despite the recent advances in diagnosis and treatment, CAH is still a potentially lethal condition. However, the mean age of death seemed to increase during the decades, from 21 years during the 1980s to 57 years in 2010. Therefore, further improvements are necessary both in the management of CAH and in the education of patients.

Clinical outcome, hormonal status, gonadotrope axis and testicular function in 219 adult men born with classic 21-hydroxylase deficiency. A French national survey

Bouvattier C, Esterle L, Renoult-Pierre P, Brac de la Perrière A, Illouz F, Kerlan V, Pascal-Vigneron V Drui D, Christin-Maitre S, Galland F, Brue T, Reznik Y, Schillo F, Pinsard D, Piguel X, Chabrier G, Decoudier B, Emy P, Tauveron I, Raffin-Sanson M-L, Bertherat J, Kuhn J-M, Caron P, Cartigny M, Chabre O, Dewailly D, Morel Y, Touraine P, Tardy-Guidollet V, Young J
University Paris-Sud, Assistance Publique Hôpitaux de Paris, Paris, France
J Clin Endocrinol Metab 2015;100(6):2303–2313

Background: The health outcome of congenital adrenal hyperplasia (CAH) due to 21-hydroxylase deficiency has been widely studied in children and women but less so in men. The aim of this study was to assess the clinical outcome in adult men with CAH, with particular emphasis on the gonadotrope axis, testicular function and fertility.
Patients and Methods: In a retrospective observational study, data from 219 men with CAH (age: 18–70 years; 73.6% salt wasters, 26.4% simple virilisers) were obtained from French metropolitan teaching hospitals. Testicular sonography was performed in 164 men and sperm analysis was performed in 71 men.

Results: The mean final height of men with CAH was 7.8cm shorter than the reference population. Obesity was more common but mean blood pressure was lower than in the reference population. None of the patients was diabetic. ACTH and renin levels were markedly elevated. Serum progesterone, 17-hydroxyprogesterone (17-OHP) and androstenedione concentrations were elevated in most cases. Hormonal profiling variously showed a normal gonadotropic-testicular axis, gonadotropin deficiency or primary testicular insufficiency. Testicular sonography revealed testicular adrenal rest tumours (TARTs) in 34% of patients. Serum inhibin B concentrations were lower and FSH concentrations were higher in patients with TARTs. Severe oligospermia or azoospermia was found in 42% of patients and was more prevalent in men with TART (70%) than in men with normal testes (3.6%; P<0.0001). Among men living with female partners, TARTs were more prevalent in those who had not fathered children.
Conclusions: Adult men with CAH treated in French specialised centres frequently have impaired exocrine testicular function, however, its reproductive implications are often overlooked.

Given the more obvious impact of classic CAH on female sexual development, the literature on classic CAH mainly concerns children and female patients, while data on adult outcomes of male patients are scarce. Here, the authors describe the anthropometric parameters, treatment and hormonal control in 219 well-phenotyped adult men with classic CAH, who were followed-up in endocrinology departments of French teaching hospitals. Particular emphasis was given to the gonadotropic axis, testicular function and fertility. This is the largest observational study of testicular function and fertility in adult men with CAH published to date. As in other European countries, only a minority of these patients are managed in specialised tertiary care centres. The average final height (± SD) was 167.8 ± 8.36cm, which was 7.8cm less than the average height of healthy French men (175.6cm) aged from 18 to 70 years. This indicates that treatment in childhood and adolescence is still not optimal. In addition, patients had frequent alterations of the gonadotropic-testicular axis, while TARTs were detected in approximately 50% of patients who underwent testicular ultrasonography. These findings raise concerns regarding the fertility of men with CAH, given that more than 40% of patients had extreme oligospermia or azoospermia, and that the presence of TARTs was a major risk factor indicating severe impairement of spermatogenesis. Therefore, a sperm count is recommended in adolescence, especially in postpubertal males with TARTs. As has been advocated by other groups [6], sperm cryopreservation should be considered in men with classic CAH, particularly those with TARTs.

Cortical bone mineral density in patients with congenital adrenal hyperplasia due to 21-hydroxylase deficiency

El-Maouche D, Collier S, Prasad M, Reynolds JC, Merke DP
National Institute of Dental and Craniofacial Research, National Institutes of Health (NIH), Bethesda, MD, USA
Clin Endocrinol (Oxf) 2015;82(3):330-337

Background: Patients with congenital adrenal hyperplasia (CAH) on glucocorticoid replacement therapy have bone mineral density (BMD) mostly in the osteopenic range. The aim of this study was to determine the BMD in patients with CAH at various sites, including the forearm.
Patients and Methods: 80 adult patients with CAH (47 classic, 33 nonclassic) participated in the study. BMD was measured using dual-energy-X-ray absorptiometry and was correlated with clinical and biochemical data.
Results: Reduced BMD (T-score<-1) was present in 52% of patients at hip, spine or forearm. Osteopenia was more common in classic compared with the nonclassic form of the disease (P<0.005), with the greatest difference observed in the forearm (P=0.01). Compared with the nonclassic form, patients with classic CAH had higher 17-hydroxyprogesterone (17-OHP) (P=0.005), lower dehydroepiandrosterone sulphate (DHEAS) (P=0.0002) and higher non-traumatic fracture rate (P=0.0005). DHEAS showed a positive association with BMD at the spine, radius and whole body in a multivariate analysis after adjusting for age, gender, height standard deviation, phenotype and cumulative glucocorticoid exposure.
Conclusions: Adult patients with classic CAH have lower BMD than patients with the nonclassic form of the disease, with the most affected area being the forearm. Low DHEAS may be associated with weak cortical bone independent of glucocorticoid exposure.

Classic CAH requires lifelong glucocorticoid replacement therapy. Patients with nonclassic CAH may need glucocorticoid treatment, however, often for a limited period of time. One of the side effects of glucocorticoid overtreatment is decreased BMD. Various studies on BMD in patients with CAH show conflicting results, with some reporting decreased BMD in 45–60% of patients [7,8] and others normal BMD. Excess glucocorticoid exposure has been associated with lower BMD in CAH patients [9].

Here, the authors report that BMD is lower in patients with classic CAH compared with patients with nonclassic CAH, with the greatest difference residing at the forearm. This is the first study to evaluate forearm BMD in CAH, which in turn reflects cortical bone. DHEAS was the only independent predictor of BMD at the forearm, whole body and AP spine. Future studies should include measurement of BMD at the forearm, with the aim to understand the underlying aetiology of cortical bone differences in CAH subgroups. Furthermore, other factors that may be affecting BMD in patients with CAH should be taken into consideration, including gonadal function, hyperandrogenism or chronic use of long-acting glucocorticoids.

Measurement of peripheral plasma 18-oxocortisol can discriminate unilateral adenoma from bilateral diseases in patients with primary aldosteronism

Satoh F, Morimoto R, Ono Y, Iwakura Y, Omata K, Kudo M, Takase K, Seiji K, Sasamoto H, Honma S, Okuyama M, Yamashita K, Gomez-Sanchez CE, Rainey WE, Arai Y, Sasano H, Nakamura Y, Ito S

Division of Nephrology, Endocrinology and Vascular Medicine, Department of Medicine, Tohoku University Hospital, Sendai, Japan

Hypertension 2015;65(5):1096–1102

Background: Adrenal venous sampling (AVS) is currently the only reliable method to distinguish unilateral from bilateral diseases in primary aldosteronism. The aim of this study was to determine whether peripheral plasma concentrations of 18-oxocortisol (18oxoF) and 18-hydroxycortisol could help differentiate between aldosteronoma and bilateral hyperaldosteronism.
Patients and Methods: 234 patients with primary aldosteronism [aldosteronoma (n=113) and bilateral hyperaldosteronism (n=121)], all of whom underwent computed tomography and adrenal venous sampling, were studied. 18oxoF and 18-hydroxycortisol were measured using liquid chromatography tandem mass spectrometry.
Results: Receiver operating characteristic analysis of 18oxoF discrimination of adenoma from hyperplasia demonstrated sensitivity/specificity of 0.83/0.99 at a cut-off value of 4.7ng/dL, compared with that based on 18-hydroxycortisol (sensitivity/specificity: 0.62/0.96). 18oxoF concentrations above 6.1ng/dL or of aldosterone >32.7ng/dL were found in 84% of patients with aldosteronoma but in no patient with bilateral hyperaldosteronism. Furthermore, 18oxoF concentrations below 1.2ng/dL, the lowest in aldosteronoma, were found in 43% of patients with bilateral hyperaldosteronism. Eight of the 27 with CT-undetectable micro aldosteronomas had CT-detectable contralateral adrenal nodules, the highest values of 18oxoF and aldosterone were 4.8 and 24.5ng/dL, respectively, both below their cut-off levels indicated above.
Conclusions: Peripheral plasma 18oxoF concentrations may be helpful to differentiate aldosteronomas from bilateral hyperaldosteronism, as well as to avoid unnecessary surgery for nonfunctioning adrenocortical nodules concurrent with hyperplasia or microadenoma.

Primary aldosteronism (PA) is the most frequent cause of secondary hypertension, albeit rare in childhood. PA should be detected and treated as early as possible to prevent cardiovascular and cerebrovascular complications, as well as chronic kidney disease. Adrenal venous sampling (AVS) is the only reliable method to differentiate between surgically curable unilateral aldosterone-producing adenoma (APA) and bilateral hyperaldosteronism (BHA); however, it is invasive, time-consuming, labour-intensive and expensive. A much simpler, non-invasive and less expensive diagnostic method is needed. 18-hydroxycortisol (18OHF) and 18-oxocortisol (18oxoF), which have structural characteristics of both aldosterone and cortisol in their chemical structures, are both synthesised from 11-deoxycortisol as substrate by aldosterone synthase (CYP11B2), although 18OHF can also be produced by 11-beta-hydroxylase (CYP11B1). Their production is known to be highly elevated in glucocorticoid-remediable aldosteronism. Furthermore, production of 18OHF and 18oxoF is elevated in patients with PA, especially in APA.

Here, the authors used liquid chromatography tandem mass spectrometry (LC-MS/MS) to quantify the plasma concentrations of 18oxoF and 18OHF in 261 patients with PA, who were subsequently classified based on the results of AVS into 113 patients with APA, 121 patients with BHA and 27 patients with micro-APA. They found that 18oxoF was a more reliable diagnostic parameter to differentiate between APA and BHA than 18OHF. This is the first study to demonstrate that the peripheral blood concentrations of 18oxoF measured by LC-MS/MS can differentiate between APA and BHA with a reasonable precision. These results indicate that measurement of 18oxoF in peripheral blood by LC-MS/MS should enable us to improve the clinical algorithm for PA, potentially omitting unnecessary AVS.

Clinical trials – New treatments

A phase 2 study of Chronocort, a modified-release formulation of hydrocortisone, in the treatment of adults with classic congenital adrenal hyperplasia

Mallappa A, Sinaii N, Kumar P, Whitaker MJ, Daley LA, Digweed D, Eckland DJ, Van Ryzin C, Nieman LK, Arlt W, Ross RJ, Merke DP
National Institutes of Health Clinical Center, Bethesda, MD, USA
J Clin Endocrinol Metab 2015;100(3):1137–1145

Background: Conventional glucocorticoid replacement therapy fails to mimic the physiological cortisol secretion in patients with congenital adrenal hyperplasia (CAH). The aim of this study was to characterise the pharmacokinetic profile of Chronocort, a modified-release hydrocortisone formulation, in adults with CAH.
Patients and Methods: 16 adult patients with classic CAH participated in an open-label, nonrandomised, Phase 2 study. 24-hour blood sampling was performed on conventional glucocorticoid therapy and following six months of Chronocort. Chronocort was initiated at 10mg (0700h) and 20mg (2300h), and subsequent dose titration was performed based on androstenedione and 17-hydroxyprogresterone (17-OHP) concentrations and clinical parameters.
Results: In patients with CAH, Chronocort cortisol profiles were similar to physiologic cortisol secretion. Compared with conventional therapy, six months of Chronocort resulted in a decrease in hydrocortisone dose equivalent (28 ± 11.8 versus 25.9 ± 7.1mg/d), with lower 24-hour morning and afternoon androstenedione area under the curve (AUC) and lower 24-hour and morning 17-OHP AUC.
Conclusions: Twice-daily Chronocort mimics physiologic cortisol secretion closely, and may therefore represent a new treatment approach for patients with CAH.

Current treatment of classic CAH aims to provide adequate glucocorticoid and, when necessary, mineralocorticoid replacement to prevent adrenal crises, and to suppress the excess secretion of adrenal androgens and steroid precursors. However, the currently available formulations of hydrocortisone do not simulate the normal cortisol circadian rhythm and patients may develop in tandem iatrogenic Cushing's syndrome and hyperandrogenism. The use of a delayed- and extended-release formulation of hydrocortisone represents a new treatment approach to CAH that offers the prospect of a more physiologic cortisol replacement, with increased cortisol concentrations very early in the morning.

Here, the authors show that it is possible to safely replace cortisol in a near-physiologic manner using Chronocort, an oral, modified-release hydrocortisone formulation in patients with CAH. This novel hydrocortisone formulation was well tolerated and effective in controlling androgen excess in adults with CAH when administered twice daily. At baseline, while receiving conventional glucocorticoid therapy, 24-hour sampling revealed inadequate androgen control throughout the day in most of the patients, despite receiving long-acting glucocorticoids. Chronocort provided a stable peak-to-trough ratio of plasma cortisol concentrations that more closely mimics the normal circadian rhythm compared with conventional glucocorticoid replacement therapy. However, even with the twice-daily regimen of Chronocort, cortisol concentrations were low in the evening but the ACTH and androgen concentrations remained in an acceptable range. Compared with conventional therapy at baseline, Chronocort at six months showed improved serial androstenedione and 17-OHP concentrations. This newly developed modified-release oral hydrocortisone formulation regimen given as a twice-daily dosing represents a new treatment approach for patients with CAH. Further studies are necessary to determine the long-term outcomes of Chronocort therapy.

A population-based, multifaceted strategy to implement antenatal corticosteroid treatment versus standard care for the reduction of neonatal mortality due to preterm birth in low-income and middle-income countries: the ACT cluster-randomised trial

Althabe F, Belizán JM, McClure EM, Hemingway-Foday J, Berrueta M, Mazzoni A, Ciganda A, Goudar SS, Kodkany BS, Mahantshetti NS, Dhaded SM, Katageri GM, Metgud MC, Joshi AM, Bellad MB, Honnungar NV, Derman RJ, Saleem S, Pasha O, Ali S, Hasnain F, Goldenberg RL, Esamai F, Nyongesa P, Ayunga S, Liechty EA, Garces AL, Figueroa L, Hambidge KM, Krebs NF, Patel A, Bhandarkar A, Waikar M, Hibberd PL, Chomba E, Carlo WA, Mwiche A, Chiwila M, Manasyan A, Pineda S, Meleth S, Thorsten V, Stolka K, Wallace DD, Koso-Thomas M, Jobe AH, Buekens PM

Institute for Clinical Effectiveness and Health Policy, Buenos Aires, Argentina

Lancet 2015;385(9968):629-639

Background: Administration of antenatal corticosteroids to pregnant women, who are at risk of preterm birth, is one of the most effective hospital-based interventions to reduce neonatal mortality. This study evaluated the effectiveness, feasibility and safety of implementing antenatal corticosteroid treatment in low and middle-income countries.

Patients and Methods: In this cluster-randomised prospective trial, rural and semi-urban clusters from six countries were randomly assigned to standard care or multi-faceted intervention. The intervention included components to improve identification of women at risk of preterm delivery and facilitated appropriate use of antenatal corticosteroids. The primary outcome measure was neonatal mortality on day 28. A birthweight below the fifth percentile was used as proxy for preterm birth. A secondary outcome measure was suspected maternal infection. 18-months follow up was completed in 51 intervention clusters and 50 control clusters.

Results: In the intervention clusters, 5% (n=2,520/47,394) of live births had birthweight below the fifth percentile, and in control clusters 4% (n=2,258/50,743). In the intervention clusters, antenatal corticosteroids had been administered in 45% of women who delivered a baby below the fifth percentile, compared with 10% in control clusters (P<0.0001). Among low birthweight infants, 28-day neonatal mortality was similar in the intervention group 225 per 1,000 live births and control group 232 per 1,000 live births (relative risk [RR] 0.96, 95% CI 0.87–1.06, P=0.65). However, among the whole population, newborn 28-day mortality and suspected maternal infection were higher in the intervention group compared with the control group (RR 1.12, 1.02–1.22, P=0.0127 and OR 1.44, 1.33–1.58, P<0.0001, respectively).

Conclusions: Although this intervention led to an increase in antenatal corticosteroid use, it had no effect on 28-day mortality rate in low birthweight babies. Overall mortality and suspected maternal infection seemed to increase.

Antenatal corticosteroids reduce neonatal mortality and morbidity substantially in both high-income and middle-income countries [10]. Based on this strong evidence, the UN included antenatal corticosteroids on the list of life-saving commodities for women and children (www. everywomaneverychild.org/images/UN_Commission_Report_September_2012_Final.pdf). Currently, ~80% of women at high risk of preterm birth receive antenatal corticosteroids in high-income countries compared with 10% in low-income countries [11]. Therefore, these authors aimed to identify women at high risk of preterm birth and administer antenatal corticosteroids in low-resource settings. However, the previously reported benefits of antenatal corticosteroids in preterm neonates were not confirmed here. Several determinants could play a role. In low-income countries, usually, neonatal intensive care is not available and many late preterm babies were included for whom no effect of antenatal corticosteroids is expected. Unfortunately, data on gestational age were not reliable in this study, and therefore birthweight was used as proxy. Another complicating factor was that antenatal corticosteroids were given to many women identified as at risk, although only 16% of these delivered a baby with birthweight below the fifth percentile. Furthermore, this intervention strategy increased mortality in the population overall. For every 1,000 women exposed to the multifaceted strategy, an excess of five perinatal deaths occurred compared with standard care. In addition, the strategy seemed to increase the risk of maternal infectious morbidity. These findings do not support the scale-up of this population-based multifaceted strategy to identify women at high risk of preterm birth at all levels of care and administer antenatal corticosteroids in low-resource settings.

New genes

Novel somatic mutations in the catalytic subunit of the protein kinase A as a cause of adrenal Cushing's syndrome: a European multicentric study

Di Dalmazi G, Kisker C, Calebiro D, Mannelli M, Canu L, Arnaldi G, Quinkler M, Rayes N, Tabarin A, Laure Jullié M, Mantero F, Rubin B, Waldmann J, Bartsch DK, Pasquali R, Lohse M, Allolio B, Fassnacht M, Beuschlein F, Reincke M
Medizinische Klinik und Poliklinik IV, Klinikum der Universität München, München, Germany
J Clin Endocrinol Metab 2014;99(10):E2093–2100

Background: Somatic mutations in the *PRKACA* gene, encoding the catalytic subunit of protein kinase A (PKA), have been recently found in a high proportion of sporadic adenomas associated with Cushing's syndrome. The aim of this study was to search for *PRKACA* mutations in a large cohort of patients with adrenocortical masses.
Methods and Results: This multicentre study included nine European centres. Samples were collected from 149 patients with nonsecreting adenomas, subclinical hypercortisolism, Cushing's syndrome, androgen-producing tumours, adrenocortical carcinomas and primary bilateral macronodular adrenal hyperplasias. DNA amplification by PCR of exons 6 and 7 of the *PRKACA* gene and direct sequencing were performed. *PRKACA* heterozygous mutations were found in 34% of patients with Cushing's syndrome. Two novel mutations were identified:c.600_601insGTG/p.Cys200_Gly201insVal in three patients and c.639C>G+c.638_640insATTATCCTGAGG/p.Ser213Arg+p.Leu212_ Lys214insIle-Ile-Leu-Arg in one. All the mutations involved a region implicated in the interaction between PKA regulatory and catalytic subunits. Patients with somatic mutations in the *PRKACA* gene showed higher concentrations of cortisol following dexamethasone suppression test and a smaller adenoma size compared with the subjects in whom no mutations were identified.
Conclusions: These data confirm and extend previous observations that somatic mutations in the *PRKACA* gene are specific for adrenocortical adenomas causing Cushing's syndrome.

Hypercortisolism due to a unilateral adrenocortical mass is the most common cause of ACTH-independent Cushing's syndrome and accounts for almost 30% of cases with overt Cushing's syndrome. In the last few years, the molecular basis of ACTH-independent Cushing's syndrome has been elucidated in sporadic adrenocortical tumours. Somatic mutations of the *PDE8B* gene and *PRKAR1A* gene have been detected in patients with cortisol-producing adenomas. Activating GNAS mutations have also been lately reported in patients with adrenocortical adenomas associated with Cushing's syndrome. However, these mutations explain only a small number of cases of adrenal hypercortisolism. Recently, somatic mutations of the *PRKACA* gene, encoding the catalytic subunit α (Cα) of the PKA, have been identified in more than one-third of patients with Cushing's syndrome due to sporadic adrenocortical adenomas [12].

Here, the authors analysed somatic mutations of the *PRKACA* gene in a large cohort of patients with sporadic adrenocortical tumours associated with Cushing's syndrome, and investigated the genotype-phenotype correlation in these cases. They show that somatic mutations of the *PRKACA* gene, resulting in a constitutive activation of the C-alpha subunit of the PKA, occurred in more than one-third of patients with adrenocortical adenomas associated with Cushing's syndrome. All these mutations were somatic and specific of patients with ACTH-independent Cushing's syndrome. Of note, the sequencing analysis revealed two novel mutations in exon 7 of the *PRKACA* gene never described before. This study strongly reinforces the hypothesis that an aberrant cAMP pathway could indeed lead to tumoural mass formation and increase steroid production. Although these mutations are associated with increased hormonal activity and smaller size of the adrenal mass, the clinical correlates are yet to be fully clarified. Additional studies are also needed to complete the molecular landscape of unilateral adrenocortical adenomas associated with ACTH-independent Cushing's syndrome.

New hope

Next-generation sequencing of adrenocortical carcinoma reveals new routes to targeted therapies

Ross JS, Wang K, Rand JV, Gay L, Presta MJ, Sheehan CE, Ali SM, Elvin JA, Labrecque E, Hiemstra C, Buell J, Otto GA, Yelensky R, Lipson D, Morosini D, Chmielecki J, Miller VA, Stephens PJ
Department of Pathology and Laboratory Medicine, Albany Medical College, Albany, NY, USA; Foundation Medicine, Inc., Cambridge, MA, USA
J Clin Pathol 2014;67(11):968–973

Background: Adrenocortical carcinoma (ACC) carries a poor prognosis and current systemic cytotoxic therapies result in only modest improvement in overall survival. The aim of this study was to perform a comprehensive genomic profiling of ACC samples to identify potential targets of therapy.
Patients and Methods: DNA from 29 ACC was sequenced to high, uniform coverage and analysed for genomic alterations (GAs).
Results: At least one GA was detected in 22 (76%) ACC. The most frequent GAs were in TP53 (34%), NF1 (14%), CDKN2A (14%), MEN1 (14%), CTNNB1 (10%) and ATM (10%). APC, CCND2, CDK4, DAXX, DNMT3A, KDM5C, LRP1B, MSH2 and RB1 were each altered in two cases (7%) and EGFR, ERBB4, KRAS, MDM2, NRAS, PDGFRB, PIK3CA, PTEN and PTCH1 were each altered in a single case (3%).
Conclusions: Next-generation sequencing can discover targets of therapy for relapsed and metastatic ACC and may improve the outcomes in patients with this aggressive form of cancer.

Adrenocortical carcinoma (ACC) is a malignant neoplasm of the adrenal cortex with an annual incidence of 0.7–2.0 cases per million people and a peak incidence between ages 40–50 years. ACC may occur as inherited or sporadic forms. The most common inherited predisposition is associated with the Li-Fraumeni Syndrome (LFS) and germline *TP53* mutations. In children, *TP53* germline mutations are present in 50–80% of ACC cases. Medical treatment of ACC has been based on non-randomised trials or retrospective analyses. However, the prognosis of patients with recurrent or metastatic ACC treated by chemotherapy remains poor. Here, the authors performed comprehensive DNA sequencing of ACC tumours using next-generation sequencing (NGS)-based genomic profiling in order to determine genomic alterations (GAs) that could be used to guide targeted therapies for patients with the disease. They screened 29 ACC samples. A total of 76 alterations were identified in 43 genes, with 22 cases (76%) harbouring at least one alteration. These findings indicate that NGS might be a promising tool to discover novel targets of therapy for the management of patients with ACC.

Transplantation of bovine adrenocortical cells encapsulated in alginate

Balyura M, Gelfgat E, Ehrhart-Bornstein M, Ludwig B, Gendler Z, Barkai U, Zimerman B, Rotem A, Block NL, Schally AV, Bornstein SR
University Hospital Carl Gustav Carus, Department of Medicine III, Technische Universität Dresden, Dresden, Germany
Proc Natl Acad Sci U S A 2015;112(8):2527–2532

Background: Current treatment of adrenal insufficiency is with life-long glucocorticoid replacement therapy. However, treatment is associated with side effects primarily owing to the inability to mimic physiological cortisol secretion. Therefore, patients with adrenal insufficiency could benefit from new therapeutic strategies that restore adrenal function. The aim of this study was to investigate whether it is possible to restore normal hypothalamic-pituitary-adrenal function in adrenalectomised rats using adrenal cell transplantation.

Methods: A bioartificial adrenal gland was created with 3D cell culture conditions by encapsulation of bovine adrenocortical cells (BACs) in alginate (enBACs). The enBACs were transplanted into adrenalectomised, immunodeficient and immunocompetent rats either intraperitoneally or subcutaneously enclosed in oxygenating and immunoisolating beta-Air devices.
Results: After enBACs transplantation, cortisol was detected in the plasma of the rats. Both types of grafted encapsulated cells were explanted after 21–25 days and showed preserved morphology and a functional response to ACTH stimulation.
Conclusions: Tranplantation of xenogenic bioartificial adrenal cells might be a promising option for the treatment of patients with adrenal insufficiency.

Adrenal insufficiency is a life-threatening disorder that requires life-long glucocorticoid substitution. Conventional glucocorticoid replacement therapy fails to mimic physiologic cortisol secretion and may have implications for morbidity and mortality in patients with the disease. Therefore, adrenal cell transplantation could be a preferable therapeutic alternative for patients with primary adrenal insufficiency. However, this option is not available at present due to the limited availability to human organ donors and the required chronic immunosuppression. On the other hand, transplantation of immune-isolated xenogeneic adrenal cells in biomatrices could be a promising therapeutic alternative for these patients. The most significant accomplishment of this study is the creation of long-term functional and immune-isolated artificial adrenals and their transplantation into animal models of adrenal insufficiency.

New concerns

Telomere length and cortisol reactivity in children of depressed mothers

Gotlib IH, LeMoult J, Colich NL, Foland-Ross LC, Hallmayer J, Joormann J, Lin J, Wolkowitz OM
Primary Work, Department of Psychology, Stanford University, Stanford, CA, USA
Mol Psychiatry 2015;20(5):615-620

Background: Patients with major depressive disorder (MDD) have decreased telomere length, which predisposes to medical illness. Both MDD and telomere length have been associated independently with high levels of stress, implicating dysregulation of the hypothalamic-pituitary-adrenal (HPA) axis in this relation. The aim of this study was to assess telomere length and its relation to the HPA-axis activity in individuals at risk for depression before the onset of disorder.
Patients and Methods: Telomere length and cortisol response to a laboratory stressor were assessed in 97 healthy young daughters of mothers either with recurrent episodes of depression or with no history of psychopathology.
Results: Daughters of depressed mothers had shorter telomere length than daughters of never-depressed mothers. Furthermore, shorter telomeres were associated with greater cortisol reactivity to stress.
Conclusions: Children at familial risk of developing MDD are characterised by accelerated biological ageing before they had experienced an onset of depression; this may predispose them to develop not only MDD but also other age-related medical illnesses.

Major depressive disorder (MDD) is characterised by shortened telomere length, which may underlie the association between depression and increased incidence of cardiovascular disease, diabetes, metabolic syndrome, osteoporosis and dementia [13]. Telomeres are specialised nucleoprotein structures that cap the ends of linear chromosomes. Telomere structure is critical for maintaining chromosomal stability by protecting against premature replication termination. When telomeres shorten to a critical length, the unprotected telomere ends initiate classic DNA damage responses, which may lead to apoptosis or to genomic instability. Telomeres shorten with each cell division and represent a marker of cellular ageing. Furthermore, decreased telomere length has been associated with childhood adversity, the stress of caring for an ill family member and lifetime exposure to depression.

Here, the authors assess the telomere length in individuals at high risk of developing MDD, but who have not yet experienced a depressive episode. They demonstrate that the daughters of mothers with recurrent depression have shorter telomeres compared with their low-risk counterparts, and that shorter telomere length is associated with greater cortisol reactivity to stress across the high- and low-risk groups. These findings suggest that healthy girls, who are at risk of developing MDD, are characterised by accelerated biologic ageing before the onset of depression, which may predispose them to develop age-related medical illnesses, such as cardiovascular disease, stroke, dementia, diabetes and osteoporosis. It remains important to identify and distinguish genetic and environmental mechanisms, including tissue sensitivity to glucocorticoids, which may contribute to telomere shortening.

New paradigms

Causal effects of the early caregiving environment on development of stress response systems in children

McLaughlin KA, Sheridan MA, Tibu F, Fox NA, Zeanah CH, Nelson CA
Department of Psychology, University of Washington, Seattle, WA, USA
Proc Natl Acad Sci U S A 2015;112(18):5637–5642

Background: Early-life adverse events may disrupt the stress response system. In rodents, early-life adversity leads to increased reactivity of the sympathetic nervous system (SNS) and hypothalamic-pituitary-adrenal (HPA) axis. However, in humans the data from several studies are inconsistent. The aim of this study was to evaluate the SNS and HPA axis activity in humans after early-life adversity.
Methods: In the Bucharest early intervention project, deprived, institutionally reared children, were randomised to either high-quality foster care intervention (n=48) or to remain in care as usual (n=42). Measurements were obtained at a mean age of 12.9 years. Data were compared with a sample of typically developing Romanian children (n=47).
Results: The children that were assigned to remain in institutional care exhibited blunted SNS and HPA axis responses to psychosocial stress compared with children randomised to foster care, whose stress responses approximated those of typically developing children. These intervention effects were only seen among children placed in foster care before the age of 24 and 18 months, respectively.
Conclusions: Early-life adversity seems to influence human stress response by blunting SNS and HPA-axis reactivity, which is markedly different from the effects observed in rodents. In addition, humans seem to have a sensitive period, during which environmental influence can alter the SNS and HPA axis stress response.

Exposure to adverse early-life environment is associated with a range of negative developmental outcomes, including poor mental and physical health, and atypical social functioning. These authors describe blunted SNS and HPA-axis stress response in children with mean age of 12.9 years, who were exposed to early-life adversity. This is in contrast with studies in rodents, which show increased activity of the stress response after early-life adversity. A possible mechanism that could explain this different pattern in humans is that early life hyperactivity of the stress-axis is followed by blunted response later in life. Down-regulation of corticotropin-releasing hormone (CRH) receptors in the pituitary could be due to chronic CRH hypersecretion from the hypothalamus. Chronic CRH hypersecretion leads to elevated cortisol concentrations in short term, and reduced cortisol concentrations in longer term, once the CRH receptors have been down-regulated. An alternative mechanism is the increased negative feedback sensitivity at the level of the hypothalamus after prolonged exposure to elevated cortisol concentrations early in life. Regardless of the mechanism, the pattern of decreased response of the SNS and HPA stress axis observed among previously institutionalised children is likely to have consequences for their physical and mental health, given that cortisol has important regulatory functions on inflammatory and immune responses, glucose metabolism and central nervous system function. Decreased HPA axis responsiveness has been associated with chronic fatigue and autoimmune conditions [14]. Decreased SNS responsiveness has been associated with disruptive behaviour disorders, including oppositional defiant disorder and conduct disorder [15,16]. Thus, it is likely that early-life adversity can lead to health problems later in life, possibly through altered stress-axis reactivity. Future research studies should aim to determine improvements in caregiving quality that may ameliorate the effects of adverse early environments on stress response.

Concepts revised

Leptin reverses diabetes by suppression of the hypothalamic-pituitary-adrenal axis

Perry RJ, Zhang X-M, Zhang D, Kumashiro N, Camporez J-PG, Cline GW, Rothman DL, Shulman GI
Howard Hughes Medical Institute, Yale University School of Medicine, New Haven, CT, USA
Nature Medicine 2014;20(7):759–765

Background: Leptin treatment reverses hyperglycaemia in animal models of poorly controlled type 1 diabetes. This antidiabetic leptin effect might be of use in the treatment of patients with diabetes. Although the exact mechanism through which leptin lowers plasma glucose concentrations is not clear, it has been postulated to occur through suppression of glucagon production, suppression of glucagon responsiveness or both. The aim of this study was to identify the pathways involved in the suppressive effects of leptin upon plasma glucose concentrations.
Methods: In animal models of poorly controlled diabetes, including a model of diabetic ketoacidosis, the leptin-mediated effects were studied on systemic and hepatic metabolic processes.
Results: In rats with poorly controlled diabetes, higher rates of hepatic gluconeogenesis could be attributed to hypoleptinaemia-induced activity of the hypothalamic-pituitary-adrenal (HPA) axis. HPA axis activity resulted in higher rates of adipocyte lipolysis, hepatic conversion of glycerol to glucose through a substrate push mechanism and conversion of pyruvate to glucose through greater hepatic acetyl-CoA allosteric activation of pyruvate carboxylase flux. Notably, these effects could be dissociated from changes in plasma insulin and glucagon concentrations and hepatic gluconeogenic protein expression. By infusing rats with intralipid or corticosterone, the systemic and metabolic fluxes could be mimicked. All effects could be corrected by leptin replacement.
Conclusions: Hypoleptinaemia and increased HPA-axis activity appear to be key players in lipolysis and substrate delivery to the liver, promoting hepatic gluconeogenesis and hyperglycaemia in poorly controlled diabetes.

Leptin treatment reverses hyperglycaemia in animal models of poorly controlled type 1 diabetes. This antidiabetic effect of leptin might be beneficial in the treatment of patients with diabetes. Decreased leptin concentrations trigger a series of neuroendocrine effects in the liver and adipose tissue, resulting in hyperglycaemia and ketoacidosis. Here, the authors established an important role for leptin deficiency in the pathophysiology of diabetes through an interaction of multiple organs, including the brain, adrenal glands, adipose tissue and liver. In diabetic rats, systemic administration of leptin rapidly reversed ketoacidosis and normalised blood glucose concentrations by decreasing the delivery of glycerol and fatty acids to the liver. The effects of leptin were mediated by decreasing the HPA-axis activity, thereby resulting in reduced ACTH and corticosterone concentrations, as well as reduced adipocyte lipolysis. The effects of leptin treatment occurred after only six hours of infusion without changes in plasma concentrations of insulin or glucagon and without changes in the expression of gluconeogenic enzymes in the liver. These findings indicate a new mechanism for leptin in regulating glucose homeostasis.

Reviews

Glucocorticoids and fetal programming part 1: Outcomes

Moisiadis VG, Matthews SG
Department of Physiology, University of Toronto, Toronto, ON, Canada
Nat Rev Endocrinol 2014;10(7):391–402

Fetal life is a critical period of development and has lifelong implications for health. Glucocorticoids play an important role in development and influence the regulation of genes necessary for normal growth and maturation. The fetal hypothalamic-pituitary-adrenal (HPA) axis is particularly susceptible to long-term programming by glucocorticoids, and these effects may persist throughout life. Dysfunction of the HPA axis as a result of fetal programming has been associated with impaired brain growth, altered behaviour and increased susceptibility to chronic disease, such as metabolic and cardiovascular disease. Moreover, the effects of glucocorticoid-mediated programming are evident in subsequent generations and transmission of these changes can occur through both maternal and paternal lineages.

Glucocorticoids and fetal programming part 2: Mechanisms

Moisiadis VG, Matthews SG
Department of Physiology, University of Toronto, ON, Canada
Nat Rev Endocrinol 2014;10(7):403–411

The lifelong health of an individual is shaped during critical periods of development. Glucocorticoids are critical for normal fetal development, as they are involved in the growth and maturation of many organ systems. The surge in fetal glucocorticoid concentrations that occurs in most mammalian species over the last few days of pregnancy is an important developmental switch leading to fundamental changes in gene regulation in many organs, including the brain. These changes are important for the transition to postnatal life. Exposure of the fetus to increased concentrations of glucocorticoids, which may be the result of maternal stress or treatment with synthetic glucocorticoids, can lead to long-term 'programming' of hypothalamic-pituitary-adrenal (HPA) function. Glucocorticoids act at multiple levels within the fetal brain. Accumulating evidence indicates that they can exert powerful effects on the epigenome, including DNA methylation, histone acetylation and microRNA to influence gene expression. These influences may represent a critical component of the 'programming' process, and may be partly responsible for the transgenerational effects of antenatal glucocorticoid exposure on neurologic, cardiovascular and metabolic function.

The early environment has significant impact on the lifelong health of an individual. Several studies in a range of species suggest that neurologic, endocrine, metabolic and cardiovascular function and dysfunction in adulthood have developmental origins. In addition, maternal stress during pregnancy and fetal exposure to high concentrations of synthetic glucocorticoids can result in lifelong and multigenerational effects on the HPA function. This field of research is referred to as the 'Developmental origins of health and disease'. Our understanding of the mechanisms of programming is rapidly expanding, with epigenetic processes clearly being implicated. Recent advances have enabled the investigation of the mechanisms involved in the developmental 'programming' of adult health and disease. Defining the mechanisms by which prenatal stress and fetal synthetic glucocorticoid exposure lead to lifelong changes in HPA function might improve the treatment and/or development of interventions that prevent or reverse any long-term negative consequences of fetal exposure to glucocorticoids. The first part of this Review discusses the evidence from human and animal studies that synthetic and endogenous glucocorticoids affect fetal programming. The second part of the Review focuses on the mechanisms underlying fetal glucocorticoid programming. It discusses the epigenetic modifications, the effects of maternal stress and synthetic glucocorticoids and the mechanisms of transgenerational programming.

Circadian clock control of endocrine factors

Gamble KL, Berry R, Frank SJ, Young ME
Division of Behavioural Neurobiology, Department of Psychiatry, Department of Medicine, University of Alabama at Birmingham, Birmingham, AL, USA
Nat Rev Endocrinol 2014;10(4):215–228

Organisms experience dramatic fluctuations in demands and stresses over the course of the day. In order to maintain biological processes within physiological boundaries, mechanisms have evolved for adaptation to these daily fluctuations. Endocrine factors have a central role in homeostasis. Not only do circulating levels of various endocrine factors oscillate over the 24-hour period, but so too does responsiveness of target tissues to these signals or stimuli. Emerging evidence suggests that these daily endocrine oscillations do not occur solely in response to behavioural fluctuations associated with sleep-wake and feeding-fasting cycles, but are orchestrated by an intrinsic timekeeping mechanism known as the circadian clock. Disruption of circadian clocks by genetic and/or environmental factors seems to precipitate numerous common disorders, including the metabolic syndrome and cancer. These data suggest that strategies designed to realign normal circadian rhythmicity may have a potential role for the treatment of various endocrine-related disorders.

The temporal relationships between processes or events is critical for our understanding of the molecular basis of physiology and the pathogenesis of disease, with endocrine factors being at the heart of circadian biology. Circulating levels of various endocrine factors exhibit a time-of-day dependence. These rhythms are the result of environmental or behavioural influences, however, the endogenous circadian system contributes considerably towards the production and maintenance of these endocrine rhythms. Cell-autonomous circadian clocks modulate both the levels of endocrine factors and the tissue responsiveness to these stimuli during the course of the day. Disrupted orchestration of circadian and endocrine rhythms results in a state of circadian dys-synchrony, which predisposes subjects to medical pathology, such as cardiometabolic diseases and cancer. Here, the authors review the importance of circadian clock control of endocrine factors. They provide a general overview of known oscillation characteristics of endocrine factors and discuss the evidence regarding mediation of endocrine rhythms by circadian clocks, the pathologies associated with disruption of normal rhythmicity and the ways to restore the orchestration of circadian processes.

Adrenal insufficiency in corticosteroids use: systematic review and meta-analysis

Broersen LH, Pereira AM, Jørgensen JOL, Dekkers OM
Department of Clinical Epidemiology, Leiden University Medical Centre, Leiden, The Netherlands
J Clin Endocrinol Metab 2015;100(6):2171–2180

Background: Glucocorticoids are widely used therapeutically, but a life-threatening side-effect of chronic use is adrenal insufficiency. The aim of this study was to determine the prevalence and predictors of adrenal insufficiency in patients receiving glucocorticoid treatment.
Methods: Seven electronic databases (PubMed, MEDLINE, EMBASE, COCHRANE, CENTRAL, Web of Science and CINAHL/Academic Search Premier) were searched to identify potentially relevant studies. Original studies testing adult corticosteroid users for adrenal insufficiency were eligible.
Results: Seventy-four articles were included with a total of 3,753 participants. Stratified by administration form, the percentages of patients with adrenal insufficiency ranged from 4.2% for nasal administration (95% CI: 0.5–28.9) to 52.2% for intra-articular administration (95% CI: 40.5–63.6). Stratified by disease, the percentages ranged from 6.8% for asthma with inhalation corticosteroids only (95% CI: 3.8–12.0) to 60.0% for haematological malignancies (95% CI: 38.0–78.6). Among patients with asthma, the risk varied according to the dose from 2.4% (95% CI: 0.6–9.3) (low dose) to 21.5% (95% CI: 12.0–35.5) (high dose), and according to treatment duration from 1.4% (95% CI: 0.3–7.4) (<28 days) to 27.4% (95% CI: 17.7–39.8) (>1 year).
Conclusions: The prevalence of adrenal insufficiency after discontinuation of glucocorticoid is high. Although higher doses and longer duration of treatment are associated with the highest risk, there was no administration form, dosing, treatment duration or underlying disease for which adrenal insufficiency can be excluded with certainty. In clinical practice, especially for those patients with nonspecific symptoms after cessation, the threshold for testing should be low.

Chronic pharmacologic use of glucocorticoids suppresses the hypothalamic-pituitary-adrenal (HPA) axis and causes iatrogenic central adrenal insufficiency. Adrenal insufficiency is a serious, potentially life threatening condition. Therefore, patients may require glucocorticoid replacement therapy after chronic use of synthetic glucocorticoids. This systematic review and meta-analysis estimated the percentage of patients who develop adrenal insufficiency following the use of corticosteroids. It showed that there is no administration form, disease, dose group or treatment duration for which the risk of adrenal insufficiency can be safely excluded. Although the percentage of patients with adrenal insufficiency after corticosteroids use declines over time, a substantial number of patients remained adrenal insufficient after six months. Given the frequent use of glucocorticoids in clinical practice, it is particularly important to identify patients at risk of adrenal insufficiency following chronic use of

pharmacologic doses of glucocorticoids. Therefore, clinicians should 1) inform patients about the risk and symptoms of adrenal insufficiency; 2) consider formally testing patients after discontinuation of high-dose or long-term treatment with glucocorticoids; and 3) have a low threshold for formally testing patients with nonspecific symptoms after cessation of chronic glucocorticoid therapy.

References

1. Swirski FK, Nahrendorf M. Leukocyte behavior in atherosclerosis, myocardial infarction, and heart failure. Science 2013;339(6116):161–166.
2. Tall AR, Yvan-Charvet L, Westerterp M, Murphy AJ. Cholesterol efflux: a novel regulator of myelopoiesis and atherogenesis. Arterioscler. Thromb Vasc Biol 2012;32(11):2547–2552.
3. Nader N, Chrousos GP, Kino T. Interactions of the circadian CLOCK system and the HPA axis. Trends Endocrinol Metab 2010;21(5):277–286.
4. Charmandari E, Chrousos GP, Lambrou GI, Pavlaki A, Koide H, Ng SS, et al. Peripheral CLOCK regulates target-tissue glucocorticoid receptor transcriptional activity in a circadian fashion in man. PLoS One 2011;6(9):e25612.
5. Swerdlow AJ, Higgins CD, Brook CG, Dunger DB, Hindmarsh PC, Price DA, et al. Mortality in patients with congenital adrenal hyperplasia: a cohort study. J Pediatr 1998;133(4):516–520.
6. Claahsen-van der Grinten HL, Otten BJ, Stikkelbroeck MM, Sweep FC, Hermus AR. Testicular adrenal rest tumours in congenital adrenal hyperplasia. Best Pract Res Clin Endocrinol Metab 2009;23(2):209–220.
7. Bachelot A, Plu-Bureau G, Thibaud E, Laborde K, Pinto G, Samara D, et al. Long-term outcome of patients with congenital adrenal hyperplasia due to 21-hydroxylase deficiency. Horm Res 2007;67(6):268–276.
8. Falhammar H, Filipsson H, Holmdahl G, Janson PO, Nordenskjöld A, Hagenfeldt K, et al. Fractures and bone mineral density in adult women with 21-hydroxylase deficiency. J Clin Endocrinol Metab 2007;92(12):4643–4649.
9. Chakhtoura Z, Bachelot A, Samara-Boustani D, Ruiz JC, Donadille B, Dulon J, et al. Impact of total cumulative glucocorticoid dose on bone mineral density in patients with 21-hydroxylase deficiency. Eur J Endocrinol 2008;158(6):879–887.
10. Roberts D, Dalziel S. Antenatal corticosteroids for accelerating fetal lung maturation for women at risk of preterm birth. Cochrane Database Syst Rev 2006;(3):CD004454.
11. Darmstadt GL, Bhutta ZA, Cousens S, Adam T, Walker N, de Bernis L, for the Lancet Neonatal Survival Steering Team. Evidence-based, cost-effective interventions: how many newborn babies can we save? Lancet 2005;365(9463):977–988.
12. Beuschlein F, Fassnacht M, Assié G, Calebiro D, Stratakis CA, Osswald A, et al: Constitutive activation of PKA catalytic subunit in adrenal Cushing's syndrome. N Engl J Med 2014;370:1019–1028.
13. Wolkowitz OM, Epel ES, Reus VI, Mellon SH. Depression gets old fast: do stress and depression accelerate cell ageing? Depress Anxiety 2010;27(4):327–338.
14. Heim C, Ehlert U, Hellhammer DH. The potential role of hypocortisolism in the pathophysiology of stress-related bodily disorders. Psychoneuroendocrinology 2000;25(1):1–35.
15. Crowell SE, Beauchaine TP, Gatzke-Kopp L, Sylvers P, Mead H, Chipman-Chacon J. Autonomic correlates of attention-deficit/hyperactivity disorder and oppositional defiant disorder in preschool children. J Abnorm Psychol 2006;115(1):174–178.
16. Boyce WT, Quas J, Alkon A, Smider NA, Essex MJ, Kupfer DJ. MacArthur Assessment Battery Working Group of the MacArthur Foundation Research Network on Psychopathology and Development. Autonomic reactivity and psychopathology in middle childhood. Br J Psychiatry 2001;179:144–150.

Oncology and Chronic Disease

Stefania Pedicelli, Sara Ciccone and Carla Bizzarri

Unit of Endocrinology and Diabetes 'Bambino Gesù' Children's Hospital, IRCCS, Rome, Italy

Advancements in radiation therapy, chemotherapy, surgery and multimodal treatment have dramatically improved childhood cancer survival, but cancer and its treatment may have immediate or delayed adverse effects on the endocrine system.

We highlight published papers that investigate the clinical effects of childhood cancer treatments on growth, pubertal development, bone health and fertility. Obesity and early and progressive insulin resistance leading to metabolic syndrome and diabetes mellitus are increasingly recognised complications of cancer treatment. Moreover, transition from paediatric to adult care represents an emerging topic of discussion, as some data suggest that a high proportion of childhood cancer survivors with hormonal defects do not receive replacement therapy in adulthood.

This year, the potential role of substitutive therapy with growth hormone (GH) on cancer recurrence or second malignancy occurrence, in patients with hypothalamic/pituitary GH deficiency induced by surgery and/or irradiation, has been re-evaluated and the conclusions seem to be reassuring.

Concepts revised: growth hormone and neoplastic risk

Growth hormone exposure as a risk factor for the development of subsequent neoplasms of the central nervous system: a report from the Childhood Cancer Survivor Study

Patterson BC, Chen Y, Sklar CA, Neglia J, Yasui Y, Mertens A, Armstrong GT, Meadows A, Stovall M, Robison LL, Meacham LR
Department of Pediatrics Emory University/Aflac Cancer and Blood Disorders Center of Children's Healthcare of Atlanta, Atlanta, GA, USA
bcpatte@emory.edu
J Clin Endocrinol Metab 2014;99(6):2030-2037

Background: Irradiation of the hypothalamic-pituitary area may cause growth hormone (GH) deficiency in paediatric cancer survivors, but the role of GH treatment on cancer recurrences or second malignancies is still debated. This study assessed the effects of GH therapy as an independent risk factor for subsequent neoplasms (SNs) of central nervous system (CNS), focusing on meningioma and glioma.
Methods: Participants were diagnosed between 1970–1986 and treated at 26 institutions in the United States and Canada. Eligible diagnoses included leukaemia, CNS tumours (all histologies), Hodgkin lymphoma, non-Hodgkin lymphoma, kidney tumour, neuroblastoma, soft tissue sarcoma or bone tumour. Benign neoplasms, such as meningioma and craniopharyngioma, were excluded. Baseline and multiple follow-up questionnaires assessed a wide range of health outcomes. Based on verified self-reports, 338 GH-treated and 11,760 GH-untreated patients were enrolled. Subsequent new primary CNS tumours were considered. Therapeutic treatments were determined through medical records, while use of oestrogen/progestin was self-reported.
Results: Regardless of GH treatment status, most new CNS tumours (94.5% of meningiomas; 79.2% of gliomas) occurred in patients exposed to cranial radiation (CR). Meningioma developed in 3% of GH-treated survivors and 1.2% of GH-untreated survivors, gliomas in 1.8% of GH-treated and 0.4% of GH-untreated survivors. Incidence of meningioma continued up to 35 years after diagnosis in all patients with prior CR and was associated with younger age at diagnosis, female gender, higher CR dose and longer time elapsed since CR. Most gliomas occurred within 20 years and were associated with higher CR dose and with a shorter time elapsed since CR. GH treatment was not associated with higher rates of meningioma or glioma in subjects with prior CR (irrespective of GH dose and adjusted for age at follow-up, sex, age at primary diagnosis, CR/time since CR, intrathecal methotrexate, length of oestrogen and/or progesterone treatment and alkylating

agents exposure). The rate ratio in GH-treated survivors for any CNS SNs was 1.0 (0.8 for meningioma; 1.9 for glioma) and for death due to any subsequent CNS neoplasm was 1.6 (95% CI 0.5–4.9, P=0.39).
Conclusions: GH-treated childhood cancer survivors have no increase in risk of new primary CNS SNs, in particular glioma and meningioma. Risk of CNS SNs was independently associated with CR dose, time from CR exposure, age at cancer diagnosis and sex.

The Childhood Cancer Survivor Study (CCSS) is a cohort study with prospective follow-up of 14,358 childhood cancer survivors diagnosed prior to age 21 years and surviving cancer for at least five years. Previous reports from this cohort described a small increase in the overall risk for subsequent neoplasia correlated with GH treatment. The relative risk was initially estimated to be 3.21 (95% CI 1.88–5.46), but with longer duration of follow-up was later revised to 2.15 (95% CI 1.3–3.5) [1,2]. In both reports, meningioma was the most common new neoplasm. Meningiomas express both GH and IGF-I receptors and, both in vitro and in vivo, meningioma cell growth is promoted by IGF-I and decreased by GH receptor antagonists [3]. Gliomas also express GH and IGF-I receptors and IGF-I has been shown to increase glioma tissue cell growth [4]. This new study describes a longer follow-up than previous reports and considers only second neoplasms (SNs) of central nervous system (CNS). Notably, cranial radiation (CR) is a confounding factor, because children exposed to CR are more likely to have GH deficiency and to require GH therapy, but they also show an increased risk of subsequent CNS neoplasms. Decisions regarding GH treatment in cancer survivors depend on many factors and the risk of SNs is one of the most relevant concerns. Further longitudinal studies on new cohorts are needed to better evaluate whether dose and duration of GH therapy and age at start of GH treatment may influence the risk of SNs and whether GH treatment has effects on different common neoplasms, such as breast or colon cancer. This could allow the development of international guidelines on GH treatment in cancer survivors.

Incidence of primary cancers and intracranial tumour recurrences in GH-treated and untreated adult hypopituitary patients: analyses from the Hypopituitary Control and Complications Study

Child CJ, Conroy D, Zimmermann AG, Woodmansee WW, Erfurth EM, Robison LL
Lilly Research Laboratories, Erl Wood Manor, Windlesham, Surrey, UK
cjc@lilly.com
Eur J Endocrinol 2015;172(6):779–790

Background: It is unclear if treatment with growth hormone (GH) is related to an increased risk of cancer. Studies in childhood cancer survivors treated with GH suggest an increased incidence of second neoplasia, while cancer risk data in GH deficient adults show conflicting results.
Methods: Adult patients with GH deficiency (GHD) were recruited between 1996–2012 from Austria, Belgium, Canada, Czech Republic, Denmark, France, Germany, Hungary, Iceland, Italy, Japan, Norway, Slovakia, Spain, Sweden, The Netherlands, UK and USA, to a study sponsored by Eli-Lilly. Risks of all-site primary cancer and risk data of specific cancers (breast, prostate, and colorectal) were analysed. The recurrence rates for pituitary adenomas and craniopharyngiomas were also investigated. Standardised incidence ratios (SIRs) were calculated by comparison to the general population using GLOBOCAN data, published by the International Agency for Research on Cancer. Neoplasm rates in GH-treated and untreated patients were compared.
Results: The study enrolled 9,686 patients with at least one follow-up visit; 8,418 GH-treated, 1,268 untreated. 3,668 GH-treated patients and 720 untreated patients had a history of pituitary adenoma, while 956 GH-treated patients and 102 untreated patients had a history of craniopharyngioma. Mean follow-up time was 4.8 ± 3.5 years. Primary cancers were identified in 225 GH-treated patients and 45 untreated patients (SIR=0.82, 95% CI 0.71–0.93). Cancer risk was not different between GH-treated and untreated patients (relative risk (RR)=1.00, 95% CI 0.70–1.41). Adjusted RR for recurrence was 0.91 (0.68–1.22) for pituitary adenoma and 1.32 (0.53–3.31) for craniopharyngioma. SIRs for GH-treated patients were 0.59 for breast, 0.80 for prostate and 0.62 for colorectal cancers. Cancer cases were identified in 205/6,732 GH-treated patients with adult onset GHD (SIR=0.78) and in 20/1,642 patients with childhood-onset GHD (SIR=1.0).
Conclusions: No increased risk for all-site cancers, breast, prostate or colorectal primary cancers in GH-treated patients was found. GH treatment did not increase the risk of recurrence in patients with history of pituitary adenoma or craniopharyngioma.

The mitogenic and proliferative effects of GH and insulin-like growth factors (IGFs) have been reported by experimental analyses. Epidemiological studies have shown a positive correlation between circulating levels of IGF-I and risk of developing breast, prostate and colorectal cancers. Furthermore, patients with acromegaly have an increased risk of colorectal cancer incidence and mortality [5]. This study reports the results of a company-sponsored register, designed to determine the long-term safety of GH replacement in adults with GH deficiency treated with recombinant human GH (Humatrope® Eli-Lilly). The relatively short duration of follow up (4.8 years) and the inclusion also of patients with only one follow up visit clearly limit the findings. It would be highly desirable to conduct such studies on larger longitudinal cohorts, independent of industry funding. Interestingly, even if the potential effect of the length of GH therapy was not analysed, the reported risks of primary and recurrent neoplasms seem to be similar in adult-onset and childhood-onset GH deficiency, suggesting a negligible effect of the duration of GH therapy on cancer risk.

Late effects of tumour therapy: broaden existing knowledge

Ovarian insufficiency and pubertal development after hematopoietic stem cell transplantation in childhood

Bresters D, Emons JAM, Nuri N, Ball LM, Kollen WJW, Hannema SE, Bakker-Steeneveld JDJ, van der Bom JG, Oostdijk W
Leiden University Medical Center, Willem-Alexander Children's Hospital, P.O. Box 9600, 2300 RC Leiden, The Netherlands
d.bresters@lumc.nl
Pediatr Blood Cancer 2014;61(11):2048-2053

Background: Ovarian insufficiency (OI) is a common late effect of haematopoietic stem cell transplantation (HSCT), resulting in impaired pubertal development and growth during childhood. Both irradiation and gonadotoxic agents are implicated. This study aimed to assess the cumulative incidence and risk factors for OI after HSCT.
Methods: 109 consecutive female patients, who underwent HSCT for both neoplastic and non-neoplastic diseases before 19 years of age, were studied. All survived at least two years after HSCT and were aged at least 10 years at the time of the study. OI was defined as elevated gonadotropin levels (FSH and LH >10U/L) and low estradiol levels (<40pmol/L), along with the absence of spontaneous puberty after age 12 years, or the absence of menses in pubertal or post-pubertal females.
Results: At a median follow-up time of 7.2 years, 56% had OI. Eight additional patients, who had been diagnosed with OI and started on hormone replacement therapy, showed spontaneous recovery of ovarian function during follow-up. In 44%, hormonal induction of puberty was indicated. OI incidence was higher in girls who were pubertal or post-pubertal at the time of HSCT (RR: 4.42 for pubertal HSCT and 22.08 for post-pubertal HSCT, compared with prepubertal HSCT). The highest incidence of OI was found in patients with malignant diseases (68%), followed by benign haematological conditions (39%) and immunodeficiency/inborn errors of metabolism (33%). Patients undergoing irradiation as a conditioning regimen had a similar rate of OI as those treated with chemotherapy. A trend for association with OI was found for busulfan in patients conditioned with chemotherapy only. With the limitations of small sample size and changes of doses over time, the gonadotoxic effect of busulfan seemed not to be dose-related.
Conclusions: Girls who were post-pubertal at the time of HSCT show the highest incidence of OI, shortly after HSCT. The role of additional risk factors, as conditioning regimen, was not confirmed.

Haematopoietic stem cell transplantation (HSCT) is now a common treatment for both neoplastic and non-neoplastic haematological conditions. Ovarian insufficiency (OI) seems to be the most common endocrine complication of HSCT. Actually, the sample size of this study seems to be too small to analyse the effect of different primary diagnoses and conditioning regimens on OI occurrence and the finding that older age is the main risk factor for OI is similar to previous studies. The lower incidence of OI in girls who were prepubertal at the time of HSCT is probably due to the higher resistance of prepubertal ovary tissue to gonadotoxic treatments. These findings are fundamental to correctly inform families about the late risks of HSCT and to give indications for fertility preservation. The young age of these women at diagnosis of OI is an indication for hormone replacement therapy in order to prevent osteoporosis, improve cardiovascular health and general well-being. However, it should be considered that a few data suggest that chronic oestrogen/progestin replacement therapy may increase the risk of breast cancer, in women with OI carrying an increased risk for secondary neoplasia (such as HSCT survivors) [6].

Dynamics of fertility impairment in childhood brain tumour survivors

Pfitzer C, Chen CM, Wessel T, Keil T, Sörgel A, Langer T, Steinmann D, Borgmann-Staudt A
Department of Paediatric Oncology/Haematology, Charité – Universitätsmedizin Berlin, Campus V rchow-Klinikum, Klinik für Pädiatrie m. S. Onkologie/Hämatologie/Stammzelltransplantation, Augustenburger Platz 1, Mittelallee 6a, Berlin, Germany
J Cancer Res Clin Oncol 2014;140(10):1759–1767

Background: Fertility impairment and recovery after chemo- and radiotherapy have been reported in both male and female childhood cancer survivors, but little is known about the dynamics. The aim of this study was to analyse the development of fertility impairment and possible recovery in childhood brain tumour survivors.
Methods: 144 survivors of childhood brain tumour, treated in two German Paediatric Oncology Centres between 2000–2005, were included in this longitudinal study. Fertility parameters were retrieved from medical records up to 12 years after diagnosis. Patients with a history of relapse were excluded. Patients older than 13 years with FSH ≥15IU/L and/or LH ≥15IU/L and/or amenorrhoea or testicular volume <5ml at age 14, or <8ml at age 15, or <10ml at age 16, or <12ml at age 17 were defined as infertile. Subgroups according to cancer therapy were defined as: 1) cranial or craniospinal irradiation ≥30Gy; 2) gonadotoxic chemotherapy without irradiation; 3) no chemotherapy or radiotherapy.
Results: Median FSH concentrations at different time points were persistently higher in participants with age ≥13 years receiving cranial or craniospinal irradiation ≥30Gy (n=23), compared with patients not receiving chemotherapy or radiotherapy (n=29); in particular mean FSH concentrations were 8.3 versus 4.1IU/L two years after the initial treatment; 8.9 versus 4.2IU/L after eight years; and 7.1 versus 3.5IU/L after 10 years. Altogether, 6.0 years after diagnosis 11/65 women reported the occurrence of amenorrhoea. Five of these women later presented a recovery of regular menstrual cycles without hormone therapy. The chance of fertility recovering increased with time since diagnosis (P=0.074). Patients receiving cranial or craniospinal irradiation ≥30Gy showed signs of fertility impairment throughout whole period of observation.
Conclusions: Signs of fertility impairment, such as amenorrhoea and elevated FSH concentrations, were found at variable time points between one and 12 years after radiation and chemotherapy. Declines in elevated FSH concentrations over time could indicate either progressive atrophy of the pituitary gland after irradiation of more than 30Gy, or recovery of fertility.

This paper describes the important finding that hypogonadism and impaired fertility in childhood brain tumour survivors are sometimes reversible with time, although those patients who received cranial irradiation ≥30Gy usually show a permanent damage. Decreasing FSH levels, after the initial increase, may represent either a sign of progressive (radiation-induced) atrophy of the pituitary gland or recovery from the initial fertility impairment mainly due to spinal irradiation in female survivors, but also related to the gonadotoxic effect of different chemotherapeutic agents. Furthermore, we must consider that cancer survivors treated with both gonadotoxic therapeutic agents and cranial irradiation may often show a 'mixed' form of hypogonadism. In this condition, primary gonadal failure due to gonadotoxic chemotherapy and central hypogonadism due to irradiation may coexist. Levels of gonadal steroids are low, but gonadotropin levels are not clearly elevated, due to a concurrent impairment of pituitary function [7–9]. Thus, the evaluation of pubertal development and gonadal function has to take into account not only the gonadotropin and steroid levels, but also the increase of gonadal volumes, the progression of sexual characteristics and the pubertal growth pattern.

Early and progressive insulin resistance in young, non-obese cancer survivors treated with hematopoietic stem cell transplantation

Bizzarri C, Pinto RM, Ciccone S, Brescia LP, Locatelli F, Cappa M
Unit of Endocrinology and Diabetes, Bambino Gesù Children's Hospital, IRCCS, Rome, Italy
Pediatr Blood Cancer 2015;62(9):1650–1655

Background: Patients receiving haematopoietic stem cell transplantation (HSCT) during childhood are at increased risk of cardiovascular disease. Early identification of insulin resistance, metabolic syndrome (MS) and abnormal

glucose tolerance in these patients could represent a useful tool for preventing cardiovascular disorders.
Methods: 45 survivors of haematological malignancies (age: 13.9 ± 4.8 years) treated with HSCT before age 18 years were compared with 90 matched healthy controls in a single-centre, cross-sectional study. Clinical, imaging and laboratory data including oral glucose tolerance tests (OGTT) were collected. Patients with hormonal defects were included only after the start of replacement therapy and the achievement of an adequate hormone balance. The control group was represented by healthy children undergoing assessment of glucose tolerance status in the context of a family screening for diabetes mellitus (DM), or for the occasional finding of hyperglycaemia.
Results: Seven of 45 patients (15.6%) showed abnormal glucose tolerance on OGTT, 1/45 (2.2%) was obese and none fulfilled the criteria for MS. Only one post-pubertal female, with DM on OGTT, also showed impaired fasting glucose (120mg/dL). A waist/height ratio >0.5 was more common in patients with abnormal glucose tolerance (85.7%) than in patients with normal glucose tolerance (42.1%) or controls (23.3%). Patients with abnormal glucose tolerance were more likely to have received total body irradiation (TBI) as conditioning regimen and had longer time elapsed since HSCT.
Conclusions: Patients treated with HSCT may develop insulin resistance early after transplantation even if they do not fulfil MS criteria. They show central fat accumulation without obesity. The main determinants of the increased metabolic risk are TBI and time elapsed from HSCT. Evaluation of MS and glucose tolerance should be part of the routine hormonal follow-up.

These findings suggest that the metabolic risk in patients treated with haematopoietic stem cell transplantation (HSCT) is primarily related to the development of an early insulin-resistant state. The proportion of patients with abnormal glucose tolerance was higher than in a previous study of young Italian subjects with simple obesity (18.4% versus 12.4%) [10]. Notably, patients treated with HSCT did not show overt obesity but had an early redistribution of fat tissue with central fat accumulation. It has been suggested that a waist/height ratio >0.5 is more useful than BMI or waist circumference as a marker of preclinical metabolic abnormalities in cancer survivors [11]. In children treated with HSCT, it is essential to correct waist circumference for height because these patients frequently show impaired linear growth. As described for young obese subjects, the assessment of fasting glucose alone is not sufficient to detect early abnormalities of glucose metabolism. The evaluation of metabolic syndrome (MS) and glucose tolerance should be part of routine follow-up, in order to prevent chronic complications related to insulin resistance. The development of prevention strategies aimed at decreasing body fat and increasing muscle mass in these patients is highly recommended. Further studies are needed to better define the early changes in body composition associated with increased metabolic risk.

Predictors of being overweight or obese in survivors of pediatric acute lymphoblastic leukaemia (ALL)

Zhang FF, Rodday AM, Kelly MJ, Must A, MacPherson C, Roberts SB, Saltzman E, Parsons SK
Department of Nutrition Science, Friedman School of Nutrition Science and Policy, Tufts University, Boston, MA USA
Pediatr Blood Cancer 2014;61(7):1263–1269

Background: An increased prevalence of obesity has been reported in survivors of paediatric ALL.
Methods: 83 children with ALL diagnosed between 1985–2010 were included in this retrospective study. Body mass index (BMI) was analysed at diagnosis, at end of induction, at end of consolidation, every six months during maintenance and yearly for up to five years post-treatment.
Results: Mean BMI Z-score at diagnosis was 0.2. A BMI >85th percentile was found in 21% of patients at diagnosis, 40% of patients at treatment completion and 40% of patients five years post-treatment. BMI Z-score increased during induction and in the first six months of maintenance and remained stable in the other points. Patients with high BMI Z-score at diagnosis showed a higher risk of being overweight/obese at the end of the treatment.
Conclusions: The risk of obesity is increased in children with ALL. Most of weight gain is observed at the beginning of treatment and then it is maintained during a five-year post-treatment follow-up.

Several studies have reported that childhood cancer survivors are more commonly overweight or obese than their peers. A recent meta-analysis synthesised the literature of the past 35 years on 1,742 paediatric ALL acute lymphoblastic leukaemia (ALL) survivors [12]; the overall BMI Z-score corresponded to the 80th percentile, suggesting paediatric ALL survivors have a substantially higher BMI than the reference population. The high prevalence of obesity was independent of cranial irradiation, gender and age at diagnosis. The strongest evidence for an increased risk of obesity in paediatric ALL survivors came from studies that evaluated recent survivors (less than five years after the completion of treatment) who were children and preadolescents at the time of study evaluation. High doses of steroids are clearly implicated not only in the first phase of treatment, when most of the weight gain is observed, but the adverse effects seem to persist even after the completion of therapy. Weight gain soon after the diagnosis of leukaemia should not be overlooked, due to the linked cardiovascular risk. Lifestyle interventions are needed early after the completion of treatment, targeting weight control.

Metabolic syndrome in hematologic malignancies survivors: a meta-analysis

Li C, Liu P, Liu L, Zhang X, Yang P, Sheng H, Bu L, Li H, Qu S
Department of Endocrinology, Shanghai Tenth People's Hospital, School of Medicine, Tongji University, Shanghai, China
lihong_endo@tongji.edu.cn; lh_endo@163.com
Med Oncol 2015;32(1):422–429

Background: Several studies have suggested an increased prevalence of metabolic syndrome (MS) in survivors of haematologic malignancies (HM).
Methods: A systematic review and meta-analysis was performed to evaluate the risk of metabolic syndrome among HM survivors. Subgroup analyses stratified by type of HM, treatment modality, criteria of MS assessment and individual components of MS. Seven cross-sectional studies with a total of 3,550 participants were included.
Results: Compared with healthy control groups, HM survivors showed an increased risk of MS (OR 2.03; 95% CI 1.23–3.35). In the subgroup analyses, a positive association was observed for haematopoietic stem cell transplantation (OR 2.40; 95% CI 1.71–3.35), but not for other major cancer treatment modalities. Further subgroup analysis by individual MS components showed a higher risk of arterial hypertension (OR 1.67; 95% CI 1.10–2.53) and central obesity (OR 1.43; 95% CI 1.02–2.01).
Conclusions: This meta-analysis confirms that HM survivors are at an increased risk of MS. Physicians should regularly monitor the metabolic status of these patients.

Recently, haematologic malignancies (HM) survivors have been reported to frequently develop metabolic syndrome (MS) and diabetes mellitus, even if it is still unclear whether there is a causal relationship between MS and early cardiovascular events in these patients. These emerging complications were poorly valued in the past, probably because they were not considered as life-threatening conditions. This meta-analysis not only confirms the association between HM survival and MS, but also reveals the specific role of haematopoietic stem cell transplantation (HSCT). Unlike other complications of HSCT, MS components seem to be, at least partially, modifiable. It has been demonstrated that exercise improves body composition in children treated with HSCT [13]. Modification of lifestyle habits aimed to decrease body fat and increase lean mass is highly recommended as prevention of later complications.

Important for clinical practice: surveillance strategies

Is outcome of differentiated thyroid carcinoma influenced by tumor stage at diagnosis?

Clement SC, Kremer LC, Links TP, Mulder RL, Ronckers CM, van Eck-Smit BL, van Rijn RR, van der Pal HJ, Tissing WJ, Janssens GO, van den Heuvel-Eibrink MM, Neggers SJ, van Dijkum EJ, Peeters RP, van Santen HM
Department of Pediatric Oncology, Emma Children's Hospital/Academic Medical Center, University of Amsterdam, Amsterdam, The Netherlands
s.c.clement@amc.uva.nl
Cancer Treat Rev 2015;41(1):9–16

Background: There is no international consensus on surveillance strategies for differentiated thyroid carcinoma (DTC) after radiotherapy for childhood cancer survivors (CCS). Neck palpation shows low sensitivity to detect thyroid cancer, particularly for early stage disease. Neck ultrasound, performed routinely during long term follow up in CCS, could allow early DTC detection, but its relevance is debated since the prognosis of DTC is excellent, even when detected in advanced stage.

Methods: A multidisciplinary working group analysed whether detection of DTC at an early stage reduces: 1) recurrence, irrespective of treatment modality 2) mortality, irrespective of treatment modality 3) surgical complications, such as hypoparathyroidism and recurrent nerve injury 4) severe adverse effects of radioactive iodine treatment, in particular second primary malignancies. The literature was systematically reviewed and conclusions were categorised by level of evidence (A: high, B: moderate-low, C: very low).

Results: Available data on secondary (radiation-induced) DTC in CCS patients were very limited. No differences were found between patients with secondary DTC compared with patients with sporadic DTC regarding: presence of lymph node and distant metastasis, multi-focality, bilateral tumours or extra-thyroidal extension at diagnosis, recurrent disease and mortality. The working group therefore justified to extrapolate evidence from patients with sporadic DTC to CCS with secondary DTC. In children, detection of DTC at an early stage (less distant metastasis and extrathyroid extension) is associated with lower recurrence and mortality (level C), but not other morbidities. In adults, stronger evidence was found that earlier DTC stage represents a favourable prognostic factor for recurrence (level B) and mortality (level A). Additionally, more extensive surgery increased the risk of transient hypoparathyroidism (level A) and higher doses of radioiodine increased the risk of second malignancies (level B).

Conclusions: There is weak evidence that early identification of DTC is beneficial for children, even considering that the overall outcome of these tumours is excellent.

This paper emphasises the very small body of evidence on the value of neck ultrasonography as a surveillance strategy for secondary thyroid cancer in childhood cancer survivors (CCS). Several long-term follow-up guidelines, mostly from outside Europe, recommend only physical examination of the thyroid gland by palpation on yearly basis, in subjects with high risk based on previous treatments (irradiation). Whenever a thyroid nodule is suspected by physical examination, the subject is referred to an endocrinologist for further diagnostic work-up (namely ultrasound, and if appropriate fine needle aspiration with cytology). Neck ultrasound is an effective, non-invasive and relatively inexpensive diagnostic tool. Even if published clinical evidences are scarce and the prognosis of advanced differentiated thyroid carcinoma remains good, in our opinion clinicians should consider supporting neck palpation with ultrasound, as a screening test for differentiated thyroid carcinoma (DTC), at least in clinical settings in which this technique is feasible. On the other hand, it is well known that ultrasound might be too sensitive in detecting thyroid nodules and this could result in needless fine needle aspirations. It is thus essential that clinical experience continues to guide the decision to perform fine needle aspiration of thyroid nodules.

Important for clinical practice: prevention of long-term consequences of chronic disease

Compromised peak bone mass in patients with inflammatory bowel disease – a prospective study

Laakso S, Valta H, Verkasalo M, Toiviainen-Salo S, Mäkitie O
Children's Hospital, Helsinki University Central Hospital and University of Helsinki, Helsinki, Finland
saila.laakso@helsinki.fi
J Pediatr 2014;164(6):1436–1443.e1

Background: Inflammatory bowel disease (IBD) may impair normal growth, pubertal development and bone health, due to chronic inflammation, malnutrition and steroid treatment. This study evaluates peak bone mass attainment in children and adolescents with IBD and identifies risk factors for suboptimal bone mass attainment.

Methods: A prospective study of 47 children and adolescents (24 males) with ulcerative colitis (n=30) or Crohn's disease (n=17) was conducted. Lumbar spine areal bone mineral density (aBMD) and height-adjusted whole body less head bone mineral content (BMC) were assessed by dual-energy X-ray absorptiometry (DXA) and corrected for bone age.
Results: At the time of IBD diagnosis, 25 patients were prepubertal, 20 were pubertal and two were post-pubertal. At a median follow-up 5.4 years, pubertal development was complete in 75% of patients. Despite clinical inactivity of the disease in 70%, no patient showed recovery of BMD or BMC Z-scores at follow-up. Lumbar spine aBMD Z-scores, whole body less head BMC and bone age–adjusted Z-scores decreased in patients who were pubertal at baseline and post-pubertal at follow-up. Post-pubertal patients had lower aBMD and BMC Z-scores compared with prepubertal and pubertal patients. Low lumbar spine aBMD (Z-score <-1.0) was associated with completed puberty, underweight and greater lifetime cumulative weight-adjusted prednisolone dose. Three patients (6%) showed vertebral fractures. One-fourth had insufficient serum levels of 25-hydroxyvitamin D (<50nmol/L), but these did not differ from those with higher serum levels in lumbar spine aBMD or whole body less head BMC adjusted Z-score.
Conclusions: Longitudinal follow-up during puberty shows that IBD has a significant negative impact on bone health. Suboptimal peak bone mass attainment may have life-long consequences.

During childhood and adolescence, bone mass increases to attain peak values by the end of the second or the beginning of the third decade of life. The highest rate of mineral accumulation occurs during puberty. Inflammation, malnutrition and glucocorticoid treatment contribute to impaired bone health in patients with inflammatory bowel disease (IBD). Two previous longitudinal studies using peripheral quantitative computed tomography showed suboptimal accrual of trabecular volumetric bone mineral density (vBMD) and bone geometry, with greater increases in vBMD in prepubertal and early pubertal subjects compared with more mature subjects [14,15]. Follow-up durations in those studies were short (one and 2.6 years, respectively) and bone health in young adults with childhood-onset IBD remains uncertain.

The current study reports a longer follow-up (5.4 years) and confirms that, despite modern treatments, suboptimal bone mass accrual during puberty is still common in adolescents with IBD. This may potentially lead to symptomatic osteoporosis during early adulthood. The high proportion of patients with insufficient vitamin D levels (25%) highlights the need for vitamin D supplementation in all patients with malabsorption and/or chronic glucocorticoid therapy, with the aim of optimal vitamin D status during the pubertal bone mass accrual. On the other hand, the lack of correlation between vitamin D levels and bone quality parameters questions the clinical significance of these low levels.

A prospective longitudinal study of growth and pubertal progress in adolescents with inflammatory bowel disease

Mason A, Malik S, McMillan M, McNeilly JD, Bishop J, McGrogan P, Russell RK, Ahmed SF
Child Health, School of Medicine, University of Glasgow Royal Hospital for Sick Children, Yorkhill, Glasgow, UK
faisal.ahmed@glasgow.ac.uk
Horm Res Paediatr 2015;83(1):45-54

Background: Early-onset inflammatory bowel disease (IBD) may delay puberty due to hypogonadotropic hypogonadism, abnormal sex steroid synthesis or hormone resistance. The consequent growth retardation may adversely impact final height.
Methods: 63 adolescents >10 years old, with IBD and without history of endocrine disorders, additional chronic inflammatory disease or congenital short stature, were followed over 12 months. Median age at diagnosis of Crohn's disease (CD) or ulcerative colitis/IBD unclassified (UC) was 11 years and age at study entry was 13.4 years. Anthropometry, pubertal stage, bone age, biochemical markers of growth and disease activity, treatment, nutritional support and quality of life were evaluated.
Results: 22% of children with CD had deficits in one or more growth parameters; median height SDS (HtSDS) was -0.13. The median difference between the chronological and bone age was 0.3 years (range -2.5 to 3.0). Sitting height at baseline and at 12 months was lower in IBD subjects than the normal population (P<0.001). Erythrocyte sedimentation rate (ESR) was the only marker of activity disease

associated with height velocity (HV) and height SDS variation (ΔHtSDS). Delayed attainment of peak HV in girls and attenuation of the peak HV in boys were found. Overall quality of life was not associated with HtSDS; only the body image domain was inversely related to HtSDS. At baseline median IGF-I SDS corrected for bone age was lower than the normal population (P=0.008). In contrast baseline median IGFBP-3 SDS corrected for bone age was higher than the normal population (P=0.002) and was positively associated with ALS levels (r=0.34, P=0.009). Median baseline IGF-I/IGFBP-3 ratio was negatively associated only with ESR (r=-0.33, P=0.016), but not with BMI or any marker of growth or disease activity (including CRP, albumin and haematocrit).
Conclusions: Boys with CD are more likely than girls to have a mild reduction in stature and an abnormal growth during adolescence, especially in the presence of active disease, but this does not seem to affect pubertal onset or progression. The described impact of IBD on final height is probably, in part, related to a diminished pubertal growth spurt.

Growth deceleration and delayed/impaired pubertal growth are still common issues in childhood-onset inflammatory bowel disease (IBD). Intact and functioning GH and sex hormone axes must be present for normal growth during puberty. The production by the liver of the three subunits of the 150-kDa complex consisting of IGF-I, IGFBP-3 and ALS is primarily under the control of GH. In healthy children, the molar ratio between IGF-I and IGFBP-3 reflects free, biologically-active IGF-I. Both IGF-I and IGFBP-3 increase during puberty but they show differential patterns, IGF-I increasing 5-fold while IGFBP-3 increases only 2.5-fold. This results in a higher IGF-I/IGFBP-3 molar ratio, reflecting increased free IGF-I levels when growth velocity is high [16]. This study provides a prospective clinical and biochemical analysis of growth and puberty in children with IBD. The strength of the study is its comprehensive evaluation of pubertal growth not only by clinical assessment but also by bone age and growth factor analysis. The low IGF-I/IGFBP-3 ratio, considering the absence of concurrent nutritional impairment, probably indicates an adverse effect of chronic inflammation on GH/IGF-I axis functioning.

Important for clinical practice: transition from paediatric to adult care

Anterior hypopituitarism in adult survivors of childhood cancers treated with cranial radiotherapy: a report from the St. Jude Lifetime Cohort Study

Chemaitilly W, Li Z, Huang S, Ness KK, Clark KL, Green DM, Barnes N, Armstrong GT, Krasin MJ, Srivastava DK, Pui CH, Merchant TE, Kun LE, Gajjar A, Hudson MM, Robison LL, Sklar CA
Department of Pediatric Medicine, Division of Endocrinology, St Jude Children's Research Hospital, Memphis, TN, USA
wassim.chemaitilly@stjude.org
J Clin Oncol 2015;33(5):492–500

Background: The risk of anterior pituitary deficiencies (APDs) in childhood cancer survivors (CCS) treated with cranial radiotherapy (CR) increases with dose and time elapsed from irradiation.
Methods: 748 adult CCS (394 men, mean age 34.2 years) treated with CR were included in this retrospective study. Anthropometric/clinical data, baseline hormonal profile, bone mineral density (BMD), exercise tolerance (six-minute walk test) and frailty (evaluated by low muscle mass, self-reported exhaustion, low energy expenditure, slow walking speed and muscle weakness) were analysed. Mean follow-up time was 27.3 years (range 10.8–47.7 years). GH deficiency was diagnosed by IGF-I level <-2 SDS. LH/FSH deficiency was diagnosed in men with total testosterone <200ng/dL plus LH <7IU/L and FSH <9.2IU/L, and in women aged <40 years by amenorrhea, estradiol levels <17pg/mL plus FSH <11.2IU/L. TSH deficiency was diagnosed by FT4 <0.9ng/dL plus TSH <4mUI/L. ACTH deficiency was diagnosed by morning cortisol level <5mcg/dL.
Results: The estimated point prevalence of APDs were: GH deficiency 46.5%, LH/FSH deficiency 10.8%, TSH deficiency 7.5% and ACTH deficiency 4%. The cumulative incidence of APDs increased with follow-up and 51.4% showed at least one APD. GH deficiency and LH/FSH deficiency were untreated in 99.7% and 78.5% of the affected adults, respectively. CR dose 22 to 29.9Gy was associated with GH deficiency; ≥22Gy with LH/FSH deficiency; and ≥30Gy with TSH and ACTH deficiencies. Untreated

GH deficiency was associated with decreased muscle mass and exercise tolerance. Untreated LH/FSH deficiency was associated with hypertension, dyslipidaemia, low bone mineral density and slow walking. Both GH deficiency and LH/FSH deficiency were independently associated with abdominal obesity, muscle weakness and low energy expenditure.
Conclusions: APDs are frequent in CSS treated with CR and their prevalence increases with time. GH deficiency is the most common defect, occurring after a relatively low radiation dose. Lifelong screening for APDs is recommended and the detrimental impact of untreated pituitary dysfunction on cardiovascular health and quality of life should be considered.

The risk of anterior pituitary deficiencies (APDs) in childhood cancer survivors (CCS) treated with cranial radiotherapy (CR) is known to increase in a time- and dose-dependent fashion. Nevertheless, extended long-term follow-up data are scarce and the impact of potentially undiagnosed or untreated deficiencies on overall health is not easily quantifiable. This large retrospective study screened for pituitary dysfunction in an established cohort of adult CCS exposed to CR. The long duration of follow-up is a major strength. The most surprising finding is the extremely high proportion of untreated patients with GH deficiency or central hypogonadism (99.7% and 78.5%, respectively). While the concerns over possible neoplastic risk might explain the decision not to treat GH deficiency, on the other hand it remains difficult to understand the high proportion of patients with untreated hypogonadism. The analysis of the correlation between untreated APDs (in particular GH deficiency and LH/FSH deficiency) and overall wellbeing and cardiovascular health is of particular interest and deserves further study.

Adult testicular volume predicts spermatogenetic recovery after allogeneic HSCT in childhood and adolescence

Wilhelmsson M, Vatanen A, Borgstro B, Gustafsson B, Taskinen M, Saarinen-Pihkala UM, Winiarski J, Jahnukainen K
Astrid Lindgren Children's Hospital, Department of Women's and Children's Health Q2:08, Karolinska University Hospital, Karolinska Institutet, Stockholm, Sweden
mari.wilhelmsson@ki.se
Pediatr Blood Cancer 2014;61(6):1094–1100

Background: Recovery of spermatogenesis in patients treated with haematopoietic stem cell transplantation (HSCT) is associated with age <25 years and no exposure to total body irradiation (TBI); it also depends on treatment before HSCT and chronic graft-versus-host disease (GvHD). Semen analysis, inhibin B and gonadotropins predict male fertility. Considering that 70–80% of adult testicular volume (ATV) consists of functional seminiferous tubules, this study evaluated the association between ATV and sperm production in a retrospective cohort with a longitudinal follow-up.
Methods: 106 males, receiving allogenic HSCT under the age of 18, who were pubertal or post-pubertal at the last follow-up visit, were studied. Chronic GvHD, time of spontaneous puberty, use of testosterone substitutive therapy, testicular volume, fathered pregnancies, serum gonadotropin levels were considered. Sub-groups were identified by diagnosis, Tanner stage and conditioning regimen [total body-irradiation (TBI), busulfan without TBI or total lymph-node irradiation (BU), cyclophosphamide (CY) and chemotherapy with total lymph-node irradiation and without TBI (TNI)].
Results: HSCT survivors showed small ATV (11 ± 6.2ml). Only two males had fathered children. ATV was smaller in leukaemia survivors, in patients undergoing HSCT in prepubertal years and in patients receiving TBI (compared with patients receiving BU or CY). TBI conditioning, being prepubertal at HSCT and single fraction TBI were independent determinants of ATV. Semen analysis, performed in 31 patients, was more often normal in non-leukaemia survivors, chemotherapy based conditioning, larger testicular volume and lower serum FSH levels. Similarly, higher FSH levels were found in leukaemia patients, in conditioning regimen with TBI and in single fraction TBI. Non-leukaemia diagnosis and adult testicular volume ≥15ml were factors independently associated with non-azoospermic semen analysis.
Conclusions: Conditioning before initiation of puberty caused small ATV. Larger ATV and lower serum levels of FSH among patients conditioned with busulfan or cyclophosphamide compared with TBI, suggest that chemotherapy-based conditioning may be less harmful than TBI for long term testicular function. Fractionated irradiation had less effect on fertility than single dose irradiation, in terms of both testicular volume and FSH levels.

The testicular germinal epithelium, where spermatogenesis occurs, is more vulnerable to radiation and chemotherapy than the Leydig cells, which secrete testosterone. Rapidly dividing germ cells are highly sensitive to toxic treatments. Spermatogenetic recovery of the surviving spermatogonia is a slow process and permanent infertility occurs when the reserve of spermatogonial stem cells is completely depleted. This study, with a mean follow-up of 13 years, provides useful information about the correlations between adult testicular volume (ATV) and semen profile in haematopoietic stem cell transplantation (HSCT) survivors. Male infertility is an important concern in these patients. It is confirmed that busulfan is less harmful than total body irradiation (TBI) for long-term testicular function. Semen analysis is the best predictor of male fertility, but it is not feasible in younger patients. ATV is more easily evaluated by the use of an orchidometer and is acceptable to young patients. Given the positive correlation between normal semen analysis, larger testicular volume and lower serum FSH levels found in this study, ATV may represent a useful tool to early predict fertility problems and drive further investigations.

Bone mineral density among long-term survivors of childhood acute lymphoblastic leukemia: results from the St. Jude Lifetime Cohort Study

Gurney JG, Kaste SC, Liu W, Srivastava DK, Chemaitilly W, Ness KK, Lanctot JQ, Ojha RP, Nottage KA, Wilson CL, Li Z, Robison LL, Hudson MM
Department of Epidemiology and Cancer Control, St. Jude Children's Research Hospital, Memphis, TN, USA
jggurney@memphis.edu
Pediatr Blood Cancer 2014;61(7):1270–1276

Background: Bone mineral density (BMD) deficits in children treated for acute lymphoblastic leukaemia (ALL) may be related both to treatments with methotrexate, glucocorticoid and/or cranial-craniospinal irradiation and to direct effects of ALL. The aim of this study was to determine the prevalence of BMD deficit in adult survivors of childhood ALL and to identify risk factors.
Methods: 845 subjects, aged 18 and older, treated for ALL at a single centre at least 10 years before, were studied. Trabecular volumetric BMD was evaluated by quantitative computed tomography (QCT) of the first and second lumbar vertebrae and expressed as Z-scores.
Results: Median age at ALL diagnosis was five years and median age at BMD evaluation was 31 years. BMD Z-score was >-1 in 70.5% of adults, between -1 to -2 in 23.8%, and <-2 in 5.7%. Endocrine dysfunctions were not associated with BMD. Cranial and cranio-spinal irradiations were associated with a higher risk of BMD Z-score ≤-1 (OR 2.05 and 1.88, respectively), more evident in women (P=0.01). 400 subjects had previously been tested for BMD for medical surveillance. At a median follow up 8.5 years, 67% of those who previously had a BMD Z-score <-2 improved. The strongest risk factor for persistent BMD deficit was high dose (>24Gy) cranial or cranio-spinal irradiation, with greater susceptibility in women.
Conclusions: Only 5.7% of ALL survivors had a BMD Z-score diagnostic for osteoporosis; 67% of patients with Z-score ≤-2 at first evaluation improved.

This study highlights the importance of preventing bone damage in patients treated for childhood acute lymphoblastic leukaemia (ALL), especially in those receiving high dose cranial or cranio-spinal radiotherapy, the primary predictor of suboptimal bone mineral density (BMD) found here. Notably, clinically low BMD was uncommon in this sample of adult survivors of childhood ALL and BMD Z-scores improved from adolescence to young adulthood. Considering that cranial and cranio-spinal irradiation is now used less frequently than in the past, concerns about persistently low BMD among adult childhood ALL survivors may be unwarranted. Strengths of the study include the large sample size and the long follow-up period between BMD evaluations. An additional strength is the use of quantitative computed tomography (QCT) rather than dual energy X-ray absorptiometry (DXA). QCT has several advantages over DXA: QCT measures trabecular bone, which is more sensitive to disease related bone change; QCT allows direct measurement of volumetric BMD, while DXA can only measure areal BMD and requires calculations for volumetric BMD that may be confounded by bone size; QCT does not overestimate BMD in obese individuals, while DXA BMD values are elevated in obese subjects because soft tissue attenuates X-ray beams [17]. The limits of this study, as the authors admit, are its cross-sectional design and lack of consideration of growth hormone deficiency, gonadal insufficiency, baseline BMD and ethnic background.

Impact of rituximab on height and weight in children with refractory steroid-dependent nephrotic syndrome

Sato M, Ito S, Ogura M, Kamei K
Division of Nephrology and Rheumatology, National Center for Child Health and Development, Tokyo, Japan
ito-shu@ncchd.go.jp
Pediatr Nephrol 2014;29(8):1373–1379

Background: Children with steroid-dependent nephrotic syndrome (SDNS) often show height growth retardation and obesity. Rituximab (RTX) may represent a promising therapeutic option to overcome steroid dependency. The aim of this study was to examine the impact of RTX on linear growth and obesity in children with SDNS.
Methods: 13 children with SDNS who were refractory to treatment with multiple immunosuppressive agents received RTX infusions. Mean follow-up from the first administration of RTX was 2.3 years. Height standard deviation score (SDS) and obesity index from prior to the initial RTX infusion throughout the last visit were assessed according to Japanese children's growth charts. The obesity index was calculated as: 100 x (body weight – standard body weight)/standard body weight (normal range: -20% to +20%).
Results: 10 of 13 patients (77%) showed a significant improvement of height SDS from -1.6 before RTX to -0.8 after RTX (P=0.03). Height SDS of seven of the eight patients with below-average height at first RTX improved from -2.6 to -1.4 SDS with RTX therapy. At the same time, the obesity index of 12 patients significantly improved (16.9% versus 3.1%; P=0.004). Following RTX therapy, the number of relapses and the mean prednisolone dose decreased.
Conclusions: Treatment with RTX may contribute to the improvement of height growth and obesity indexes in patients with SDNS suffering from severe side effects of steroid therapy.

The adverse impacts of chronic steroid therapy and chemotherapy on linear growth, body composition and bone health is well known. The severity of the damage is related to the total steroid dose. Rituximab is an anti-CD20 monoclonal antibody belonging to the emerging class of drugs defined as 'biologic' agents, acting directly against lymphocyte clones and cytokines implicated in the different tissue-specific autoimmune processes. This study is interesting but the sample size is very small and the follow-up is relatively short to draw definitive conclusions. Further studies are needed to assess whether the positive short-term effects on height SDS are accompanied by improved final height. Further issues that need to be clarified relate to the potentially severe side effects of 'biologic' agents (mostly serious infections) and their impacts on growth and general health. If the benefits of rituximab are confirmed in larger controlled studies, it could represent a valuable option to avoid the detrimental effects of chronic steroid therapy in children.

Infliximab maintains durable response and facilitates catch-up growth in luminal pediatric Crohn's disease

Church PC, Guan J, Walters TD, Frost K, Assa A, Muise AM, Griffiths AM
The Hospital for Sick Children, Toronto, ON, Canada
anne.griffiths@sickkids.ca
Inflamm Bowel Dis 2014;20(7):1177–1186

Background: Since 2000, infliximab (anti-TNF-alpha antibody) has been used for induction and maintenance of remission in children with moderate/severe luminal inflammatory Crohn's disease (CD) unresponsive to conventional immunomodulators, but paediatric long-term study are lacking. This report evaluates the impact of infliximab on linear growth and analyses factors associated with nonresponse to infliximab.
Methods: Clinical records of 195 children with luminal inflammatory CD, treated with infliximab as primary indication (with or without immunomodulators) since January 2000 to December 2011, were retrospectively reviewed. Activity disease index, auxological parameters, biochemical markers of inflammation, levels of infliximab and antibodies (Ab) to this drug (in case of loss of responsiveness) were assessed during a median follow-up time of 21.4 months.

Results: 81% of patients experienced complete response. The response was associated with male gender and shorter CD duration at the time of infliximab initiation. Males at Tanner stage 4/5 were more likely to respond than females at Tanner stage 4/5 (odds ratio=3.82). During the first years of follow-up, 35% required an individualised regimen modification and 16/157 complete responders experienced loss of response due to development of infliximab Ab. Combination therapy with immunomodulators decreased the risk of loss of responsiveness (hazard ratio=0.25; P=0.014). Children with Tanner stage 1/2 at induction had a higher decrease in height Z-score from diagnosis, but showed a height Z-score improvements during the two years after the start of infliximab therapy (P=0.001); this increase was maintained up to four-year post-induction.
Conclusions: Rate of clinical response in children treated with infliximab is high, especially in patients with shorter duration of the disease and in males with advanced puberty. Combination therapy after infliximab induction is useful to sustain the response and an earlier initiation of treatment is associated with an improvement of height growth.

Infliximab is a 'biologic' agent that acts as a TNF-blocker. It has been recently introduced in the treatment of inflammatory bowel disease (IBD) and other chronic inflammatory and autoimmune diseases. The short-term efficacy of infliximab to induce and maintain clinical remission in luminal inflammatory paediatric Crohn's disease (CD) is well established. Data concerning long-term maintenance of response of biologic agents are particularly important in children, considering their longer life expectancy, during which effective CD treatment is needed. This study, although retrospective, comprises the largest paediatric cohort reported to date. It confirms the efficacy and safety of infliximab in achieving clinical remission of luminal CD and in facilitating linear growth. The results on height gains need to be confirmed and compared with those obtained in children treated with previous therapeutic regimens. Finally, considering the early loss of response due to development of anti-infliximab antibodies, the real effect on adult height should be defined, before proposing the use of infliximab not only in patients who are unresponsive to conventional immunomodulators, but also as a first-line treatment.

New evidence

Diencephalic syndrome in childhood craniopharyngioma – results of German multicentre studies on 485 long-term survivors of childhood craniopharyngioma

Hoffmann A, Gebhardt U, Sterkenburg AS, Warmuth-Metz M, Müller HL
Department of Pediatrics, Zentrum für Kinder-und Jugendmedizin, Klinikum Oldenburg, Medical Campus University Oldenburg, Oldenburg, Germany
mueller.hermann@klinikum-oldenburg.de
J Clin Endocrinol Metab 2014;99(11):3972-3977

Background: Childhood craniopharyngioma (CP) is commonly associated with hypothalamic obesity. Atypical CP manifestations include the diencephalic syndrome (DS) characterised by failure to thrive or to maintain a normal body mass index (BMI).
Methods: This multicentre German study retrospectively analysed the 21 of 485 (4.3%) childhood CP patients with a BMI <-2SD at diagnosis. Anthropometric data were acquired from routine child health surveillance visits at birth, three to 10 days, three to four weeks, three to four months, six to seven months, 10 to 12 months, 21 to 24 months, 3.5 to four years and five years of age. BMI and height were further evaluated at CP diagnosis and at defined intervals after diagnosis. DS was identified in 11/21 children by demonstrated hypothalamic involvement. In these patients (DS-CP) clinical manifestations, weight gain before and after CP diagnosis and MRI appearances were analysed and compared with CP with normal weight at diagnosis (NW-CP) and obese CP patients (O-CP).
Results: Tumour size and location (at diagnosis) were similar in DS-CP and other CP patients. The weight difference between with DS-CP and NW-CP patients was first observed at age five years. DS-CP patients

still had a lower weight than O-CP patients at two years after CP treatment, but not at later follow-up. After eight to 12 years, low or high BMI SDS at diagnosis had no relevance. All CP patients were obese (median BMI +3.98 SD). No preventive effect of low weight at diagnosis on later obesity was evident.
Conclusions: DS is a rare clinical manifestation of childhood CP and is a differential diagnosis of failure to thrive. DS at the time of diagnosis in CP with hypothalamic involvement does not preclude progressive weight gain after diagnosis and treatment. Long-term follow-up reveals that all CP patients with hypothalamic involvement eventually develop obesity.

Craniopharyngioma (CP) is a rare intracranial embryonic neoplasm arising from remnants of Rathke's pouch. It shows low-grade histological malignancy, but due to its sellar and parasellar location may affect hypothalamic and pituitary function. The most common c inical manifestations at presentation include visual and endocrine impairments. Primary hypothalamic involvement and treatment-related hypothalamic lesions, resulting in pathological eating behaviour and obesity, may adversely affect prognosis and quality of life in survivors. Diencephalic syndrome (DS) is a rare clinical condition presenting in early infancy and characterised by profound emaciation with the absence of subcutaneous adipose tissue despite adequate or slightly reduced food intake, normal linear growth, alertness and euphoria. DS is usually associated with supratentorial midline space-occupying lesions involving the hypothalamus. Considering the rarity of CP, the strength of this study is its relatively large series of patients that allows the recognition of DS as a rare clinical manifestation of CP. As the authors state, results are limited due to the retrospective design. Assessments of tumour properties were confined to the small subgroup of patients with MRI scans of sufficient quality. This study suggests that DS at the time of diagnosis does not preclude progressive weight gain after treatment of CP with hypothalamic involvement. Obesity in these patients seems to be more related to treatment than to the initial tumour-related hypothalamic injury.

Bone turnover in long-term survivors of childhood acute lymphoblastic leukemia

Watsky MA, Carbone LD, An Q, Cheng C, Lovorn EA, Hudson MM, Pui CH, Kaste SC
Department of Cell Biology & Anatomy, Georgia Regents University, Augusta, GA, USA
skaste@stjude.org
Pediatr Blood Cancer 2014;61(8):1451–1456

Background: Impairment of bone mineral density (BMD) has been documented in acute lymphoblastic leukaemia (ALL) survivors. This study aimed to determine the impact of anthropometric, demographic and lifestyle factors on bone turnover markers in ALL survivors and their relationship with treatment and BMD.
Methods: 418 patients in continuous complete remission for at least five years were enrolled. None had received supplementation with calcium or vitamin D during the three months prior to study entry. Age at diagnosis, treatment history, physical activity, anthropometric measures and nutritional intakes were collected. Volumetric lumbar spine (LS)-BMD Z-score was determined by computed tomography (CT) scanner. Serum bone-specific alkaline phosphatase (BALP) and osteocalcin (OC) were considered as markers of bone formation; urinary N-telopeptide indexed to creatinine (NTX/Cr) was considered as a marker of bone resorption.
Results: Median age at diagnosis was 4.6 years and median age at study entry was 17 years. BALP and OC were higher in males than in females (60.8 versus 34.1 and 22.4 versus 15.1, respectively; $P<0.001$). Age and Tanner stage were inversely related to all markers ($P<0.001$), while BMI was inversely associated with OC and BTX/Cr. No relation was found between biomarkers and lifestyle factors, ALL treatment, dietary intake and LS-BMD Z-score. Lifestyle habits (as physical activity, tobacco use or dietary supplementation with calcium and vitamin D) were not associated with bone turnover indexes.
Conclusions: Long-term bone turnover in ALL survivors is not affected by different ALL treatments and it is not related to volumetric LS-BMD. Bone formation markers are related to age, pubertal stage and sex, as observed in healthy children. In contrast to healthy children, BMI is inversely related to OC and NTX/Cr and not related to BALP.

In adults, high bone turnover predicts low bone mineral density (BMD). However, the relationship between bone turnover and skeletal health outcomes in children is not clear. Bone turnover markers in children reflect not only bone remodelling but also new endochondral bone formation, longitudinal and diameter growth. The pubertal growth spurt is associated with marked increases in bone turnover markers concurrently with peak height velocity. Gender, nutritional status and pubertal stage are physiologic factors regulating bone turnover in healthy children. Vitamin D deficiency, premature birth and malnutrition may adversely impact bone turnover. The analysis of biochemical markers of bone turnover may provide insight into the impact of disease states, including cancer and chronic inflammatory diseases, on bone mass accrual. Bone turnover has been reported to be increased in children with acute lymphoblastic leukaemia (ALL) during glucocorticoid treatment and high intravenous doses of methotrexate have been reported to enhance osteoclastic activity [18]. In contrast, this study demonstrates that these immediate effects on bone turnover in ALL are temporary and ALL survivors had a long-term bone turnover similar to that of healthy children. The study was conducted in a single institution on a large population in follow up. The analysis of several biomarkers and volumetric BMD by computed tomography adds further value. A potential limitation is that data on bone turnover at diagnosis were lacking.

References

1. Sklar CA, Mertens AC, Mitby P, Occhiogrosso G, Qin J, Heller G, et al. Risk of disease recurrence and second neoplasms in survivors of childhood cancer treated with growth hormone: a report from the Childhood Cancer Survivor Study. J Clin Endocrinol Metab 2002;87:3136–3141.
2. Ergun-Longmire B, Mertens AC, Mitby P, Qin J, Heller G, Shi W, et al. Growth hormone treatment and risk of second neoplasms in the childhood cancer survivor. J Clin Endocrinol Metab 2006;91:3494–3498.
3. Friend KE, Radinsky R, McCutcheon IE. Growth hormone receptor expression and function in meningiomas: effect of a specific receptor antagonist. J Neurosurg 1999;91:93–99.
4. Friend KE, Khandwala HM, Flyvbjerg A, Hill H, Li J, McCutcheon IE. Growth hormone and insulin-like growth factor-I: effects on the growth of glioma cell lines. Growth Horm IGF Res 2001;11:84–91.
5. Crofton PM, Ahmed SF, Wade JC, Stephen R, Elmlinger MW, Ranke MB, et al. Effects of intensive chemotherapy on bone and collagen turnover and the growth hormone axis in children with acute lymphoblastic leukaemia. J Clin Endocrinol Metab 1998;83:3121–3129.
6. Kenney LB, Yasui Y, Inskip PD, Hammond S, Neglia JP, Mertens AC, et al. Breast cancer after childhood cancer: A report from the Childhood Cancer Survivor Study. Ann Intern Med 2004;141:590–597.
7. Nishi Y, Hamamoto K, Fujita N, Okada S. Empty sella/pituitary atrophy and endocrine impairments as a consequence of radiation and chemotherapy in long-term survivors of childhood leukaemia. Int J Hematol 2011;94:399–402.
8. Landier W, Armenian S, Bhatia S. Late effects of childhood cancer and its treatment. Pediatr Clin North Am 2015;62:275–300.
9. Gan HW, Spoudeas HA. Long-term follow-up of survivors of childhood cancer (SIGN Clinical Guideline 132). Arch Dis Child Educ Pract Ed 2014;99:138–143.
10. Brufani C, Ciampalini P, Grossi A, Fiori R, Fintini D, Tozzi A, et al. Glucose tolerance status in 510 children and adolescents attending an obesity clinic in Central Italy. Pediatr Diabetes 2010;11:47–54.
11. Neville KA, Cohn RJ, Steinbeck KS, Johnston K, Walker JL. Hyperinsulinemia impaired glucose tolerance, and diabetes mellitus in survivors of childhood cancer: Prevalence and risk factors. J Clin Endocrinol Metab 2006;91:4401–4407.
12. Zhang FF, Kelly MJ, Saltzman E, Must A, Roberts SB, Parsons SK. Obesity in pediatric ALL survivors: a meta-analysis. Pediatrics 2014;133:e704–715.
13. Chamorro-Vina C, Ruiz JR, Santana-Sosa E, Gonzalez Vicent M, Madero L, Perez M, et al. Exercise during hematopoietic stem cell transplant hospitalisation in children. Med Sci Sports Exerc 2010;42:1045–1053.
14. Dubner SE, Shults J, Baldassano RN, Zemel BS, Thayu M, Burnham JM, et al. Longitudinal assessment of bone density and structure in an incident cohort of children with Crohn's disease. Gastroenterology 2009;136:123–130.
15. Werkstetter KJ, Pozza SB, Filipiak-Pittroff B, Schatz SB, Prell C, Bufler P, et al. Long-term development of bone geometry and muscle in paediatric inflammatory bowel disease. Am J Gastroenterol 2011;106:988–998.
16. Juul A, Dalgaard P, Blum WF, Bang P, Hall K, Michaelsen KF, et al. Serum levels of insulin-like growth factor (IGF)-binding protein-3 (IGFBP-3) in healthy infants, children, and adolescents: the relation to IGF-I, IGF-II, IGFBP-1,IGFBP-2, age, sex, body mass index, and pubertal maturation. J Clin Endocrinol Metab 1995;80:2534–2542.
17. Link TM. Osteoporosis imaging: State of the art and advanced imaging. Radiol 2012;263:3–17.
18. Atkinson SA. Vitamin D status and bone biomarkers in childhood cancer. Pediatr Blood Cancer 2008;50:479–482.

Type 1 Diabetes Mellitus

Wieland Kiess

Hospital for Children and Adolescents, Centre for Pediatric Research, University of Leipzig, Leipzig, Germany

The prevalence and incidence of type 1 diabetes (T1DM) in children and adolescents is increasing in many countries. Outside the learned societies and the medical community this global epidemic has been largely neglected. Still, diabetes complications present a challenge to the individuals affected and their families as well as to the health care systems worldwide. Acute complications include episodes of hypoglycaemia which might lead to impaired cognitive development especially at a young age [1]. Chronic and long-term complications comprise diabetic macro- and microvascular complications including diabetic nephropathy, diabetic retinopathy, diabetic neuropathy and possibly also psychosocial sequelae. There is a large body of research that is being made available every year in regards to basic aspects of the aetio-pathogenesis of T1DM including its immunology. In addition, and importantly, modern new technologies applying continuous blood glucose monitoring, insulin pumps and computerised decision-making may make coping with the disease easier and lessen the pathologic burden in the long term. Stem cell biology and systems biology approaches may eventually lead to effective prevention or cure from the disease [1].

Basic science discoveries – generation of functional beta cells

Generation of functional human pancreatic beta cells in vitro

Pagliuca FW, Millman JR, Gürtler M, Segel M, Van Dervort A, Ryu JH, Peterson QP, Greiner D, Melton D

Department of Stem Cell and Regenerative Biology, Harvard Stem Cell Institute, Harvard University, 7 Divinity Avenue, Cambridge, MA, USA

dmelton@harvard.edu

Cell 2014;159(2):428–439

Background: The generation of insulin-producing pancreatic beta cells from stem cells in vitro would provide an unprecedented cell source for drug discovery and cell transplantation therapy in diabetes. However, insulin-producing cells previously generated from human pluripotent stem cells (hPSC) lack many functional characteristics of bona fide beta cells.
Results: Stem-cell-derived beta cells (SC-beta) were generated that express markers found in mature beta cells, flux Ca(2+) in response to glucose, package insulin into secretory granules and secrete quantities of insulin comparable to adult beta cells in response to multiple sequential glucose challenges in vitro. Furthermore, these cells secrete human insulin into the serum of mice shortly after transplantation in a glucose-regulated manner, and transplantation of these cells ameliorates hyperglycaemia in diabetic mice.
Conclusions: The authors report a scalable differentiation protocol that can generate hundreds of millions of glucose-responsive beta cells from hPSC in vitro.

Stem cell biology is being developed at an impressive speed. Our understanding of tissue-specific cell lineage and the genes and transcription factors that are involved in regulating stem cell differentiation into functional tissue is being supplemented by approaches to generate reliable sources for self-renewing progenitor cells. If one was to reliably and stably produce insulin-producing beta cells from stem cells and transplant them into the human body, a first step towards a cure of T1DM could be envisaged. However, key challenges still remain including the production of sufficient numbers of cells for research and transplantation and finally for clinical use in a large number of affected patients with T1DM. Recent approaches to this problem have shown that the presence of organ- and stage-specific mesenchyme improves the generation of progenitors, from endoderm to endocrine cells. Alternatively, utilisation of three-dimensional culture may improve the efficiency and yield of directed differentiation. There are still a vast number of persistent challenges that will need to be overcome before personalised cell-based therapy becomes a feasible strategy [2].

Basic science discoveries – insulin sensitisation

Endocrinisation of FGF1 produces a neomorphic and potent insulin sensitiser

Suh JM, Jonker JW, Ahmadian M, Goetz R, Lackey D, Osborn O, Huang Z, Liu W, Yoshihara E, van Dijk TH, Havinga R, Fan W, Yin YQ, Yu RT, Liddle C, Atkins AR, Olefsky JM, Mohammadi M, Downes M, Evans RM
Gene Expression Laboratory, Salk Institute for Biological Studies, La Jolla, CA, USA
Nature 2014;513:436–439

Background: Fibroblast growth factor 1 (FGF1) is an autocrine/paracrine regulator whose binding to heparan sulphate proteoglycans effectively precludes its circulation. Although FGF1 is known as a mitogenic factor, FGF1 knockout mice develop insulin resistance when stressed by a high-fat diet, suggesting a potential role in nutrient homeostasis.
Methods: The authors tested parenteral delivery of a single dose of recombinant FGF1 (rFGF1) in a diabetic mouse model.
Results: Chronic pharmacological treatment with rFGF1 increased insulin-dependent glucose uptake in skeletal muscle and suppressed the hepatic production of glucose to achieve whole-body insulin sensitisation. The sustained glucose lowering and insulin sensitisation attributed to rFGF1 were not accompanied by the side effects of weight gain, liver steatosis and bone loss associated with current insulin-sensitising therapies. The glucose-lowering activity of FGF1 could be dissociated from its mitogenic activity and was mediated predominantly via FGF receptor 1 signalling.
Conclusions: Administration of recombinant FGF1 results in potent, insulin-dependent lowering of glucose levels that is dose-dependent but does not lead to hypoglycaemia. The findings indicate an unexpected, neomorphic insulin-sensitizing action for exogenous non-mitogenic human FGF1 with therapeutic potential for the treatment of insulin resistance and type 2 diabetes.

It has been shown that an intact PPARγ-FGF1 axis is required for adaptive adipose remodelling and metabolic homeostasis [3]. Although feast and famine cycles illustrate that remodelling of adipose tissue in response to fluctuations in nutrient availability is essential for maintaining metabolic homeostasis, the underlying mechanisms remain poorly understood. Fibroblast growth factor 1 (FGF1) was identified as a critical transducer in this process in mice. The FGF1 axis is linked to the nuclear receptor PPARγ (peroxisome proliferator activated receptor γ), which is the adipocyte master regulator and the target of the thiazolidinedione class of insulin sensitising drugs. FGF1 is the prototype of the 22-member FGF family of proteins and has been implicated in a range of physiological processes, including development, wound healing and cardiovascular changes. It is thought that FGF1 is highly induced in adipose tissue in response to a high-fat diet and that mice lacking FGF1 develop an aggressive diabetic phenotype coupled to aberrant adipose expansion when challenged with a high-fat diet. Further analysis of adipose depots in FGF1-deficient mice revealed multiple histopathologies in the vasculature system, an increased inflammatory response, aberrant adipocyte size distribution and ectopic expression of pancreatic lipases. In conclusion, adipose induction of FGF1 upon feeding is regulated by PPARγ acting through an evolutionarily conserved promoter proximal PPAR response element within the FGF1 gene. Therefore, new physiologic mechanism of and new targets for insulin sensitisation will become known [3].

Immunology of T1DM – B-lymphocyte depletion

B-lymphocyte depletion with rituximab and beta-cell function: two-year results

Pescovitz MD, Greenbaum CJ, Bundy B, Becker DJ, Gitelman SE, Goland RS, Gottlieb PA, Marks JB, Moran A, Raskin P, Rodriguez H, Schatz DA, Wherrett DK, Wilson DM, Krischer JP, Skyler JS; Type 1 Diabetes TrialNet Anti-CD20 Study Group
University of Miami Diabetes Research Institute, Miami, FL, USA
Diabetes Care 2014;37(2):453–459

Background: The authors previously reported that selective depletion of B-lymphocytes with rituximab, an anti-CD20 monoclonal antibody, slowed decline of beta-cell function in recent-onset type 1 diabetes mellitus

(T1DM) at one year. Subjects were followed further to determine whether there was persistence of effect.
Methods: 87 subjects (aged eight to 40 years) were randomly assigned to, and 81 received, infusions of rituximab or placebo on days one, eight, 15 and 22. The primary outcome-baseline-adjusted mean 2-h area under the curve (AUC) serum C-peptide during a mixed-meal tolerance test (MMTT) at one year-showed higher C-peptide AUC with rituximab versus placebo. Subjects were further followed with additional MMTTs every six months.
Results: The rate of decline of C-peptide was parallel between groups but shifted by 8.2 months in rituximab-treated subjects. Over 30 months, AUC, insulin dose and HbA_{1c} were similar for rituximab and placebo. However, in evaluating change in C-peptide over the entire follow-up period, the rituximab group means were larger as compared within assessment times with the placebo group means using a global test (P=0.03). Odds ratio for loss of C-peptide to <0.2nmol/L following rituximab was 0.565 (P=0.064). B-lymphocytes recovered to baseline values by 18 months. Serum IgG levels were maintained in the normal range but IgM levels were depressed.
Conclusions: Like several other immunotherapeutic approaches tested, in recent-onset T1DM, rituximab delays the fall in C-peptide but does not appear to fundamentally alter the underlying pathophysiology of the disease.

Despite the fact that T-lymphocytes, interleukin-1 and antigen-presenting cells and macrophages have been implicated in the aetiopathogenesis of diabetes, antibody producing cells and B-cells in general have also been in the focus of research related to the immunology of diabetes. Selective depletion of B-cells might slow down the decline of beta-cell function in developing diabetes. In a recent report, the complexity of diabetes immunology has been demonstrated using elegant experiments with non-obese diabetes (NOD) mice, which are often used as an experimental model of type I diabetes (TID). Treatment with complete Freund's adjuvant (CFA) in pro-diabetic NOD mice inhibited diabetes progression by activating CD1d-specific natural killer (NK) T cells and inducing interleukin (IL)-17 secretion in innate immune cells. A combined treatment of IFA and L. Monocytogenes, a microbe that infects the liver and is primarily combatted by NK and cytotoxic T lymphocytes, was able to effectively delay TID development in the NOD mice. Increased levels of regulatory T cells were detected. Furthermore, IFA + L. monocytogenes mice exhibited higher levels of IgG2a, although no notable T-helper 1 cell response was observed when compared with the CFA or IFA control treated mice. Therefore both NK cells, T-helper cells, macrophages and B-lymphocytes act together in protecting and attacking intact beta-cells of the pancreas [4]. The first antibody-based therapeutic strategies to interfere with B-lymphocyte biology in order to slow progression of diabetes or even prevent immune cells to cause the disease have been designed and appropriate clinical studies are clearly under way.

Immunology of T1DM – regulatory T-cells

Therapy of type 1 diabetes with CD4(+)CD25(high)CD127-regulatory T cells prolongs survival of pancreatic islets – results of one year follow-up

Marek-Trzonkowska N, Myśliwiec M, Dobyszuk A, Grabowska M, Derkowska I, Juścińska J, Owczuk R, Szadkowska A, Witkowski P, Młynarski W, Jarosz-Chobot P, Bossowski A, Siebert J, Trzonkowski P
Department of Clinical Immunology and Transplantology, Medical University of Gdańsk, Dębinki 7, 80-210 Gdańsk, Poland
ptrzon@gumed.edu.pl
Clin Immunol 2014;153(1):23–30

Background: It is hypothesised that CD4(+)CD25(+)FoxP3(+) regulatory T cells (Tregs) can prevent destruction of pancreatic islets protecting from type 1 diabetes (T1DM).
Methods: Here the authors describe the results of one year follow-up of 12 T1DM children treated with autologous expanded ex vivo Tregs. Patients received either a single or double Tregs infusion up to the total dose of $30x10^6$/kg.
Results: No severe adverse effects were observed. The treatment did not impair post-immunisation antibody responses. Tregs infusion was followed by increase in Tregs number in peripheral blood. Most

of the patients responded to the therapy with increase in C-peptide levels (8/12 and 4/6 after the first and the second dose, respectively). Tregs administration resulted also in lower requirement for exogenous insulin (8/12 treated patients versus 2/10 untreated controls in remission) with two children completely insulin independent at one year.
Conclusions: Repetitive administration of Tregs is safe and can prolong survival of beta-cells in T1DM.

Autoimmune diabetes mellitus (DM) results from the destruction of pancreatic islet cells by activated T lymphocytes. T-cells are thought to being primed by activated dendritic cells (DC). Individualised therapy with ex-vivo DC manipulation and reinfusion has been proposed as a treatment for T1DM. In situ modulation of the DC phenotype in the host would be readily accessible and therefore feasible in large numbers of affected individuals. The expression of negative regulatory molecules, such as programmed death ligand 1 (PD-L1) and interleukin-1 receptor-associated kinase M (IRAK-M), are markedly increased upon DC treatments in rodents and in vivo transfer of treated DC into prediabetic NOD mice delays pancreatic insulitis. Pharmaceutical modulation of DC maturation and function in situ, and modulation of T-cell responses may represent a futuristic opportunity to treat autoimmune disease in general and diabetes in particular [5].

Immunology of T1DM – prevention

Hydrolyzed infant formula and early β-cell autoimmunity: a randomised clinical trial

Knip M, Akerblom HK, Becker D, Dosch HM, Dupre J, Fraser W, Howard N, Ilonen J, Krischer JP, Kordonouri C, Lawson ML, Palmer JP, Savilahti E, Vaarala O, Virtanen SM; TRIGR Study Group
Children's Hospital, University of Helsinki, Helsinki, Finland
if.iknisleh@pink.leakim
JAMA 2014;311:2279–2287

Background: The disease process leading to clinical type 1 diabetes (T1DM) often starts during the first years of life. Early exposure to complex dietary proteins may increase the risk of beta-cell autoimmunity in children at genetic risk for T1DM. Extensively hydrolysed formulas do not contain intact proteins. This study aimed to test the hypothesis that weaning to an extensively hydrolysed formula decreases the cumulative incidence of diabetes-associated autoantibodies in young children.
Methods: A double-blind randomised clinical trial of 2,159 infants with HLA-conferred disease susceptibility and a first-degree relative with T1DM recruited from May 2002 to January 2007 in 78 study centres in 15 countries; 1,078 were randomised to be weaned to the extensively hydrolysed casein formula and 1,081 were randomised to be weaned to a conventional cows' milk-based formula. The participants were observed to April 16, 2013. The participants received either a casein hydrolysate or a conventional cows' milk formula supplemented with 20% of the casein hydrolysate.
Main outcomes: Primary outcome was positivity for at least two diabetes-associated autoantibodies out of four analysed. Autoantibodies to insulin, glutamic acid decarboxylase and the insulinoma-associated-2 (IA-2) molecule were analysed using radiobinding assays and islet cell antibodies with immunofluorescence during a median observation period of 7.0 years (mean, 6.3 years).
Results: The absolute risk of positivity for two or more islet autoantibodies was 13.4% among those randomised to the casein hydrolysate formula (n=139) versus 11.4% among those randomised to the conventional formula (n=117). The unadjusted hazard ratio for positivity for two or more autoantibodies among those randomised to be weaned to the casein hydrolysate was 1.21 (95% CI, 0.94–1.54), compared with those randomised to the conventional formula, while the hazard ratio adjusted for HLA risk, duration of breastfeeding, vitamin D use, study formula duration and consumption and region was 1.23 (95% CI, 0.96–1.58). There were no clinically significant differences in the rate of reported adverse events between the two groups.
Conclusions: Among infants at risk for T1DM, the use of a hydrolysed formula, when compared with a conventional formula, did not reduce the incidence of diabetes-associated autoantibodies after seven years. These findings do not support a benefit from hydrolysed formula.

Toward primary prevention of type 1 diabetes

Skyler JS
Division of Endocrinology, Diabetes, & Metabolism, Pediatrics, and Psychology, University of Miami Miller School of Medicine, Miami, FL, USA
JAMA 2015;313:1520–1521

Background: There is a very urgent need for interventions for primary prevention of type 1 diabetes (T1DM) in children at genetically high risk. The incidence of T1DM has been progressively increasing during the past several decades, particularly among children younger than five years. At the same time, there has been substantial progress in understanding the pathogenesis of the disease and identifying those at risk of progressing to T1DM. *Results/Conclusions:* In children at genetic risk, diabetes-related autoantibodies appear, followed by the evolution of metabolic abnormalities and the eventual clinical appearance of the disease. If individuals identified by genetic markers subsequently undergo seroconversion and develop two or more diabetes-related autoantibodies, their risk of progression to T1DM is 75% over 10 years and appears to be almost inevitable over 20 years. However, attempts at both primary prevention, before seroconversion, and secondary prevention, in those with diabetes-related autoantibodies, have not been successful. The interventions evaluated to date have been limited to those deemed extremely safe, because such interventions would be used in at-risk individuals who may or may not actually progress to T1DM.

Numerous research groups around the world have tried to design interventions to prevent T1DM in high risk individuals. However, a large number attempts at primary prevention (that is, before seroconversion of subjects who are genetically at risk), as well as secondary prevention (that is, in those who already show antibodies against insulin and beta-cell specific proteins) have not been successful. Knip et al. describe the first outcomes of the large-scale TRIGR trial, which was based on the observations that beta-cell autoimmunity develops early in postnatal life and appears to be higher in infants exposed to cow's milk protein. The findings of this a priori prespecified endpoint, humoral beta-cell autoimmunity, dash the hopes raised by the initial pilot study. However, this impressively large and well-conducted trial is powered to assess effects of the intervention on the development of T1DM by 10 years of age, and we remain hopeful for those findings.

Once clinical diabetes has occurred, immunologic therapies will be targeted to prevent further damage to the pancreas and the insulin producing beta-cell in particular (secondary prevention). In the setting of antigen-specific therapy in allergy and type 1 diabetes, assays to monitor the immunological mechanisms of disease have been improving in recent years. Emerging advances in antigen-specific biomarkers have the potential to dramatically impact our understanding of T cell-mediated autoimmune diseases and inform more targeted immunotherapies against diabetes [6]. An ideal immunotherapy should inhibit the autoimmune attack, avoid systemic side effects and allow beta-cell regeneration. To re-establish tolerance to beta cells in T1DM, synthetic antigen-specific immunotherapy involving anti-apoptotic pathways have been developed. Specifically, phosphatidylserine-liposomes loaded with insulin peptides have been generated to simulate apoptotic cells recognition by antigen presenting cells [7]. Meanwhile, other recent studies suggest that parasite infections could trigger immune reactions capable of preventing immune reactions targeted against beta cells. Therefore, exposure towards helminths or against helminth antigens may be new principles of immune prevention of T1DM [8].

Molecular basis of diabetes complications – osteopontin

Osteopontin is a strong predictor of incipient diabetic nephropathy, cardiovascular disease, and all-cause mortality in patients with type 1 diabetes

Gordin D, Forsblom C, Panduru NM, Thomas MC, Bjerre M, Soro-Paavonen A, Tolonen N, Sandholm N, Flyvbjerg A, Harjutsalo V, Groop PH; FinnDiane Study Group
Diabetes Care 2014;37:2593–2600

Background: Osteopontin (OPN) is a multifunctional protein suggested to be a player in the arterial disease of patients with type 2 diabetes. However, its role for complications in patients with type 1 diabetes

(T1DM) is unknown. This aimed to investigate the associations between OPN and diabetic vascular complications and all-cause mortality in patients with T1DM.
Methods: Serum OPN was measured in 2,145 adults with T1DM without end-stage renal disease (ESRD; dialysis or transplantation) as part of the Finnish Diabetic Nephropathy (FinnDiane) Study. Data on renal status, cardiovascular disease (CVD) and all-cause mortality during follow-up were verified from medical files, hospital discharge registries and the Finnish National Death Registry, respectively. The median follow-up time was 10.5 (interquartile range 8.9–11.8) years.
Results: Serum OPN was higher at baseline in patients who developed incident microalbuminuria (16.0 ± 0.9 versus 14.1 ± 0.2microgram/L; P=0.04), progressed to ESRD (28.3 ± 1.7 versus 15.4 ± 0.2microgram/L; P<0.001), suffered an incident CVD event (20.2 ± 1.2 versus 15.5 ± 0.2microgram/L; P<0.001) or died (23.3 ± 1.4 versus 15.8 ± 0.2microgram/L; P<0.001) during follow-up. In multivariate Cox regression analysis, OPN was independently associated with the development of incident microalbuminuria, an incident CVD event and death, after adjustments for associated risk factors. Even after calculating reclassification indexes, OPN was predictive of CVD and all-cause mortality beyond the Framingham risk score covariates and hs-CRP.
Conclusions: Serum OPN is a strong predictor of incipient diabetic nephropathy, a first-ever CVD event and all-cause mortality in patients with T1DM. Serum OPN may be of clinical significance for the risk prediction of CVD events in patients with T1DM.

Biomarkers in autoimmune disease have been eagerly sought. For example, substantial effort has been made to identify biomarkers for multiple sclerosis that can improve disease diagnosis, predict disease progression and improve clinical outcomes. However, to date, few of these findings have proven clinically useful. Amongst the biomarkers used in multiple sclerosis research (such as miRNA and mRNA, myelin reactive T cells, Kir4.1 antibodies, osteopontin and microbiome associated lipopeptides) osteopontin has also been implicated in the aetiopathogenesis of diabetes [9]. Whether or not osteopontin will turn out to be useful in identifying people who are at risk to develop diabetes and whether or not new therapies will include osteopontin biologicals remains uncertain at present.

Molecular basis of diabetes complications - soluble receptor for AGE

Circulating concentrations of soluble receptor for AGE are associated with age and AGER gene polymorphisms in children with newly diagnosed type 1 diabetes

Salonen KM, Ryhänen SJ, Forbes JM, Härkönen T, Ilonen J, Laine AP, Groop PH, Knip M; Finnish Pediatric Diabetes Register
Children's Hospital, University of Helsinki and Helsinki University Central Hospital, Helsinki, Finland
Diabetes Care 2014;37(7):1975-1981

Background: This study analysed the relationship among soluble receptor for advanced glycation end products (sRAGEs), the clinical phenotype, HLA genotype and risk-associated single nucleotide polymorphisms (SNPs) in the AGER gene in a large population of Finnish children with newly diagnosed type 1 diabetes (T1DM).
Methods: Samples from 2,115 clinically phenotyped children <15 years of age in whom T1DM was diagnosed and 316 control subjects were analysed for sRAGEs. Three SNPs of AGER, previously associated with HLA-DR/DQ haplotype independent diabetes risk (rs2070600, rs9469089 and rs17493811), were analysed in 1,390 affected subjects.
Results: Children with T1DM and control subjects had similar sRAGE concentrations (1,171 versus 1,153pg/mL, P=0.48). There was a correlation between age at diagnosis and serum sRAGE concentrations (r=0.10, P<0.001) among the patients but not among the control subjects. Children <2 years of age had the lowest concentrations in the diabetic population (1,027 versus 1,181pg/mL, P<0.001) and the highest among the control subjects (1,329 versus 1,140pg/mL, P=0.04). Ketoacidosis at diagnosis was associated with reduced concentrations (1,086 versus 1,190pg/mL, P<0.001). HLA DR3/DR4 heterozygosity and the DR3 allele were associated with reduced sRAGE concentrations. The predisposing AA genotype of rs2070600 was associated with decreased sRAGE concentrations, while the protective CC genotype of rs9469089 was linked to increased concentrations.

Conclusions: Age and AGER polymorphisms are associated with the circulating sRAGE concentration among children with T1DM. The observations of reduced sRAGE concentrations in young children, in those with ketoacidosis and in carriers of the high-risk HLA DR3/DR4 genotype suggest that decreased sRAGE concentration reflects a more aggressive disease phenotype.

Metabolic control and serum lipids are related to the concentration of advanced glycation end products (AGEs) in the serum of children and adolescents with T1DM, as determined by fluorescence spectroscopy and nepsilon-(carboxymethyl)lysine ELISA [10]. It is now clear that soluble receptor for advanced glycation end products (sRAGEs) is also related to diabetes comorbidities and genetically linked to severity of disease. This does not come as a surprise as AGEs are a complex and heterogenous group of proteins that are formed by non-enzymatic glycation in a series of reactions and play a role in the pathogenesis of diabetes-related complications. Clinical studies have shown that serum levels of AGEs are correlated with clinical stages of diabetes complications such as retinopathy and nephropathy, and it is now clear that sRAGE concentrations are reduced in those with ketoacidosis.

Clinical care - clinic-integrated, low-intensity treatment

Randomised clinical trial of clinic-integrated, low-intensity treatment to prevent deterioration of disease care in adolescents with type 1 diabetes

Holmes CS, Chen R, Mackey E, Grey M, Streisand R
Department of Psychology, Pediatrics and Psychiatry, Virginia Commonwealth University, Richmond, VA Center for New Designs in Leadership and Scholarship, Georgetown University, Washington, DC, USA
cholmes@richmond.edu
Diabetes Care 2014;37(6):1535–1543

Background: This study aimed to evaluate the efficacy of two office-based treatments designed to prevent deterioration in glycaemic control in young adolescents with type 1 diabetes in a randomised clinical trial. An individualised, more intensive family teamwork coping skills program was compared with a diabetes education treatment.
Methods: A baseline assessment was followed by four brief treatment sessions and immediate post-testing over the course of 1.5 years. Families of 226 early adolescents (ages 11–14) were randomised to receive either individualised coping skills education or diabetes education as adjunctive treatment to quarterly medical appointments. Continued follow-up occurred at 3.5-month intervals for a long-term follow-up of up to three years. A post hoc usual care group facilitated comparisons of glycaemic control.
Results: Growth curve analysis showed that both treatment groups successfully prevented deterioration in adolescent disease care and simultaneously improved adolescent and parent quality of life that included indicators of more effective communication and reduced adherence barriers-without a concomitant increase in diabetes-related or general family conflict. However, contrary to expectation, the education group was more efficacious than the coping group in improvement of disease adherence and glycaemic control over a three-year follow-up.
Conclusions: Low-intensity office-based quarterly treatment can maintain or improve disease care adherence in early adolescence when provided to adolescent/parent dyads. Better outcomes are achieved when treatment goals and techniques match the needs of the targeted population.

Puberty is related to deterioration of glycaemic control and new concepts to keep metabolic control in good order during adolescence are required. The issue of transition from peadiatric to adult care is also of utmost importance and remains a challenge where the outcome is often unknown. In one study 52.5% of patients changed their health care provider at least once after transition. The mean frequency of changes was 1.47, and there was a decrease in clinic attendance rate after transition (8.5 ± 2.3/years versus 6.7 ± 3.2/years). Patients criticised the lack of arrangements, poor information about transfer and the specific age for transition (18 years) set by legislation. The transfer was considered a negative experience by 58 patients. The establishment of transition clinics and closer cooperation between specialists in peadiatric and adult medicine is mandatory [11].

Insulin analogs - are they worth it? Yes!

Grunberger G
Grunberger Diabetes Institute, Bloomfield Hills, MI, USA
grunberger@comcast.net
Diabetes Care 2014;37(6):1767-1770

Insulin analogs - is there a compelling case to use them? No!

Davidson MB
Department of Internal Medicine, Charles R. Drew University, Los Angeles, CA, USA
mayerdavidson@cdrewu.edu
Diabetes Care 2014;37(6):1771-1774

Background: The availability of insulin analogues has offered insulin replacement strategies that are proposed to more closely mimic normal human physiology. Specifically, there are a considerable number of reports demonstrating that prandial insulin analogues (lispro, aspart, glulisine) have pharmacokinetic and pharmacodynamic profiles closer to normal, with resulting faster onset and offset of insulin effect when compared with regular human insulin. In addition, basal insulin analogues (glargine, detemir) have been reported to offer longer duration of action, less variability, more predictability, less hypoglycaemia (especially nocturnal) and a favourable effect on weight. However, an argument against use of analogue insulins as compared with use of regular or NPH insulin is one that states that the effectiveness and risk of hypoglycaemia are the only two valid clinical outcomes that should be used to compare the analogue and human insulins. Thus, there remains a debate in some circles that analogue insulins are no more effective than human insulins, yet at a much higher financial cost. To provide an in-depth understanding of both sides of the argument, we provide a discussion of this topic as part of this two-part point-counterpoint narrative.

Results: In the counterpoint narrative presented here, Dr. Davidson provides his argument and defends his opinion that outside of a few exceptions, analogue insulins provide no clinical benefit compared with human insulins but cost much more. In the preceding point narrative, Dr. Grunberger provides a defense of analogue insulins and their value in clinical management and suggests that when evaluating the 'cost' of therapy, a much more global assessment is needed.

Modern insulins, old paradigms and pragmatism have been outlined by many authors: choosing wisely when deciding how to treat T1DM is still an individual choice and individualised medicine needs to be revisited. There is a clinical imperative to improve metabolic control in the treatment of patients with T1DM, but in doing so, hypoglycaemia should also be avoided. Insulin analogues and the assumption they would better mimic the pharmacokinetic profile of endogenous insulin secretion emerged as a magic bullet in the treatment of patients with T1DM but these assumptions are not always evidence-based. However, although insulin analogues have pharmaceutical properties, such as pharmacodynamic stability, reproducibility of action and a more physiological timing of action, which could possibly facilitate insulin use, the results obtained in clinical practice have not at all been as positive as one might have expected and as the pharmaceutical industry has led us to believe. Like all clinical decisions, the decision regarding which insulin would be better for the patient should be, if at all possible, evidence based [12].

Clinical care – diabetes self-care

Real-time support of pediatric diabetes self-care by a transport team

Franklin BE, Crisler SC Jr, Shappley R, Armour MM, McCommon DT, Ferry RJ Jr
Division of Pediatric Endocrinology, Department of Pediatrics, University of Tennessee Health Science Center, Memphis, TN, USA
bob@uthsc.edu
Diabetes Care 2014;37(1):81–87

Background: The study seeks to improve access for underserved patients via novel integration of Pedi-Flite (a critical care transport team) and to validate whether this safely enhances diabetes care and effectively expands the endocrine workforce.
Methods: The authors retrospectively analysed pager service use in a cohort of established diabetic patients (n=979) after inception of Pedi-Flite support. Outcomes included incidence and severity of recurrent diabetic ketoacidosis (DKA) and cost savings generated from reduced referrals to the emergency department (ED) and on-call endocrinologist. Descriptive statistics were generated to characterise the study population and ED visits for DKA, and logistic regression models to examine associations of pager use and likelihood of ED visitation and non-elective inpatient admission from an ED for DKA.
Results: Pager users comprised 30% of the patient population. They were younger but had more established diabetes than nonusers. While pager users were 2.75 times more likely than non-users to visit the ED for DKA ($P<0.0001$), their visits were less likely to lead to inpatient admissions (odds ratio 0.58; $P<0.02$). More than half (n=587) of all calls to the pager were resolved without need for further referral. Estimates suggest that 439 ED visits and 115 admissions were avoided at a potential cost savings exceeding 760,000 USD.
Conclusions: Integration of a transport service provides a novel, cost-effective approach to reduce disparities in diabetes care. Advantages include scalability, applicability to other disease areas and settings and low added costs. These findings enrich an emerging evidence base for telephonic care-management models supported by allied health personnel.

Diabetic acidosis still poses great risks for morbidity and mortality especially in young children [13]. Very often circumstances of manifestation, family and cultural background, financial resources and the health care system determine quality of care and the danger of ketoacidosis to occur either at manifestation or later during the disease course. This paper reports evidence in favour of telephone-based emergency hotlines and pager systems, which are now being widely used to reduce hospital admissions and critical incidences in children with T1DM [14].

New associations and chronic complications – chronic fatigue

Chronic fatigue in type 1 diabetes: highly prevalent but not explained by hyperglycemia or glucose variability

Goedendorp MM, Tack CJ, Steggink E, Bloot L, Bazelmans E, Knoop H
Expert Centre for Chronic Fatigue, Radboud University Nijmegen Medical Centre, Nijmegen, The Netherlands
hans.knoop@radboudumc.nl
Diabetes Care 2014;37(1):73–80

Background: Fatigue is a classical symptom of hyperglycaemia, but the relationship between chronic fatigue and diabetes has not been systematically studied. This study aimed to investigate the prevalence, impact and potential determinants of chronic fatigue in patients with type 1 diabetes mellitus (T1DM).
Methods: Out of 324 randomly selected T1DM outpatients, 214 participated in this cross-sectional observational study. Participants were compared with age- and sex-matched population-based controls. Chronic fatigue, functional impairments, current health status, comorbidity, diabetes-related factors and

fatigue-related cognitions and behaviours were assessed with questionnaires, and HbA_{1c} values and comorbidity were assessed with medical records. 66 patients underwent continuous glucose monitoring combined with an electronic fatigue diary for five days. Acute fatigue and four glucose parameters were determined: mean, variability and relative time spent in hypoglycaemia and hyperglycaemia.
Results: T1DM patients were more often chronically fatigued (40%; 95% CI 34–47%) compared with matched controls (7%; 95% CI 3–10%; P<0.001). Chronically fatigued patients had more functional impairments. Fatigue was the most troublesome symptom. Age, depression, pain, sleeping problems, low self-efficacy concerning fatigue, and physical inactivity were associated with chronic fatigue. Chronically fatigued patients spent slightly less time in hypoglycaemia (proportion 0.07 ± 0.06 versus 0.12 ± 0.10; P=0.025). Glucose parameters were not related to acute fatigue.
Conclusions: Chronic fatigue is highly prevalent and clinically relevant in T1DM. Its significant relationship with cognitive behavioural variables and weak association with blood glucose levels suggests that behavioural interventions could be helpful in managing chronic fatigue in T1DM.

Neurobehavioural symptoms are frequently reported in patients with diabetes. Fatigue symptoms and cognitive performance have been studied in one particular study using a dimensional approach. Specific dimensions of fatigue were assessed using the Multidimensional-Fatigue-Inventory (MFI). Cognitive performance on tests of choice reaction time, pattern recognition memory and spatial planning was evaluated using the Cambridge-Neuropsychological-Automated-Battery (CANTAB). Body mass index (BMI) and glycated-haemoglobin (HbA_{1c}) concentrations were collected, as well as information on diabetes complications and disease duration. Patients with type 2 diabetes, regardless of insulin treatment status, exhibited higher scores of fatigue, primarily in the dimensions of general and physical fatigue as well as reduced activity. Cognitive alterations, in the form of longer reaction times and impaired spatial planning, were also detected in type 2 diabetic patients treated with insulin. These alterations were overall unrelated to glucose control, as reflected in HbA_{1c} levels, and were not explained by complications and duration of diabetes. Interestingly and importantly, no specific alteration was measured in type 1 diabetic patients who exhibited fatigue scores and cognitive performance comparable to healthy participants. While associated with fatigue, increased BMI did not account for the relationship of type 2 diabetes with general fatigue and physical fatigue. BMI, however, modulated the association of type 2 diabetes with reduced activity and the association of insulin-treated type 2 diabetes with psychomotor slowing. These findings reveal specific fatigue and cognitive symptoms in patients with type 2 diabetes but not in individuals with autoimmune disease/ T1DM and suggest the involvement of differential pathophysiological processes possibly involving increased body weight and body weight perception [15].

New associations and chronic complications – multiple sclerosis

Higher relative risk for multiple sclerosis in a pediatric and adolescent diabetic population: analysis from DPV database

Bechtold S, Blaschek A, Raile K, Dost A, Freiberg C, Askenas M, Fröhlich-Reiterer E, Molz E, Holl RW
Department of Pediatrics, Medical University Munich, Munich, Germany
susanne.bechtold@med.uni-muenchen.de
Diabetes Care 2014;37(1):96-101

Background: Type 1 diabetes (T1DM) and multiple sclerosis (MS) are typical autoimmune diseases in children and young adults. This study aimed to assess the co-occurrence of T1DM and MS by estimating the relative risk (RR) for MS in a peadiatric and adolescent diabetic population and look for possible influencing factors.
Methods: Within the Diabetes Patienten Verlaufsdokumentation (DPV)-Wiss Project, from January 1995 to October 2012, data from 56,653 patients with T1DM were collected in 248 centres in Germany and Austria. Published data on German and Mid-European MS prevalence were taken for comparison. Multivariable regression analysis was used to identify confounders for co-occurrence of T1DM and MS.
Results: The RR for MS in patients with T1DM was 3.35–4.79 (95% CI 1.56–7.21 and 2.01–11.39,

respectively). Immigration status in all patients (P<0.05) and the presence of thyroid antibodies in male patients only (P=0.05) were identified as influencing factors on MS incidence. The month-of-birth pattern revealed that spring and summer births were more frequent in the population with T1DM and MS compared with those with T1DM only.

Conclusions: There is a higher risk of co-occurrence of MS in a peadiatric and adolescent T1DM population. Immigration status and thyroid antibodies in male patients were independent risk indicators for MS. Diabetic patients born during spring and summer had a higher risk for the development of MS. The authors suggest that environmental factors may modulate the risk for the co-occurrence of T1DM and MS.

It is interesting to note that associations between T1DM and other autoimmune diseases point to common causes and basic pathophysiological principles shared by autoimmune diseases in general. However, what molecules may be causative, whether or not genetic predisposition paves the way for immune alterations in general and how TH1 and TH2 helper cells interact to trigger autoimmune processes in the pancreas is largely unknown. It is therefore important to use large databases such as the DPV co-ordinated by the University of Ulm in Germany to search for such associations. This database consists of three basic modules: the diabetes documentation software DPV, semi-annual benchmarking for diabetes units (QC-DPV) and a data pool for diabetes research (DPV-SCIENT). The documentation system is available for general practices as well as for hospitals and it supports the daily routine work of the diabetes team. The system covers a superset for all-important datasets of quality initiatives in Germany. Longitudinal analyses of quality indicators related to diabetes are integrated. The vast majority of all patients less than 20 years of age with T1DM in Germany are now documented in DPV [16].

New associations and chronic complications – depression

Depression in adults in the T1D Exchange clinic registry

Trief PM, Xing D, Foster NC, Maahs DM, Kittelsrud JM, Olson BA, Young LA, Peters AL, Bergenstal RM, Miller KM, Beck RW, Weinstock RS; T1D Exchange Clinic Network
Jaeb Center for Health Research, Tampa, FL, USA
t1dstats@jaeb.org
Diabetes Care 2014;37(6):1563–1572

Background: Little is known about the frequency of depression in adults with type 1 diabetes (T1DM) or its relationship to diabetes outcomes. The T1DM Exchange clinic registry allows exploration of depression in a large, heterogeneous sample.

Methods: Participants ≥18 years old (n=6,172; median age 34 years; median diabetes duration 16 years; 55% female; and 89% non-Hispanic white) completed the eight-item Patient Health Questionnaire (PHQ-8), a validated, reliable measure of current depression. Probable major depression was defined in four ways: PHQ-8 ≥10, PHQ-8 ≥12, per diagnostic algorithm and as a continuous variable. Characteristics and clinical outcomes of those with and without depression were compared using logistic and linear regression models.

Results: Between 4.6 to 10.3% of participants were classified as having probable major depression, depending on the definition. Participants classified as depressed were more likely to be female, non-white race/ethnicity, to have a lower household income and lower education level, to exercise less often, to miss insulin doses and to have one or more complications (neuropathy, nephropathy, treatment for retinopathy or cardiovascular/cerebrovascular disease) (all P<0.01). HbA_{1c} was higher in the depressed versus not depressed groups (8.4 ± 1.7% [68 ± 8.6mmol/mol] versus 7.8 ± 1.4% [62 ± 15.3mmol/mol]; P<0.001). Occurrence of one or more diabetic ketoacidosis events (11 versus 4%; P<0.001) and one or more severe hypoglycaemic events (18 versus 9%; P<0.001) in the past three months was higher among depressed participants.

Conclusions: In the T1DM Exchange Clinic Registry, adults with probable major depression have worse clinical outcomes than those not depressed. Whether identification and treatment of depression improves diabetes outcomes requires study. Depression is common in T1DM and better identification and treatment of this comorbid condition is needed.

Depression is often associated with poor glycaemic control in patients with type 2 diabetes mellitus (T2DM). For example, data from a 24-month, prospective, observational study that evaluated glycaemic response in patients with T2DM who initiated insulin therapy (n=985) in five European countries were related to secondary measures which included patient-reported diagnosis of depression at baseline, severity of depressed/anxious mood (EuroQol [EQ]-5D item) and diabetes-related distress (Psychological Distress domain of the Diabetes Health Profile, DHP-18). Patients with higher depression parameters or distress at baseline had higher rates of microvascular complications at baseline. Patients with a diagnosis of depression or high diabetes-related distress had higher HbA_{1c} than patients without. These data stress the fact that a history of diagnosed depression, diabetes-related distress or depressed mood are associated with a higher rate of microvascular complications and higher HbA_{1c} in adults with type 2 diabetes [17]. These data need to be extrapolated into T1DM and the relationship between depressive symptoms and metabolic control in young children with T1DM should be studied carefully.

New associations and chronic complications - eating disorders

Eating disorders in girls and women with type 1 diabetes: a longitudinal study of prevalence, onset, remission, and recurrence

Colton PA, Olmsted MP, Daneman D, Farquhar JC, Wong H, Muskat S, Rodin GM
Department of Psychiatry, University Health Network, Toronto, ON, Canada; Department of Psychiatry, University of Toronto, Toronto, ON, Canada
Diabetes Care 2015;38(7):1212-1217

Background: Girls and women with type 1 diabetes (T1DM) are at increased risk for developing eating disorders (EDs), and these disorders are associated with serious diabetes-related medical complications. This study describes the longitudinal course of disturbed eating behaviour (DEB) and EDs in a cohort with T1DM.
Methods: 126 girls with T1DM receiving care for diabetes at The Hospital for Sick Children in Toronto participated in a series of seven interview-based assessments of ED behaviour and psychopathology over a 14-year period, beginning in late childhood. Survival analysis was used. Mean age was 11.8 ± 1.5 years at time one and 23.7 ± 2.1 years at time seven.
Results: At time seven, 32.4% (23/71) met the criteria for a current ED, and an additional 8.5% (6/71) had a subthreshold ED. Mean age at ED onset (full syndrome or below the threshold) was 22.6 years (95% CI 21.6–23.5), and the cumulative probability of onset was 60% by age 25 years. The average time between onset of ED and subsequent ED remission was 4.3 years (95% CI 3.1–5.5), and the cumulative probability of remission was 79% by six years after onset. The average time between remission of ED and subsequent recurrence was 6.5 years (95% CI 4.4–8.6), and the cumulative probability of recurrence was 53% by six years after remission.
Conclusions: In this longitudinal study, EDs were common and persistent, and new onset of ED was documented well into adulthood. Further research regarding prevention and treatment for this vulnerable group is urgently needed.

Clinical characteristics and outcome of 467 patients with a clinically recognised eating disorder identified among 52,215 patients with type 1 diabetes: a multicentre German/Austrian study

Scheuing N, Bartus B, Berger G, Haberland H, Icks A, Knauth B, Nellen-Hellmuth N, Rosenbauer J, Teufel M, Holl RW; DPV Initiative; German BMBF Competence Network Diabetes Mellitus
Institute of Epidemiology and Medical Biometry, Central Institute for Biomedical Technology, University of Ulm, Ulm, Germany
Diabetes Care 2014;37(6):1581-1589

Background: This study aimed to compare clinical characteristics and outcome of type 1 diabetes mellitus (T1DM) between patients with and without a clinically recognised eating disorder (ED).
Methods: 52,215 T1DM patients aged eight to <30 years from the prospective diabetes data acquisition

system DPV were analysed. 467 patients had an additional diagnosis of ED according to DSM-IV criteria (anorexia nervosa [AN], n=141 [female: 94.3%]; bulimia nervosa [BN], n=62 [90.3%]; and EDs not otherwise specified, including binge-eating disorder [EDNOS], n=264 [74.2%]). Groups were compared using multivariable regression. Cox proportional hazard ratios were calculated for the association between ED and retinopathy.
Results: After adjustment for age, sex and duration of diabetes, patients with ED had higher HbA_{1c} (no ED versus AN, BN or EDNOS, respectively: 8.29 ± 0.01% [67.1 ± 0.1mmol/mol] versus 8.61 ± 0.15% [70.6 ± 1.6mmol/mol], 9.11 ± 0.23% [76.1 ± 2.5mmol/mol] or 9.00 ± 0.11% [74.9 ± 1.2mmol/mol]) and a higher rate of pathological insulin injection sites (48.4 versus 64.3, 64.1 or 62.1%). Furthermore, ketoacidosis (5.7 ± 0.1 versus 12.1 ± 2.1, 18.0 ± 4.1 or 12.9 ± 1.6 events per 100 person-years) and hospitalisation (54.9 ± 0.3 versus 89.3 ± 6.0, 132.0 ± 12.7 or 91.0 ± 4.4 per 100 person-years) were more common and duration of hospital stay was longer (4.81 ± 0.01 versus 11.31 ± 0.21, 18.05 ± 0.48 or 8.44 ± 0.13 days per year). All P values were <0.05. Patients with BN and EDNOS had a 2.5-fold (95% CI 1.3–4.8) and a 1.4-fold (0.8–2.3) higher risk for retinopathy, whereas AN patients had no increased risk (0.9 [95% CI 0.4–2.3]).
Conclusions: Diabetes health care professionals should be aware of comorbid EDs in peadiatric/young-adult T1DM patients. An ED diagnosis is associated with worse metabolic control and higher rates of diabetes complications.

Eating disorders (ED) are highly prevalent in young women with T1DM. EDs are characterised by a persistent disturbance of eating that impairs health or psychosocial functioning. They are associated with increased rates of medical complications and mortality. Insulin omission is a unique purging behaviour available to individuals with T1DM. The standard treatment regimen for T1DM requires a major focus on food and eating patterns. Moreover, intensive insulin therapy is associated with increasing body weight. These factors, combined with the psychological burden of chronic disease management and depression, may contribute to ED. The comorbidity of ED in T1DM patients is associated with poorer glycaemic control and consequently higher rates of diabetes complications. Early recognition and adequate treatment of ED in T1DM is essential. However, research on treatment for diabetes and co-occurring eating disorders is sparse. Outcomes from multidisciplinary residential treatment for women with T1DM and eating disorders and the impact of treatment duration on outcomes has been studied. Treatment produced significant reductions in blood glucose, eating disorder symptoms and psychological concerns. Longer treatment duration was associated with greater improvements in psychological symptoms [18,19,20].

New associations and chronic complications - musculoskeletal complications

Musculoskeletal complications in type 1 diabetes

Larkin ME, Barnie A, Braffett BH, Cleary PA, Diminick L, Harth J, Gatcomb P, Golden E, Lipps J, Lorenzi G, Mahony C, Nathan DM; Diabetes Control and Complications Trial/Epidemiology of Diabetes Interventions and Complications Research Group
Massachusetts General Hospital Diabetes Research Center, Harvard University, Boston, MA, USA
Diabetes Care 2014;37(7):1863-1869

Background: The development of periarticular thickening of skin on the hands and limited joint mobility (cheiroarthropathy) is associated with diabetes and can lead to significant disability. This study aimed to describe the prevalence of cheiroarthropathy in the well-characterised Diabetes Control and Complications Trial/Epidemiology of Diabetes Interventions and Complications (DCCT/EDIC) cohort and examine associated risk factors, microvascular complications and the effect of former DCCT therapy (intensive [INT] versus conventional [CONV]) on its development.
Methods: This cross-sectional analysis was performed in 1,217 participants (95% of the active cohort) in EDIC years 18/19 after an average of 24 years of follow-up. Cheiroarthropathy, defined as the presence of any one of the following: adhesive capsulitis, carpal tunnel syndrome, flexor tenosynovitis, Dupuytren's contracture or a positive prayer sign, was assessed using a targeted medical history and standardised physical examination. A self-administered questionnaire (Disabilities of the Arm, Shoulder and Hand [DASH]) assessed functional disability.

Results: Cheiroarthropathy was present in 66% of subjects (64% of the INT group and 68% of the CONV group; P=0.1640) and was associated with age, sex, diabetes duration, skin intrinsic fluorescence, HbA_{1c}, neuropathy and retinopathy (P<0.005 for each). DASH functional disability scores were worse among subjects with cheiroarthropathy (P<0.0001).
Conclusions: Cheiroarthropathy is common in people with type 1 diabetes of long duration (-30 years) and is related to longer duration and higher levels of glycaemia. Clinicians should include cheiroarthropathy in their routine history and physical examination of patients with type 1 diabetes because it causes clinically significant functional disability

A recent study reported that the prevalence of juvenile idiopathic arthritis (JIA) is high in young people with T1DM. Diabetes onset was earlier in children with JIA (7.2 years versus 8.3 years, P=0.04). Children with JIA were smaller (SDS: -0.22 versus 0.09, P=0.004). Correspondingly, weight SDS was lower in patients with JIA (-0.02 versus 0.22, P=0.01). Surprisingly, HbA_{1c} was somewhat lower in children with JIA, possibly because of a more intensive treatment or a latent haemolysis caused by the inflammation (21). These data show that great care has to be taken when caring for children and adolescents with T1DM and co-morbidities must also be looked for in respect to musculoskeletal diseases [21].

Acute complications - neurological consequences of diabetic ketoacidosis

Neurological consequences of diabetic ketoacidosis at initial presentation of type 1 diabetes in a prospective cohort study of children

Cameron FJ, Scratch SE, Nadebaum C, Northam EA, Koves I, Jennings J, Finney K, Neil JJ, Wellard RM, Mackay M, Inder TE; DKA Brain Injury Study Group
Department of Endocrinology and Diabetes, Royal Children's Hospital, Murdoch Children's Research Institute, University of Melbourne, Melbourne, VIC, Australia
Diabetes Care 2014;37(6):1554-1562

Background: This study aimed to investigate the impact of new-onset diabetic ketoacidosis (DKA) during childhood on brain morphology and function.
Methods: Patients aged six to 18 years with and without DKA at diagnosis were studied at four time points: <48 hours, five days, 28 days and six months post-diagnosis. Patients underwent magnetic resonance imaging (MRI) and spectroscopy with cognitive assessment at each time point. Relationships between clinical characteristics at presentation and MRI and neurologic outcomes were examined using multiple linear regression, repeated-measures and ANCOVA analyses.
Results: 36 DKA and 59 non-DKA patients were recruited between 2004–2009. With DKA, cerebral white matter showed the greatest alterations with increased total white matter volume and higher mean diffusivity in the frontal, temporal and parietal white matter. Total white matter volume decreased over the first six months. For grey matter in DKA patients, total volume was lower at baseline and increased over six months. Lower levels of N-acetylaspartate were noted at baseline in the frontal grey matter and basal ganglia. Mental state scores were lower at baseline and at five days. Of note, although changes in total and regional brain volumes over the first five days resolved, they were associated with poorer delayed memory recall and poorer sustained and divided attention at six months. Age at time of presentation and pH level were predictors of neuroimaging and functional outcomes.

Neurological complications of diabetic ketoacidosis (DKA) are associated with significant mortality and morbidity. Acute cerebral infarction (CI) and extra pontine myelinolysis (EPM) at onset of T1DM still occur despite the fact that clinical management is being performed according to generally accepted guidelines. Putative risk factors that may predispose for the development of acute cerebrovascular complications are known. Not only cerebral oedema but also other severe neurological complications such as CI should be suspected when neurological deterioration occurs during DKA. [22]. In addition, and most importantly, as is shown here by Cameron and colleagues in Melbourne, neurologic sequelae of T1DM are of clinical relevance, may occur at any time and are based on alterations of brain geometry, connectivity and substance.

Acute complications - hypoglycaemia

A randomised trial of a home system to reduce nocturnal hypoglycaemia in type 1 diabetes

Maahs DM, Calhoun P, Buckingham BA, Chase HP, Hramiak I, Lum J, Cameron F, Bequette BW, Aye T, Paul T, Slover R, Wadwa RP, Wilson DM, Kollman C, Beck RW; In Home Closed Loop Study Group
Jaeb Center for Health Research, Tampa, FL, USA
Diabetes Care 2014;37(7):1885-1891

Background: Overnight hypoglycaemia occurs frequently in individuals with type 1 diabetes (T1DM) and can result in loss of consciousness, seizure or even death. The authors conducted an in-home randomised trial to determine whether nocturnal hypoglycaemia could be safely reduced by temporarily suspending pump insulin delivery when hypoglycaemia was predicted by an algorithm based on continuous glucose monitoring (CGM) glucose levels.
Methods: Following an initial run-in phase, a 42-night trial was conducted in 45 individuals aged 15–45 years with T1DM in which each night was assigned randomly to either having the predictive low-glucose suspend system active (intervention night) or inactive (control night). The primary outcome was the proportion of nights in which ≥1 CGM glucose values ≤60mg/dL occurred.
Results: Overnight hypoglycaemia with at least one CGM value ≤60mg/dL occurred on 196 of 942 (21%) intervention nights versus 322 of 970 (33%) control nights (odds ratio 0.52 [95% CI 0.43–0.64]; P<0.001). Median hypoglycaemia area under the curve was reduced by 81%, and hypoglycaemia lasting >2 hours was reduced by 74%. Overnight sensor glucose was >180mg/dL during 57% of control nights and 59% of intervention nights (P=0.17), while morning blood glucose was >180mg/dL following 21% and 27% of nights, respectively (P<0.001), and >250mg/dL following 6% and 6%, respectively. Morning ketosis was present <1% of the time in each arm.
Conclusions: Use of a nocturnal low-glucose suspend system substantially reduced overnight hypoglycaemia without an increase in morning ketosis.

Hypoglycaemic episodes are the most frequent acute complication of insulin treatment for T1DM. In particular, overnight hypoglycaemia occurs frequently in individuals with T1DM and can result in loss of consciousness, seizure or even death. Any systematic approach to reduce the frequency of hypoglycaemia should therefore be welcomed and therapeutic strategies have to include measures to reduce the severity and number of hypoglycaemic episodes especially in the young child with T1DM.

New technologies - outpatient closed-loop control

Safety of outpatient closed-loop control: first randomised crossover trials of a wearable artificial pancreas

Kovatchev BP, Renard E, Cobelli C, Zisser HC, Keith-Hynes P, Anderson SM, Brown SA, Chernavvsky DR, Breton MD, Mize LB, Farret A, Place J, Bruttomesso D, Del Favero S, Boscari F, Galasso S, Avogaro A, Magni L, Di Palma F, Toffanin C, Messori M, Dassau E, Doyle FJ
Center for Diabetes Technology and Department of Medicine, Division of Endocrinology, University of Virginia, Charlottesville, VA, USA
boris@virginia.edu
Diabetes Care 2014;37(7):1789-1796

Background: The aim of this study was to assess the effect size of hypoglycaemia risk reduction on closed-loop control (CLC) versus open-loop (OL) sensor-augmented insulin pump therapy in supervised outpatient setting.
Methods: 20 with type 1 diabetes (T1DM) initiated the study at the Universities of Virginia, Padova and Montpellier and Sansum Diabetes Research Institute; 18 completed the entire protocol. Each patient

participated in two 40-hour outpatient sessions, CLC versus OL, in randomised order. Sensor (Dexcom G4) and insulin pump (Tandem t:slim) were connected to Diabetes Assistant (DiAs)-a smartphone artificial pancreas platform. The patient operated the system through the DiAs user interface during both CLC and OL; study personnel supervised on site and monitored DiAs remotely. There were no dietary restrictions; 45-minute walks in town and restaurant dinners were included in both CLC and OL; alcohol was permitted.

Results: The primary outcome-reduction in risk for hypoglycaemia as measured by the low blood glucose (BG) index (LGBI)-resulted in an effect size of 0.64, P=0.003, with a twofold reduction of hypoglycaemia requiring carbohydrate treatment: 1.2 versus 2.4 episodes/session on CLC versus OL (P=0.02). This was accompanied by a slight decrease in percentage of time in the target range of 3.9–10 mmol/L (66.1 versus 70.7%) and increase in mean BG (8.9 versus 8.4 mmol/L; P=0.04) on CLC versus OL.

Conclusions: CLC running on a smartphone (DiAs) in outpatient conditions reduced hypoglycaemia and hypoglycaemia treatments when compared with sensor-augmented pump therapy. This was accompanied by marginal increase in average glycaemia resulting from a possible overemphasis on hypoglycaemia safety.

New technologies – real-time continuous glucose monitoring

Real-time continuous glucose monitoring among participants in the T1D Exchange clinic registry

Wong JC, Foster NC, Maahs DM, Raghinaru D, Bergenstal RM, Ahmann AJ, Peters AL, Bode BW, Aleppo G, Hirsch IB, Kleis L, Chase HP, DuBose SN, Miller KM, Beck RW, Adi S; T1D Exchange Clinic Network
Jaeb Center for Health Research, Tampa, FL, USA
t1dstats@jaeb.org
Diabetes Care 2014;37(10):2702-2709

Background: This study aimed to assess the frequency of continuous glucose monitoring (CGM) device use, factors associated with its use and the relationship of CGM with diabetes outcomes (HbA_{1c}, severe hypoglycaemia [SH] and diabetic ketoacidosis [DKA]).

Methods: Survey questions related to CGM device use one year after enrollment in the T1D Exchange clinic registry were completed by 17,317 participants. Participants were defined as CGM users if they indicated using real-time CGM during the prior 30 days.

Results: 9% of participants used CGM (6% of children <13 years old, 4% of adolescents 13 to <18 years, 6% of young adults 18 to <26 years and 21% of adults ≥26 years). CGM use was more likely with higher education, higher household income, private health insurance, longer duration of diabetes and use of insulin pump (P<0.01 all factors). CGM use was associated with lower HbA_{1c} in children (8.3% versus 8.6%, P<0.001) and adults (7.7% versus 7.9%, P<0.001). In adults, more frequent use of CGM (≥6 days/week) was associated with lower mean HbA_{1c}. Only 27% of users downloaded data from their device at least once per month and ≤15% of users reported downloading their device at least weekly. Among participants who used CGM at baseline, 41% had discontinued within one year.

Conclusions: CGM use is uncommon but associated with lower HbA_{1c} in some age-groups, especially when used more frequently. Factors associated with discontinuation and infrequent use of retrospective analysis of CGM data should be considered in developing next-generation devices and education on CGM use.

MD-Logic overnight control for 6 weeks of home use in patients with type 1 diabetes: randomised crossover trial

Nimri R, Muller I, Atlas E, Miller S, Fogel A, Bratina N, Kordonouri O, Battelino T, Danne T, Phillip M
The Jesse Z. and Sara Lea Shafer Institute for Endocrinology and Diabetes, National Center for Childhood Diabetes, Schneider Children's Medical Center of Israel, Petah Tikva, Israel Sackler Faculty of Medicine, Tel Aviv University, Tel Aviv, Israel
mosheph@post.tau.ac.il
Diabetes Care 2014;37(11):3025-3032

Background: This study aimed to evaluate the effect of the MD-Logic system on overnight glycaemic control at patients' homes.
Methods: Twenty-four patients (aged 12–43 years; average HbA_{1c} 7.5 ± 0.8%, 58.1 ± 8.4mmol/mol) were randomly assigned to participate in two overnight crossover periods, each including six weeks of consecutive nights: one under closed loop and the second under sensor-augmented pump (SAP) therapy at patients' homes in real-life conditions. The primary end point was time spent with sensor glucose levels below 70mg/dL (3.9mmol/L) overnight.
Results: Closed-loop nights reduced time spent in hypoglycaemia (P=0.02) and increased the percentage of time spent in the target range of 70–140mg/dL (P=0.003) compared with nights when the SAP therapy was used. The time spent in substantial hyperglycaemia above 240mg/dL was reduced by a median of 52.2% (interquartile range [IQR] 4.8, 72.9%; P=0.001) under closed-loop control compared with SAP therapy. Overnight total insulin doses were lower in the closed-loop nights compared with the SAP nights (P=0.04). The average daytime glucose levels after closed-loop operation were reduced by a median of 10.0mg/dL (IQR -2.7, 19.2; P=0.017) while lower total insulin doses were used (P=0.038). No severe adverse events occurred during closed-loop control; there was a single event of severe hypoglycaemia during a control night.
Conclusions: The long-term home use of automated overnight insulin delivery by the MD-Logic system was found to be a feasible, safe and an effective tool to reduce nocturnal hypoglycaemia and improve overnight glycaemic control in subjects with type 1 diabetes

While a cure for T1DM is still not possible, the primary goal of T1DM treatment is to attain near-normal glucose values. This remains out of reach for most children and adolescents with T1DM despite intensified insulin treatment in the form of insulin analogues, educational interventions, continuous glucose monitoring and sensor augmented insulin pumps. As outlined above, the main and most devastating problem is risk of hypoglycaemia. Additionally, patients' burn-out often develops with years of tedious day-to-day diabetes management, rendering available diabetes-related technology less efficient.

Over the past 40 years, attempts have been made towards computer-programmed insulin delivery in the form of closed loop. Automated insulin delivery may reduce human error in glycaemic control and considerably lessened the burden of routine self-management [23]. In a recent randomised, open-label, prospective controlled trial outpatient overnight glucose control with dual-hormone artificial pancreas, single-hormone artificial pancreas or conventional insulin pump therapy in children and adolescents with T1DM was studied [24]. Additional benefits of the dual-hormone (insulin and glucagon) artificial pancreas was compared with the single-hormone (insulin alone) artificial pancreas in outpatient unrestricted conditions. The time spent at a glucose concentration lower than 4.0mmol/L was median 0% (IQR 0.0–2.4) during nights with the dual-hormone artificial pancreas, 3.1% (0.0-6.9) during nights with the single-hormone artificial pancreas (P=0.032) and 3.4% (0–11.0) during nights with conventional pump therapy (P=0.0048 compared with dual-hormone artificial pancreas and P=0.32 compared with single-hormone artificial pancreas). 15 hypoglycaemic events (<3.1mmol/L for 20 min measured by sensor then confirmed with capillary glucose <4.0mmol/L) were noted during nights with conventional pump therapy compared with four events with the single-hormone system and no events with the dual-hormone system. None of the assessed outcomes varied with the order in which children and young adults were assigned interventions. These very recent data show that progress has indeed been made towards a functional and safe closed-loop artificial pancreas.

References

1. Kiess W, Gorski T, Penke M, Klamt S, Kapellen TM. Diabetes mellitus in children and adolescents – a global epidemic which has become neglected. J Pediatr Endocrinol Metab 2015;28:247–250.
2. Chmielowiec J, Borowiak M. In vitro differentiation and expansion of human pluripotent stem cell-derived pancreatic progenitors. Rev Diabet Stud 2014;11:19–34.
3. Jonker JW, Suh JM, Atkins AR, Ahmadian M, Li P, Whyte J, et al. A PPARγ-FGF1 axis is required for adaptive adipose remodelling and metabolic homeostasis. Nature 2012;485:391–394.
4. Wang HP, He ZG. Treatment with incomplete Freund's adjuvant and Listeria monocytogenes delays diabetes via an interleukin-17-secretion-independent pathway. Exp Ther Med 2015;9:1934–1938.
5. Hayashi T, Yao S, Crain B, Promessi VJ, Shyu L, Sheng C, et al. Induction of tolerogenic dendritic cells by a PEGylated TLR7 ligand for treatment of type 1 diabetes. PLoS One 2015;10:e0129867.
6. Odegard JM, Nepom GT, Wambre E. Biomarkers for antigen immunotherapy in allergy and type 1 diabetes. Clin Immunol 2015: S1521–6616(15)00218-1 (Epub ahead of print) doi:10.1016/j.clim.2015.05.023.
7. Pujol-Autonell I, Serracant-Prat A, Cano-Sarabia M, Ampudia RM, Rodriguez-Fernandez S, Sanchez A, et al. Use of autoantigen-loaded phosphatidylserine-liposomes to arrest autoimmunity in type 1 diabetes. PLoS One 2015;10:e0127057.
8. Méndez-Samperio P1, de-la-Rosa-Arana JL. Prevention of type 1 diabetes through parasite infection. Immunotherapy 2015;7(6):595–598.
9. Housley WJ, Pitt D, Hafler DA. Biomarkers in multiple sclerosis. Clin Immunol 2015 Jul 2. pii: S1521–6616(15)00219–3. (Epub ahead of print) doi:10.1016/j.clim.2015.06.015.
10. Galler A, Müller G, Schinzel R, Kratzsch J, Kiess W, Münch G. Impact of metabolic control and serum lipids on the concentration of advanced glycation end products in the serum of children and adolescents with type 1 diabetes, as determined by fluorescence spectroscopy and nepsilon-(carboxymethyl)lysine ELISA. Diabetes Care 2003;26:2609–2615.
11. Busse FP, Hiermann P, Galler A, Stumvoll M, Wiessner T, Kiess W, et al. Evaluation of patients' opinion and metabolic control after transfer of young adults with type 1 diabetes from a paediatric diabetes clinic to adult care. Horm Res 2007;67:132–138.
12. Schaan BD, Scheffel RS. Modern insulins, old paradigms and pragmatism: choosing wisely when deciding how to treat type 1 diabetes. Diabetol Metab Syndr 2015;7:35.
13. Kapellen T, Vogel C, Telleis D, Siekmeyer M, Kiess W. Treatment of diabetic ketoacidosis (DKA) with 2 different regimens regarding fluid substitution and insulin dosage (0.025 vs. 0.1 units/kg/h). Exp Clin Endocrinol Diabetes 2012;120:273–276.
14. Kapellen TM, Dost A, Leludas C, Kiess W. Patient acceptance and use of an emergency telephone hotline service in peadiatric diabetes care. Diabetes Care 1998;21:1365.
15. Lasselin J, Layé S, Barreau JB, Rivet A, Dulucq MJ, Gin H, et al. Fatigue and cognitive symptoms in patients with diabetes: relationship with disease phenotype and insulin treatment. Psychoneuroendocrinology 2012;37:1468–1478.
16. Grabert M, Schweiggert F, Holl RW. A framework for diabetes documentation and quality management in Germany: 10 years of experience with DPV. Comput Methods Programs Biomed 2002;69:115–121.
17. Ascher-Svanum H, Zagar A, Jiang D, Schuster D, Schmitt H, Dennehy EB, et al. Associations between glycaemic control, depressed mood, clinical depression, and diabetes distress before and after insulin initiation: an exploratory, post hoc analysis. Diabetes Ther 2015 Jul 10 (Epub ahead of print).
18. Moosavi M, Kreisman S, Hall L. Intentional hypoglycaemia to control bingeing in a patient with type 1 diabetes and bulimia nervosa. Can J Diabetes. 2015;39:16–17.
19. Dickens YL, Haynos AF, Nunnemaker S, Platka-Bird L, Dolores J. Multidisciplinary residential treatment of type 1 diabetes mellitus and co-occurring eating disorders. Eat Disord 2015;23:134–143.
20. Sivertsen B, Petrie KJ, Wilhelmsen-Langeland A, Hysing M. Mental health in adolescents with type 1 diabetes: results from a large population-based study. BMC Endocr Disord 2014;14:83.
21. Hermann G, Thon A, Mönkemöller K, Lilienthal E, Klinkert C, Holder M, et al. Diabetes Patienten Verlaufsdokumentation-initiative; Federal Ministry of Education and Research Competence Network Diabetes Mellitus. Comorbidity of type 1 diabetes and juvenile idiopathic arthritis. J Pediatr 2015;166:930–935.
22. Petzold S, Kapellen T, Siekmeyer M, Hirsch W, Bartelt H, Siekmeyer W, et al. Acute cerebral infarction and extra pontine myelinolysis in children with new onset type 1 diabetes mellitus. Pediatr Diabetes 2011;12:513–517.
23. Battelino T, Omladič JŠ, Phillip M. Closed loop insulin delivery in diabetes. Best Pract Res Clin Endocrinol Metab 2015;29:315–325.
24. Haidar A, Legault L, Matteau-Pelletier L, Messier V, Dallaire M. Outpatient overnight glucose control with dual-hormone artificial pancreas, single-hormone artificial pancreas, or conventional insulin pump therapy in children and adolescents with type 1 diabetes: an open-label, randomised controlled trial. Lancet Diabetes Endocrinol 2015;3(8):595–604.

Obesity and Weight Regulation

Martin Wabitsch, Daniel Tews, Christian Denzer, Julia von Schnurbein, Anja Moss, Stephanie Brandt, Heike Vollbach and Pamela Fischer-Posovszky

Division of Paediatric Endocrinology and Diabetes, and Endocrine Research Laboratory, Department of Paediatrics and Adolescent Medicine, University of Ulm, Ulm, Germany

We have been very happy to get 1,350 papers out of our established search strategy in PubMed which have been saved in our 2015 Yearbook EndNote database. We have then selected 19 papers which in our mind have been the most exciting ones.

The highlights in this year chapter are publications about new developments in the leptin field, MC4R and SIM1 related mutations and a systematic review on the evaluation of conservative obesity treatment programmes. Furthermore, the present Yearbook chapter on obesity and weight regulation covers a broad research area. Obesity and weight regulation is a multidisciplinary research field.

Leptin – the voice of adipose tissue

20 years of leptin. What we know and what the future holds

O'Rahilly S

MRC Metabolic Diseases Unit, Metabolic Research Laboratories, Wellcome Trust-MRC Institute of Metabolic Science, University of Cambridge, Cambridge, UK

so104@medschl.cam.ac.uk

J Endocrinol 2014;223:E1–E3

Background: It is now the 20th anniversary of the discovery of leptin, a hormone produced by adipose tissue, which provides critical signals to the organism regarding the status of its energy stores.
Methods: This article introduces a special issue of the *Journal of Endocrinology*. The articles in this issue are dedicated to different aspects of the biology of leptin.
Results: This introductory article by Steve O'Rahilly and the following articles by some of the world leaders in leptin research, provide an excellent overview on the current knowledge of leptin biology and the exciting open research questions that are currently under investigation.
Conclusion: Leptin circulates at levels proportional to body fat and serves as an afferent signal in a negative feedback loop that regulates food intake and metabolism to maintain homeostatic control of body weight. Before the detection of leptin the existence of a system maintaining homeostatic control of energy balance was unclear. Therefore the identification of leptin has uncovered a new endocrine system that also links changes in nutrition to adaptive responses in most if not all other physiological systems.

Back in 1959 the first classic parabiosis experiments (parabiosis is a method in which two living organisms are joined together surgically and develop a shared circulatory system) were performed by Cummings and Hervey [1], providing the first evidence of a circulating factor affecting body fat stores. Coleman subsequently undertook the well-known parabiosis experiments in *ob/ob* and *db/db* mice [2], demonstrating that the *ob/ob* mouse lacks a circulation factor to which the *db/db* mouse was resistant. At the time when these experiments were performed the technical resources available were limited. Two decades later, Jeff Friedman was able to identify this circulating factor through positional genetic cloning methods in the mouse. The subsequent identification of the leptin receptor [3] and its disruption in the *db/db* mouse [4,5] were additional landmarks on the way of our current understanding of body weight regulation.

It has been subsequently shown that leptin acts in part by activating POMC neurons and inhibiting NPY/AGRP neurons besides other neural populations that also play a role, either as direct neural targets or downstream. The identification of leptin and its receptor have provided an entry point for delving into the neural mechanism that control not only body weight but also complex behaviours.

This special issue of *Journal of Endocrinology* includes articles on signalling assemblies of the leptin receptor [6], connecting leptin signalling to biological function [7], elucidating the role of leptin and the reproductive function [8,9], as well as reports on the experiences of human recombinant metreleptin in human leptin deficiency syndromes [10]. Finally, a review by DePaoli summarises clinical data on a subset of the potential utilities of leptin as a therapeutic for general or common obesity and its metabolic consequences including type 2 diabetes and non-alcoholic fatty liver disease [11]. Rosenbaum and Leibel summarise the human physiology of leptin and body weight regulation with a special emphasis on the idea of preventing the decrement in leptin induced by weight loss by leptin substitution, and thereby abrogating some of the 'energy-saving' responses to weight loss [12].

The articles together also indicate new research areas in leptin physiology that have the potential to illuminate the role of this fascinating adipose-derived hormone in a variety of biological functions and to optimise its use to benefit human health.

Biologically inactive leptin and early-onset extreme obesity

Wabitsch M, Funcke JB, Lennerz B, Kuhnle-Krahl U, Lahr G, Debatin KM, Vatter P, Gierschik P, Moepps B, Fischer-Posovszky P
Division of Pediatric Endocrinology and Diabetes, Department of Pediatrics and Adolescent Medicine, Ulm University, Ulm, Germany
martin.wabitsch@uniklinik-ulm.de; pamela.fischer@uniklinik-ulm.de
N Engl J Med 2015;372:48–54

Background: Congenital leptin deficiency is a rare cause of early-onset extreme obesity characterised by the absence of leptin in circulation. A 2-year-old boy with early-onset extreme obesity and high immunoreactive circulating levels of leptin is described here.
Methods: Leptin gene sequencing was performed on DNA from the patient. Cloning and secretion studies using HEK293 cells; binding, internalisation and competition studies; and experimental animal studies with nonmutant and D100Y leptin produced in baculovirus-infected Trichoplusia ni BTI-Tn-5B1-4 cells have been applied to investigate the pathomechanism of the disease.
Results: Overexpression studies confirmed that the mutant protein (change from aspartic acid to tyrosine at amino acid position 100 (p.D100Y)) is secreted but neither binds to nor activates the receptor. Furthermore, the mutant protein failed to reduce food intake and body weight in leptin-deficient ob/ob mice. Finally, treatment of the patient with recombinant human leptin (metreleptin) normalised eating behaviour and reduced rapidly body weight due to a reduction mainly in body fat mass.
Conclusion: A new disease entity is described here, due to a mutation in the leptin gene that is characterised by a protein lacking biological activity. Therefore, circulating leptin levels normal in relation to body fat mass do not rule out disease causing mutations in the leptin gene and might obscure the correct diagnosis.

The phenomenon of bio-inactive hormones has been described for several other protein hormones such as TSH, LH, ACTH, STH, IGF-1 and insulin. In such cases, single amino acid substitutions give rise to protein hormones that display immunoreactivity in commonly used assays but lack biological activity. This illustrates that immunoassay-based diagnostic tests may have potential limitations when a disease-causing mutation is suggested.

The clear clinical phenotype of our patient that was characterised by early-onset hyperphagia including food-seeking behaviour leading to extreme weight gain, led us to the hypothesis of a bio-inactive mutated leptin protein which would be unable to mediate the satiety signal to the central nervous system. Our experimental studies have proven this hypothesis. We have shown that the mutant leptin was unable to induce the phosphorylation of Stat3 in leptin receptor–overexpressing HEK293 cells since it was not able to bind to the receptor. In *ob/ob* mice, lacking circulating leptin, treatment with the mutant leptin had no influence on food intake or body weight development, whereas, the wild-type leptin led to a clear reduction in food intake and body weight. To examine whether the high endogenous levels of the mutated leptin would possibly interfere with exogenous supplementation with metreleptin we have performed a competition assay treating leptin receptor-overexpressing HEK293 cells with increasing concentrations of wild-type leptin (3–1000ng/ml) in the presence and/or absence of high concentrations of recombinant D100Y leptin (100 and 300ng/ml). These experiments showed that there was no competition of wild-type and mutant protein for leptin receptor activation. These results suggested that the high levels of mutated leptin in the circulation of the patient would not interfere with the metreleptin treatment. This whole set of experiments has been the necessary prerequisite for starting the treatment with metreleptin which finally has been successful.

In the meantime, we have detected further patients with biologically inactive leptin who are being treated successfully with metreleptin. We suggest that congenital leptin deficiency due to biologically inactive leptin associated with high circulating hormone levels should be considered in all patients with early-onset extreme obesity due to hyperphagia and food-seeking behaviour. Circulating levels of leptin that appear normal in relation to body mass index or fat mass do not exclude disease-causing mutations in the leptin gene. Treatment of these patients will not only result in rapid weight loss but also in an improvement of metabolic, hormonal and immunological abnormalities associated with leptin deficiency.

Transition in adolescent obesity: who cares?

Transition to adult care in adolescent obesity: a systematic review and why it is a neglected topic

Shrewsbury VA, Baur LA, Nguyen B, Steinbeck KS
Academic Department of Adolescent Medicine, The Sydney Children's Hospital at Westmead, NSW, Australia
vanessa.shrewsbury@health.nsw.gov.au
Int J Obes 2014;38:475–479

Background: Childhood obesity is a chronic disease with increasing numbers of affected children and adolescents. There is a need of transition of these patients to adult services. However, transition of obese adolescents is not yet well established, and many open questions have to be solved.
Methods: This study aimed to identify the formal transition services or transition guidelines existing internationally. Two systematic reviews of the published and 'grey' literature were performed via searches of relevant databases, search engines and websites.
Results: Only a total of six of the identified documents contained information on transition in adolescent obesity – however, the most detailed documents provided only a brief statement recommending that transition services should take place.
Conclusion: So far, transition care for obese adolescents has been neglected. There is an absence of published intervention programmes/policies and a brevity of clinical guidance. Therefore, transition of adolescents with obesity is a priority research area.

The majority of adolescents with obesity will remain overweight or obese in adulthood [13,14]. The well-established and serious long- and short-term health implications of obesity make it a priority to improve services for weight management in young people. Although the evidence basis is limited, lifestyle interventions exist that are capable of producing modest weight loss. In addition, there is a clear need for improving medical care of adolescents and young adults with obesity with respect to the diverse comorbidities related to obesity.

Therefore, this article has picked up an important, so far neglected area of medical care in adolescent medicine and transitional medicine.

Transition means the purposeful planned movement of patients from paediatric to adult services. This is necessary and is key to help young people with chronic health conditions. The aim of transitional care has been described as providing health care that is 'uninterrupted, coordinated, developmentally appropriate, psychosocial sound and comprehensive' [15]. This systematic review found no evidence of empirical research on transition of adolescence with obesity and only a few clinical statements containing brief recommendations on this topic.

In our view, there are four medical challenges which show that there is an urgent need for transition recommendations and clinical studies in the area of transition: 1) *Body weight development in obese adolescents and young adults:* The clinical experience teaches us that obese adolescents gain up to 10 to 15 kg per year in weight and this development clearly will continue until mid-adulthood. Behavioural-based programmes, in some cases pharmacological treatment and in selected cases also surgical treatment will be necessary to control weight development and to reduce comorbidity. 2) *Treatment of comorbidities:* A considerable percentage of obese adolescents have manifest comorbidities, for example, hypertension, fatty liver disease, sleep apnoea syndrome, disturbed glucose regulation, depression and others. There is a need for evidence-based treatment of these comorbidities. Only a minority of patients in transitional age-group is treated adequately [16]. 3) *Behaviour-based treatment programmes:* classical behaviour-based treatment programmes for weight management are not accepted by the majority of obese adolescents, and in addition, show high dropout rates. Therefore, new conservative treatment approaches need to be established for this age-group. 4) *Structured care for extremely obese adolescents:* This special group of patients may not profit from behaviour-based weight management programmes. Bariatric surgery may be an option in some of these patients. However, this should only be performed in clinical studies and documented in registries due to the unknown risk of these operations and the subsequent changes in physiology. In addition, these extremely obese groups especially need specified multidisciplinary care for the diverse comorbidities. Finally, this care should also aim at helping these young people to find a place in the society, such as getting into apprenticeships, as well as to access the job market.

Chronotype, BMI and dietary behaviour

Associations among late chronotype, body mass index and dietary behaviors in young adolescents

Arora T, Taheri S
Weill Cornell Medical College in Qatar, Qatar Foundation, Education City, Doha, Qatar
staheri@me.com
Int J Obes (Lond) 2015;39(1):39–44

Background: Paediatric obesity and overweight has become a serious health problem with a prevalence rate ranging between 15–40% in developed countries. Despite an enormous amount of research, so far the pathophysiology leading to obesity is not explained satisfactorily. In adults, short sleep duration and/or poor sleep quality have been shown to add to obesity development. As adolescents transition through puberty, they progressively develop a later chronotype, resulting in sleep loss. However, little is known whether chronotype is associated with body mass index (BMI) or dietary behaviours in adolescents.
Methods: A total of 511 young adolescents (11–13 years) from eight secondary schools across the Midlands region in the UK participated in the Midlands Adolescent Schools Sleep Education Study (MASSES), to assess the relationships between chronotype and BMI z-score as well as dietary habits. Height (cm) and weight (kg) were objectively measured for BMI calculation and participants completed a questionnaire to assess sleep and dietary habits. A subsample of 236 adolescents wore wrist actigraphy for seven days to estimate average sleep duration and sleep efficiency.
Results: Definitely evening chronotype was associated with an increased BMI z-score compared with definitely morning chronotype (β=0.51, P<0.01, after adjustment). Higher frequency of consuming unhealthy snacks, night-time caffeine consumption and inadequate daily intake of fruit/vegetables were also associated with later chronotype (all P≤0.01). Actigraphy estimated sleep duration was an independent predictor of BMI z-score (β=-0.36, P<0.001). Sleep efficiency did not predict BMI z-score after adjustment (β=-0.03, P=0.07).
Conclusions: This study shows that young adolescents with a later chronotype have an increased risk for a higher BMI and poorer dietary behaviours independently of sleep duration or efficiency. Sleep hygiene education may help adolescents to improve their sleeping habits.

The authors describe a highly interesting and important topic. As we come to understand that most of our physiological processes underlie a circadian rhythm, an increasing number of research projects focus on chronobiology. An important term in this area is 'circadian misalignment', meaning that daily routine is performed without concept of a person's natural rhythms (for example sleeping during daytime). It has long been shown in large population studies that reduced sleep, sleep fragmentation and also marked circadian misalignment (for example shift work) are associated with an increased risk for obesity and metabolic disturbances [17, 18]. Unsurprisingly, a late chronotype (late bedtimes) and increased misalignment due to socially enforced early wakening times (so-called 'social jet lag') are also associated with increased BMI [19] and also metabolic disturbances [20] in adults.

A number of studies have described the impact of sleep duration on obesity in adolescents, however with inconsistent results, possibly due to subjective measurements of sleep (for review see [21]). Also, none have taken chronotype or social jet lag into their considerations.

Here, the authors describe the first study of chronotype and BMI in young adolescents. Since adolescents develop a progressively later chronotype during puberty [22] this is a very important question. They recruited a large cohort and confirmed subjectively reported chronotypes by actimetry in a subsample. As in adults [19], adolescents showed a progressive increase of BMI score with greater 'evening chronotype'. However the difference in BMI-z scores between 'definitely morning' and 'definitely evening' chronotypes was not very large (-0.36 ± 0.81 versus 0.14 ± 1.06) in a cohort with a surprisingly low prevalence of overweight (8.6%). The authors also replicated a former finding that a late chronotype in adolescents is associated with unhealthy eating habits [23]. Again, as a limitation the consumption of unhealthy snacks was most likely under-reported (~50% reported 'only sometimes/rarely consume unhealthy snacks').

Still, these results are important. We cannot change the chronotype of our children and adolescents, but good sleep hygiene might enable even late chronotypes to receive more sleep. In addition, we should strive to influence the social environment that forces most adolescents to rise too early for their chronotype. Further studies are needed to confirm these findings, to assess the impact of chronotype on metabolic outcomes in adolescents and most importantly to assess long-term effects of improved sleeping habits on BMI and metabolic functions.

MC4R – the story goes on

Functional characterization of variants in MC4R gene promoter region found in obese children

Tan KM, Ooi SQ, Ong SG, Kwan CS, Chan RM, Seng Poh LK, Mendoza J, Heng CK, Loke KY, Lee YS
Department of Pediatrics, Yong Loo Lin School of Medicine, National University Health System, Singapore
paeleeys@nus.edu.sg
J Clin Endocrinol Metab 2014;99:E931–E935

Background: Mutations in the melanocortin-4 receptor (*MC4R*) gene are known to be the most common cause of human monogenetic obesity. Although the coding region of the *MC4R* gene and its variants are well characterised, only a few studies report on the promoter region. Yet the literature does not report about variants upstream of the translational site with functional relevance.
Methods: The promoter region 1,500 bp upstream of *MC4R* gene was sequenced in 267 unrelated children and adolescents with severe early-onset obesity. They were previously screened negative for variants in the coding regions of the *MC4R* and *MC3R* genes. In silico and in vitro analyses were performed. Transcriptional activities were investigated in transiently transfected cells by luciferase assay.
Results: Two novel heterozygous single nucleotide polymorphisms (SNP) (c.-105C>G and c.-803A>G) in the promotor region of the *MC4R* gene were identified in two unrelated Malay boys. In silico analysis by PROMO predicted the disruption in transcription factor binding sites. Compared with the wild type, both variants showed significantly reduced transcriptional activity (c.-105C>G: 1.14 fold; c.-803A>G

1.61 fold) in the in vitro studies. However penetrance seems to be variable among family members. Another rare but already known SNP (c. -216C>T) was found. It did not show alterations in transcriptional activity.
Conclusion: For the first time, rare variants in the promoter region of the *MC4R* gene were identified that resulted in reduced transcriptional activity. These variants were found in children with early-onset obesity.

The *MC4R* gene is located on chromosome 18q22 and encodes for a seven transmembrane G-protein coupled receptor. It is widely expressed in the brain, including hypothalamus, thalamus, cortex, brainstem and spinal cord [24,25]. Hypothalamic activation of *MC4R* reduces food intake and increases energy expenditure. Dysfunction impairs energy homeostasis, respectively body weight regulation. Since variants in the *MC4R* gene lead to the most common cause of monogenetic obesity [26], its coding region is well characterised. More than 150 different nonsense, frame shift or mis-sense mutations are currently known [27].

The promoter region of the *MC4R* gene is defined as -556 to -416 bp upstream of the MC4R translational start site. In addition a region -1,926 bp upstream to the translational start site regulates transcriptional activity [28]. *MC4R* transcription seems to be influenced by regulators like nescient helix-loop-helix-2 and Sp transcription factor family. Corresponding binding sites have been identified within this region [29,30].

So it seems plausible that genetic variation in the *MC4R* promoter region might influence expression and consequently the translation of the *MC4R* gene. Here, the authors studied the in vitro effect of SNPs in the promoter region of the MC4R gene on basal transcriptional activity. They report two novel mis-sense mutations (c.-803A>G and c.-105C>G) that reduce mRNA transcription. However, further post-transcriptional studies might elucidate the impact of these variants on the pathogenesis of severe obesity.

The effects of the variants reported here showed variable intra-familial penetrance. This phenomenon has been described for mutations in the coding region of the *MC4R* gene [31]. Both patients were heterozygous for the novel SNP and the nature of phenotype and its penetrance in homozygous individuals remain to be described.

SIM 1 – the story goes on

Mutation screen of the SIM1 gene in pediatric patients with early-onset obesity

Zegers D, Beckers S, Hendrickx R, Van Camp JK, de Craemer V, Verrijken A, Van Hoorenbeeck K, Verhulst SL, Rooman RP, Desager KN, Massa G, Van Gaal LF, Van Hul W
Department of Medical Genetics, University of Antwerp, Antwerp, Belgium
wim.vanhul@ua.ac.be
Int J Obes (Lond) 2014;38(7):1000–1004

Background: The transcription factor SIM1 (Single-minded 1) is involved in the control of food intake and in the pathogenesis of obesity. In some patients with severe obesity, rare loss-of-function SIM1 mutations have been found.
Methods: 561 severely overweight and obese children and adolescents and 453 lean adults were screened for mutations in the coding region of the SIM1 gene. To evaluate the effect of the mutations on SIM1 transcriptional activity, luciferase reporter assays were performed.
Results: Mutation analysis identified four novel non-synonymous coding variants in SIM1 in four unrelated obese individuals (p.L242V, p.T481K, p.A517V and p.D590E). For two of these variants (p.T481K and p.A517V), a decrease in SIM1 transcriptional activity was observed. In the lean control population, four other rare SIM1 variants without loss of transcriptional activity were identified (p.G408R, p.R471P, p.S492P and p.S622F).

Conclusions: In this study, the presence of rare *SIM1* variants in both an obese paediatric population and a population of lean adult controls was demonstrated. Functional in vitro analysis of SIM1 might help to distinguish pathogenic mutations from benign variants.

Identification of two novel loss-of-function SIM1 mutations in two overweight children with developmental delay

Montagne L, Raimondo A, Delobel B, Duban-Bedu B, Noblet FS, Dechaume A, Bersten DC, Meyre D, Whitelaw ML, Froguel P, Bonnefond A
European Genomic Institute for Diabetes, Lille, France
p.froguel@imperial.ac.uk, murray.whitelaw@adelaide.edu.au
Obesity (Silver Spring) 2014;22(12):2621-2624

Background: In some obese patients with developmental delay and further abnormalities including Prader-Willi-like syndrome, deletions on chromosome 6q have been found. In some of these patients, these deletions included the gene for SIM1. In addition, many of the obese patients identified with rare variants in the *SIM1* gene, showed also neurological abnormalities. The aim of the current study was to ascertain whether functional relevant *SIM1* mutations can be found in children presenting primarily with neurodevelopmental abnormalities.
Methods: *SIM1* was sequenced in 283 children presenting with developmental delay and at least overweight. The effect of the identified mutations on SIM1 transcriptional activity in stable human cell lines was assessed using luciferase gene reporter assays.
Results: Two novel mutations (p.R296G and p.S309G) in two boys with variable degrees of cognitive deficits were identified. Both mutations showed a strong loss-of-function effect on SIM1 transcriptional activity. However, the child carrying the p.R296G variant presented with more severe additional symptoms than the p.S309G carrier (obesity, compulsive eating, neonatal hypotonia versus overweight only).
Conclusions: Severe loss-of-function SIM1 mutations can be associated with a spectrum of developmental delay phenotypes and obesity. Therefore, *SIM1* sequencing should be considered in patients presenting with developmental delay, especially if they harbour further Prader-Willi-like aspects.

A further approach to unravel the pathophysiology of overweight and obesity is to search for genes causing obesity or at least rendering subjects more prone to obesity. Several new genes have been identified in the last years (see also Yearbook 2014 [32]); however, many have been identified only in very few patients or show a highly variable penetrance, so their contributions to obesity in their carriers remain unclear.

Mutations in the *SIM1* gene are perhaps the most intensively studied 'new' mutations [32]. In mice, SIM1 is important for the development and function of the paraventricular nucleus of the hypothalamus [33] and is believed to act downstream of the MC4-receptor [34]. On the population level, common SIM1 variants are associated with BMI in Pima Indians [35] and white male Americans [36] but not in a cohort of female or black Americans [36] nor in a French cohort [37].

Functional heterozygous *SIM1* mutations co-segregate with obesity only with a variable penetrance [38], however heterozygous rare variants are consistently found in patients with overweight/obesity [38–41]. Many mutation carriers also show neurological abnormalities. Zegers et al strengthen the evidence that rare variants in the SIM1 gene might cause or at least predispose to severe obesity. Unfortunately, they were unable to perform co-segregation analysis. However, they demonstrated convincingly that functional analysis of rare non-synonymous variants in the *SIM1* gene might help to distinguish between benign and pathogenic changes.

Deletions on chromosome 6q are long-known to cause neurological deficits [42]. However, affected patients harbour different length deletions, some encompassing SIM1 and others not [43]. Many, but not all, patients show a combination of behavioural and neurological changes, termed 'Prader-Willi-like syndrome' (developmental delay, learning disability, severe food-seeking, hyperphagia and obesity). Because of these known neurological abnormalities, Montagne et al took a different approach to identify *SIM1* mutations. Instead of screening severely obese patients, they screened for mutations in this gene in patients with developmental delay who in addition were at least overweight. They identified two new rare variants with a strong loss-of-function-effect. Screening for *SIM1* mutations should be considered in further patients with developmental delay, especially with PWS-like aspects. Apart from the direct clinical implications, this study also reminds us very nicely that it is often worthwhile to consider new approaches to answer common questions.

Linking back to the paper on chronotype and obesity (see Arora and Taheri above), it is intriguing to learn, that SIM1 and its partners for heterodimerisation, ARNT1 and 2, are part of the same family as the most well-known transcriptional activators of the circadian clock in mammals, CLOCK and BMAL1. Both pairs are so called basic helix-loop-helix PER-ARNT-SIM (bHLH-PAS) proteins. The Per-Arnt-Sim (PAS) domain is highly conserved throughout nature. Members of this family are often found in pathways that regulate responses to environmental changes including circadian pathways (for review see [44]). So far there is no evidence that mutations in *SIM1* gene lead to disturbances in the circadian rhythms of affected patients but this aspect might be worth a new study.

Methylphenidate and food choices

Methylphenidate decreases fat and carbohydrate intake in obese teenagers

Danilovich D, Mastrandrea LD, Cataldi L, Quattrin T
Women and Children`s Hospital of Buffalo, Department of Pediatrics, School of Medicine and Biomedical Sc ences, University of Buffalo, Buffalo, NY, USA
tquattrin@upa.chob.edu
Obesity 2014;22(3):781–785

Background: Behaviours associated with non-homeostatic feeding are regulated by the mesolimbic system and dopamine signalling. Dopamine inhibits the expression of neuropeptide Y, a promoter of food intake. Methylphenidate (MPH) alters central dopamine levels. MPH action is based on selective binding to dopamine transporter, leading to increased dopamine within neuronal synapses. The purpose of the study was to investigate the effect of a single dose of MPH on fat, carbohydrate and total energy intake in obese adolescents. Furthermore, an association between variable number repeats (VNTR) polymorphism in the 3´-untranslated region of the dopamine transporter gene (DAT1) and dose-response reduction in caloric intake was investigated.
Methods: Participants for this randomised, single-blind, placebo-controlled, within subject study were recruited from paediatric practices in the urban and suburban areas of Buffalo. Inclusion criteria were: 10–18 years, BMI $\geq 95^{th}$ percentile for age and gender, pubertal tanner stage ≥ 2; n=29 subjects fulfilled the inclusion criteria and were eligible for the study. Two standardised test meals were conducted within a window of 14–21 days. Participants arrived at the centre between 7 and 9 am. Subjects were given MPH (0.3mg/kg) or placebo and had to wait for one hour prior to test meal. Participants were offered a standard tray from which they could choose an array of breakfast options that included foods with high and low fat and carbohydrate content. Subjects were instructed to consume as much or as little as they wished. Participants were instructed not to read, talk on the phone or text-message during the test meal. Food was weighted before and after the meal. Energy intake (EI) from carbohydrates (CHO), fat and total energy was calculated. From the n=29 eligible subjects for the study, n=7 failed to initiate the study or were excluded. Data from n=22 completers (n=7 males) were analysed. At the first test meal visit, a DNA sample was collected. DAT1 VNTR polymorphism analysis was performed.
Results: Total EI following MPH treatment was lower compared with placebo ($P>0.05$). EI from CHO and fat was lower following MPH treatment compared with placebo. Total EI, EI from CHO and fat decreased with MPH in the late pubertal group (T4–T5), but not in the early pubertal group (T2–T3). There was no association between DAT1 genotype and EI responses to MPH.

MPH is a well-known treatment for ADHD in children and adults. Common side effects are appetite suppression and weight loss. In obese patients inappropriately high EI often plays a key role. The effect of a single-dose of MPH on EI and on EI from macronutrients has been investigated in adults

[45] and in obese adults [46]. A significant reduction in EI [45,46] and in fat intake [45] following MPH treatment has been described. To study whether this effect is also observable in obese adolescents, Danilovich et al designed a randomised placebo-controlled crossover study to test the effect of a single-dose of MPH. As for adults, in obese adolescents total EI as well as EI from CHO and from fat was lower on MPH compared with placebo. To sum up, MPH and possibly other agents that increase brain dopamine by blocking its reuptake and synthesis could be pharmacologic agents in the treatment of obesity by inhibiting eating behaviour.

Childhood obesity and bone strength

Bone fractures in children: is there an association with obesity?

Sabhaney V, Boutis K, Yang G, Barra L, Tripathi R, Tran TT, Doan Q
Department of Pediatrics, British Columbia Children's Hospital, Vancouver, BC, Canada
vsabhaney@cw.bc.ca
J Pediatr 2014;165:313–318

Background: Musculoskeletal sequelae of childhood obesity, such as slipped capital femoral epiphysis, Blount diseases and recurrent pain are well described. Whether childhood obesity is also associated with an increased risk of acute musculoskeletal injuries is an unresolved issue with studies reporting controversial results.
Methods: The present study is a prospective study conducted in the setting of paediatric emergency departments (ED) at two tertiary care centres. Otherwise healthy children between the age of two and 17 years presenting to the ED with non-penetrating extremity injuries were eligible for study inclusion. The main outcome measure of the study was the odds of an extremity bone fracture based on BMI category.
Results: 2,213 children were enrolled of whom n=1,078 (48.7%) were diagnosed with an extremity fracture. Adjusted for age, sex, mechanism of injury and family income level, obese children had a decreased odds (0.75, 95% confidence interval 0.58, 0.97) for fracture compared with normal weight children. Furthermore, underweight children had an increased odds for extremity fracture (1.44, 95% confidence interval 1.00, 2.07) compared with normal weight children, whereas fracture risk was not increased in overweight compared with normal weight children.
Conclusion: Obese children have a slightly lower risk for extremity fracture compared with normal weight children and underweight children may have a higher odds of sustaining a fracture compared with normal weight peers.

The authors report a minor but nonetheless statistically significant lower risk of extremity fractures among obese children compared with normal weight children. Given the controversy in published data on this topic, the large and well-characterised study population described here makes a strong case for lower fracture risk in obese children, and this also makes sense from the physiological perspective. Bone mineral density, which unfortunately was not been measured here, is proportional to BMI in children and adolescents [47]. So are there practical consequences from the study's findings? The good news is that increased fracture risk seems not to be another member of the multi-faceted family of childhood obesity's comorbidities. Although the present study did not show an effect of self-reported activity level on fracture risk, the interested reader will still suspect that children with more active lifestyles are more prone to fractures than those with a more sedentary routine. Nonetheless, measures promoting an active childhood (including experiences in tree-climbing of one sort or another) are definitely an important building block in almost all public health strategies, and especially in those aimed to prevent childhood obesity.

Genetic and functional characterization of clonally derived adult human brown adipocytes

Shinoda K, Luijten IH, Hasegawa Y, Hong H, Sonne SB, Kim M, Xue R, Chondronikola M, Cypess AM, Tseng YH, Nedergaard J, Sidossis LS, Kajimura S
Diabetes Centre, University of California, San Francisco (UCSF), San Francisco, CA, USA
skajimura@diabetes.ucsf.edu
Nat Med 2015;21(4):389-394

Background: The existence of brown adipose tissue (BAT) in human adults is nowadays widely accepted. However, the cellular origins and molecular identity of brown adipocytes in humans are still under debate, largely because of the heterogeneity in human adipose tissue depots. The aim of this study was to investigate expression patterns of brown adipocyte precursor cells on a single cell level.
Methods: Clonal cell lines were established from isolated stromal vascular cells of BAT of two different donors. Transcriptome analysis of progenitor cells and in vitro differentiated adipocytes was performed using RNA sequencing followed by comparison to gene array data of human and mouse white, beige and brown adipocyte samples.
Results: Adipocytes positive for the BAT marker UCP1 showed transcriptome signatures closely related to a recruitable (meaning 'beige') adipocytes including a set of genes which was highly enriched in UCP1 positive human adipocytes. Using a loss-of-function approach, two of these genes, potassium channel K3 (*KCNK3*) and mitochondrial tumour suppressor 1 (*MTUS1*), were found to be required for beige adipocyte differentiation and function.
Conclusions: These findings provide important information for further screens of thermogenic regulators and cell-based disease modelling.

Lineage tracing experiments performed in mice revealed that white adipocytes originate from different progenitors than brown adipocytes in the interscapular brown fat depot [48]. Moreover, another intermediate brown-like cell phenotype arising in white adipose tissue - called 'beige' adipocyte - can be distinguished from classical brown adipocytes by marker gene analysis [48]. Two studies in humans showed that all of these adipocyte types are present in humans and their relative appearance is strongly dependent on the adipose tissue location [49,50]. Brown adipocyte progenitor cells have been isolated recently from different regions in the neck. Interestingly, differentiating these cells *ex vivo* revealed molecular and functional differences compared with white adipocytes. However, heterogeneity of the samples did not allow discrimination between classical brown and beige phenotypes [51,52].

Using a clonal cell line approach in the present study allowed similar analyses based on a sample material of higher purity, leading to the observation that human brown adipocytes are more closely related to beige than to classical brown adipocytes. This is important since this suggests that brown adipocytes are not only present but also recruitable in human adults. Moreover, the identification of genes that are involved in the process of brown adipocytes recruitment could lead to strategies to improve energy metabolism by targeting brown adipose tissue differentiation.

Direct evidence of brown adipocytes in different fat depots in children

Rockstroh D, Landgraf K, Wagner IV, Gesing J, Tauscher R, Lakowa N, Kiess W, Bühligen U, Wojan M, Till H, Blüher M, Körner A
Centre for Pediatric Research Leipzig, University Hospital for Children & Adolescents, Department of Women's and Child Health, University of Leipzig, Leipzig, Germany
antje.koerner@medizin.uni-leipzig.de
PLoS One 2015;10(2):e0117841

Background: The presence of active brown adipose tissue (BAT) has been recently demonstrated, opposite to former views of being restricted to infants. In this study, the presence of brown adipocytes in adipose tissue samples of children and adolescents (0 to 18 years) is investigated in association with age, location and obesity.

Methods: Adipose tissue samples of n=131 children and n=23 adults were analysed using immunohistochemistry and mRNA expression quantification.
Results: Adipocytes positive for the BAT marker uncoupling protein 1 (UCP1) were found in 10.3% of lean children (age 0.3 to 10.7 years) and in one overweight infant while they were absent in both obese children and adults. These brown-like adipocytes were found interspersed within white adipose tissue of perirenal, visceral und subcutaneous samples. On the mRNA level, expression of UCP1, PRDM16, PGC1a and CIDEA were increased in samples with brown-like adipocytes compared with tissue without brown-like adipocytes while other brown selective markers, such as PAT2, P2RX5, ZIC1, LHX8, TMEM26, HOXC9 and TBX1 were not differentially expressed.
Conclusions: These findings indicate that brown adipocytes are still present after infancy, even in white subcutaneous and visceral adipose tissue.

This study provides important evidence on the existence of brown adipocytes in white adipose tissue (WAT) depots in children and adolescents. We know from anatomical studies in the 1970s and recent publications that brown adipose tissue (BAT) can be found in distinct areas during infancy [53,54]. While some BAT depots can be still found in adolescents and even in adults (supraclavicular, cervical, costovertebral, mediastinal and axillar), other depots vanish completely (for example, interscapular) [53]. Moreover, recent papers also suggest that BAT prevalence increases during childhood and peaks in puberty [55]. Focusing on classical white adipose tissue depots, the authors here demonstrate that brown-like adipocytes also appear in these depots, a finding that is commonly described in mice as 'browning' of adipose tissue. Moreover, these brown-like adipocytes were still present after infancy, pointing to a functional relevance of these cells in older children. However, no genetic markers of these adipocytes could be found highly expressed in UCP1 positive compared with UCP1 negative samples, questioning the relevance of these markers in the human context.

Activation of human brown adipose tissue by a β3-adrenergic receptor agonist

Cypess AM, Weiner LS, Roberts-Toler C, Franquet Elía E, Kessler SH, Kahn PA, English J, Chatman K, Trauger SA, Doria A, Kolodny GM
Joslin Diabetes Centre, Harvard Medical School, Boston, MA, USA
Cell Metab 2015;21(1):33–38

Background: Activation of brown adipose tissue has been shown to be mediated via beta-3-adrenergic receptors in mice, however this has never been demonstrated in humans. Pharmacological activation of BAT thereby increasing energy expenditure might be a potential approach to treat obesity and diabetes. This study aimed at investigating the effects of a beta-3-adrenergic on BAT activity agonist in human in vivo.
Methods: n=12 healthy adult subjects were given orally 200mg mirabegron, a beta-3-adrenergic agonist developed to treat hyperactive bladder. BAT activity was determined by ^{18}F-FDG-PET/CT and metabolic rate was calculated using indirect calorimetry. Subjects were tested under basal, placebo and treatment conditions.
Results: Compared with placebo, acute mirabegron treatment led to increase in BAT activity and also increased resting metabolic rate (RMR) by 203 ± 40kcal/day (13% increase). Moreover, changes in RMR were also predicted by BAT metabolic activity.
Conclusions: Stimulating BAT activity with a beta-3-adrenergic agonist might be a potential treatment approach targeting obesity.

Brown adipose tissue has an important impact on body weight regulation in rodents [56,57] and it has been recently demonstrated that chronic activation of BAT by cold exposure can also reduce body fat content in humans [58]. Pharmacological activation of BAT with nonspecific sympathomimetic drugs failed or are not suitable for obesity treatment due to severe side effects on the cardiovascular system [59]. Moreover, beta-3-adrenergic agonists already tested in phase 2 clinical trials were also not successful due to cross activity to the beta-1-adrenergic receptor [60].

By using a beta-3 adrenergic agonist, the authors here demonstrate that BAT can indeed be activated by this receptor pathway. Even more importantly, treatment increased energy expenditure, which underlines the physiological significance of BAT in human metabolism. Further studies have to prove that chronic pharmacological stimulation of BAT is safe and also effective.

A rationally designed monomeric peptide triagonist corrects obesity and diabetes in rodents

Finan B, Yang B, Ottaway N, Smile DL, Ma T, Clemmensen C, Chabenne J, Zhang L, Habegger K, Fischer K, Campbell JE, Sandoval D, Seeley R, Bleicher K, Uhles S, Riboulet W, Funk J, Hertel C, Belli S, Sebokova E, Conde-Knape K, Konkar A, Drucker DJ, Gelfanov V, Pfluger PT, Müller TD, Perez-Tilve D, DiMarchi RD, Tschöp MH
Institute for Diabetes and Obesity, Helmholtz Zentrum München, German Research Centre for Environmental Health, Neuherberg, Germany
brian.finan@helmholtz-muenchen.de; rdimarch@indiana.edu; tschoep@helmholtz-muenchen.de
Nat Med 2015;21(1):27–36

Background: Obesity and related metabolic disease are a major health burden not only for affected individuals, but also for healthcare systems. Current pharmacological treatments are neither safe nor efficient. Therefore there is an urgent need for novel therapeutics.
In previous work the authors had demonstrated that dual agonism for the GLP-1 receptor/glucagon receptor (GcgR) or the GLP-1R/GIP receptors (GIPR) had considerable weight-lowering effects or improved metabolic disturbances, respectively.
In this study they hypothesised that a peptide, that co-agonises all three receptors (GLP1R, GcgR, GIPR) would have even better therapeutic outcomes.
Methods: A balanced unimolecular triagonist for GLP-1R, GIPR and GcgR was rationally designed. The compound was tested in vitro and in vivo in several rodent models of obesity and diabetes.
Results: The triagonist activated all three target receptors GLP-1R, GIPR and GcgR, but displayed no cross-reactivity with other related receptors. The triagonist outperformed all exisiting dual coagonists in terms of reduction on body weight, improvement of insulin sensitivity and reversal of liver steatosis. The three different activities were required for the overall effects on metabolism as demonstrated in knockout mouse models and additional chemical/pharmacological approaches.
Conclusions: This novel unimolecular, triagonistic approach is a highly effective tool to induce weight loss and reverse obesity-induced metabolic disease.

The authors introduced for the first time a monomeric peptide activating three metabolically relevant receptors at the same time: the glucagon receptor, the GLP-1 receptor and the GIP receptor. The aim behind this rational drug design was to produce a 'super weapon' against obesity and metabolic disease. Glucagon is a peptide hormone produced by alpha cells of the pancreas, whereas glucagon-like peptide-1 (GLP-1) and gastric inhibitory polypeptide (GIP) are gut hormones.

The chemical compound was designed to be used for *in vivo* pharmacology and metabolic characterisation studies across species. Importantly, it was modified to be protected from DPP-4 mediated degradation and to make it more potent than the native hormones. By including glucagon they intended to increase energy expenditure, GLP-1R agonism was to reduce calorie intake and to ameliorate glucose control, whereas GIPR agonism was to potentiate the incretin effect and at the same time protect from the diabetogenic effect of glucagon. All in all, their plan came together. The triagonist represents the most potent pharmacotherapy against obesity and metabolic disease to date with excellent weight-lowering effects. The next important step will be to test this novel compound in clinical studies.

The new GWAS – the largest one

Genetic studies of body mass index yield new insights for obesity biology

Locke AE, Kahali B, Berndt SI, Justice AE, Pers TH, Day FR, et al
joelh@broadinstitute.org; ruth.loos@mssm.edu; espeliot@med.umich.edu
Nature 2015;518(7538):197–206

Background: Genetic factors predispose to obesity and associated disease. The aim of this study was to better understand the genetic basis of obesity.
Methods: A two-stage meta-analysis was performed in order to identify genetic loci associated with BMI in European adults. The first stage involved meta-analysis of 80 genome-wide association studies (GWAS) (n=234,069); in the second stage data from n=588,136 individuals genotyped by Metabochip from 34 additional studies were included. All in all, 322,154 individuals of European descent and 17,072 individuals of non-European descent were analysed.
Results: This study identified 97 genetic loci associated with the BMI. Out of these, 41 had already been identified earlier. Many loci had an impact on other metabolic phenotypes and five loci showed clear evidence of independent associations. The 97 loci are responsible for ~2.7% of BMI variation. The authors suggest that 21% of BMI variation is due to common genetic variation. Pathway analyses underlined the crucial role of the central nervous system in the susceptibility to obesity.
Conclusions: GWAS based on large cohorts and with improved computer technology will continue to give insights into the genetic basis of obesity and body weight regulation.

From all over the world, researchers now contribute DNA samples or analysed results from their study participants to large international genetic consortia. This is the largest genome-wide association study ever performed in the context of obesity. All in all, 339,224 DNA samples along with anthropometric data were analysed. The authors identified 97 genetic loci associated with obesity. They not only tested for associations with BMI or metabolic traits, but also used cutting-edge computational methods to identify relevant tissues, pathways or gene sets. In particular, they took advantage of the novel DEPICT approach (Data-driven Expression Prioritized Integration for Complex Traits) [61] to study if expression of genes, which are in close proximity to obesity SNPs, is enriched in specific tissues. Indeed, 27 of the 31 significantly enriched tissues were in the central nervous system. Interestingly, enrichment was not only detected in well-known areas of body weight regulation like the hypothalamus, but also in the hippocampus and the limbic system, which are involved in emotion, memory, learning and cognition. Also using DEPICT they performed gene set enrichment analysis and found out that the most strongly enriched gene sets are also related to the central nervous system, such as synaptic function or neurotransmitter signalling. Taken together, this study identified previously unknown genetic factors of obesity and once more underlines the important role of the CNS for the regulation of body weight.

Evaluation of conservative obesity treatment programmes

Weight loss in children and adolescents. A systematic review and evaluation of conservative, non-pharmacological obesity treatment programs

Mühlig Y, Wabitsch M, Moss A, Hebebrand J
Department of Child and Adolescent Psychiatry, LVR-Klinikum Essen, University of Duisburg-Essen, Essen, Germany
yvonne.muehlig@lvr.de
Dtsch Arztebl Int 2014;111:818–824

Background: Conservative behavioural-based weight-loss treatments are primarily used as methods of choice for treating obese children and adolescents, and their effectiveness has been shown in several studies. However, a detailed analysis about the amount of expected weight loss is lacking so far which was aim of this systematic review.

Methods: A systematic literature research in Medline was performed between May 2008 and December 2013. Thereby, this analysis directly follows a Cochrane meta-analysis by Oude Luttikhuis regarding interventions for treating obesity in children [62]. The identified randomised controlled trials were analysed regarding their methodological quality. Therefore, seven criteria were predefined which are the following: 1) statistical power-analysis for BMI or BMI z score, 2) intention-to-treat analysis, 3) description of randomisation procedure, 4) reporting of adverse events, 5) information about adherence, 6) information about dropout rate, 7) information about loss to follow-up.
Results: Studies (n=48) with a total of 5,025 participants and at least six months of follow-up could be included in qualitative analyses. According to eight trials that met the predefined qualitative criteria best, a weight loss of 0.05 to 0.42 BMI z score could be observed within 12 to 24 months follow-up. 85.4% (n=41) of included trials reported on dropout rates. A dropout of 25% and higher could be found in 22% (n=9) of this trials.
Conclusion: Conservative obesity treatment results in only modest degree of weight loss. This fact should be communicated to families seeking treatment.

In this systematic review, the authors objectively analysed randomised controlled trials with dietary, physical and/or behavioural intervention, at least six months of follow up and BMI or BMI z score as study endpoint via seven predefined methodological criteria. Although conservative obesity treatment was formerly reported to be effective and is still used as state of the art, only modest success in amount of weight loss could be observed in this qualitative analysis. This result implies that excessive weight cannot be normalised by the currently available conservative weight-loss programmes applying for most children and adolescents with obesity. On this basis, another therapeutic approach should therefore be chosen for (extreme) obese persons, despite the reported attainable reduction of cardiovascular comorbidities, and improvement in nutritional and exercise behaviour via conservative obesity treatment [63,64]. The focus should include coping with the health problem instead on weight-loss *per se*.

The discrimination of persons with obesity is widely experienced, for example, within the family and/or healthcare settings, and emphasises the need to help the person cope with it. Because of this and the fact that obese people have more often mental disorders [65], psychological and/or psychiatric evaluation is required as a standard component of obesity lifestyle interventions. As part of a new and better approach, the modest effectiveness and potential adverse effects of conservative weight-loss treatments should be communicated to families seeking treatment.

The meaningfulness of conservative obesity treatment is also lowered by lacking weight data of patients who were lost to follow-up. To prevent high rates of loss to follow-up and dropout, longitudinal observations over several years including intensive efforts to motivate patients to make use of the available healthcare resources over the long term are needed. The authors conclude that further clinical research should focus on determining predictive factors for therapeutic benefit and on the evaluation of coping-oriented interventions that are intended to improve the patient's quality of life and psychosocial functioning.

Adolescent girls and weight gain

Targeted prevention of excess weight gain and eating disorders in high-risk adolescent girls: a randomized controlled trial

Tanovsky-Kraff M, Shomaker LB, Wilfley DE, Young JF, Sbrocco T, Stephens M, Ranzenhofer LM, Elliott C, Brady S, Radin RM, Vannucci A, Bryant EJ, Osborn R, Berger SS, Olsen C, Kozlosky M, Reynolds JC, Yanovski JA
Medical and Clinical Psychology, Uniformed Services University of the Health Sciences, Bethesda, MD, USA
marian.tanofsky-kraff@usuhs.edu
Am J Clin Nutr 2014,100:1010-1018

Background: Obesity and eating disorders share several risk factors, therefore coordinated prevention of both conditions has been proposed. The present study investigates whether an adapted interpersonal psychotherapy programme is more efficacious for reducing excess weight gain and worsening of disordered eating compared with a health education programme in a population of adolescent girls identified to be at-risk for the development of either obesity or an eating disorder.

Methods: This is a parallel-group, randomised-controlled trial including n=113 adolescent girls (age 12–17 years) with a BMI between the 75th and 97th percentile and reporting at least one episode of loss-of-control eating (LOC). Study participants were randomised to participate either in an adapted interpersonal psychotherapy programme (IPT) or a health education programme (HE) for 12 weekly group sessions. Main outcome measures were the difference between expected versus actual BMI change, change in BMI z-score and percentage body fat (measured with DXA), as well as the number of LOC- and binge-eating episodes during follow-up. Follow-up visits occurred at the end of the programme and six and twelve months after completion of the programme.

Results: Both interventions resulted in decreases in expected BMI gain, BMI z-score and percentage body fat. Furthermore, episodes of LOC-eating, symptoms of depression and anxiety decreased in both intervention groups without significant group differences. IPT seemed to be more effective than HE in reducing objective binge-eating episodes at 12 months follow-up.

Conclusions: Health education and interpersonal psychotherapy proved to reduce expected weight gain and loss-of-control eating in a population of normal-weight to overweight girls seeking counselling on obesity prevention.

Loss-of-control eating episodes predict the development of eating disorders and aggravate depressive symptoms in children and adolescents. In the quest for effective strategies to prevent obesity in childhood and adolescence, targeting groups with more or less easily identifiable risk factors as in the present study seems to be an attractive and promising option. What is reassuring about the findings here is that even the control intervention, consisting of health education, provided enough impact in the obviously well-motivated, help-seeking group of study participants, to improve outcome measures comparably to psychotherapy group sessions at least during the short follow-up period. Basic interventions providing experiences of group cohesion and disrupting social isolation may therefore be a viable and effective way to prevent obesity and eating disorders in at-risk adolescents during critical phases of development. Given the likely better effect of group sessions of psychotherapy on the occurrence of binge-eating episodes in adolescent girls – which exert a particularly negative effect on future excess weight gain and an adverse psychological outcome – adding psychotherapeutical supervision to such targeted education programmes may be of special importance. Unfortunately, and as all too often in clinical obesity research, despite use of high-quality methods, the authors could not overcome one of the main obstacles to informing evidence-based decision and policy-making: the lack of at least mid-term (not to speak of long-term) follow-up data.

Helpful reviews

Drugs commonly associated with weight change: a systematic review and meta-analysis

Domecq JP, Prutsky G, Leppin A, Sonbol MB, Altayar O, Undavalli C, Wang Z, Elraiyah T, Brito JP, Mauck KF, Lababidi MH, Prokop LJ, Asi N, Wei J, Fidahussein S, Montori VM, Murad MH
Mayo Clinic, Knowledge and Evaluation Research Unit, Rochester, MN, USA
murad.mohammad@mayo.edu
J Clin Endocrinol Metab 2015;100:363–370

Background: Clinicians who prescribe drugs should be aware about their impact on weight development, especially in patients with obesity.

Methods: An expert panel from the Endocrine Society is charged with developing clinical practice guidelines for the management of obesity. A part of the work related to this activity has been a systematic review and meta-analysis in order to provide a summary of evidence about commonly prescribed drugs and their associations with weight loss or weight gain. The meta-analysis included randomised trials that compared an a priori selected list of drugs to placebo and measured weight change.

Results: 257 randomised trials were included enrolling more than 80,000 patients with a total of 54 different drugs. Atypical antipsychotics were associated with the most weight gain (largest effect by olanzapine (2.4 kg)). Amongst the anticonvulsants and mood stabilisers gabapentin, divalproex and carbamazepine were associated with weight gain. Significant weight loss was noted with zonisamide (7.7kg) and topiramate (3.8kg). Within the group of hypoglycaemic agents tolbutamide, pioglitazone, glimepiride, gliclazide, glyburide, glipizide, sitagliptin and nateglinide have been associated with weight gain, whereas metformin, acarbose, miglitol, pramlintide and glucagon-like peptide-1 agonists were associated with significant weight loss. Liraglutide and exenatide were also associated with weight loss depending on the dosage and the time of application. Within the group of hormones, weight gain occurred under treatment with glucocorticoids, whereas growth hormone treatment was associated with a reduction of BMI. Finally, antidepressants amitriptyline and mirtazapine were associated with weight gain, whereas bupropion and fluoxetine resulted in significant weight loss.
Conclusion: Several drugs are associated with weight changes of varying magnitude. This systematic review provides data to guide the choice of drugs when several options exist and weight management is a critical issue in the patient.

Current guidelines on various medications often have limited information about their side-effects on weight gain. There are also limited comparative data about the magnitude of effects on weight change caused by otherwise acceptable drugs. That information might allow clinicians who prescribe such medications to modify the risks of weight gain. The current review and meta-analysis therefore provides useful information about the absolute weight gain effects of various medications so that certain drugs might be avoided, replaced or sought for as appropriate to a given situation. Furthermore, the findings may help to inform pre-emptive weight loss strategies when prescribing certain drugs, as reported [66–68].

Pharmacological management of obesity: an Endocrine Society clinical practice guideline

Apovian CM, Aronne LJ, Bessesen DH, McDonnell ME, Murad MH, Pagotto U, Ryan DH, Still CD
Boston University School of Medicine and Boston Medical Centre, Boston, MA, USA
govt-prof@endocrine.org
J Clin Endocrinol Metab 2015;100:342–362

Background: Obesity is a disease. Permanent weight loss cannot be achieved exclusively with behavioural reductions in food intake and increases in energy expenditure in most patients. Worldwide there are several drugs in the group of weight loss medications on the market. There is a need of a clinical practice guideline.
Methods: The Clinical Guidelines Subcommittee of the Endocrine Society appointed a Task Force to work out evidence-based recommendations for the pharmacological management of obesity. The Task Force followed the approach recommended by the Grading of Recommendations, Assessment, Development and Evaluation (GRADE) group. The guideline was co-sponsored by the European Society of Endocrinology and The Obesity Society.
Results: Weight loss is a therapeutic goal in obese patients since it improves health and obesity-associated risk factors and comorbidities. Medications approved for chronic weight management can be useful adjuncts to lifestyle change for patients who have been unsuccessful with diet and exercise alone. Recommendations are provided for the care of patients with obesity with a focus on pharmacological treatment options.
Conclusion: This Endocrine Society clinical practice guideline summarises the effects of currently available drugs for weight management and comprises recommendations for prescribing such drugs. Most of the drugs have not yet been proved for the use in children and adolescents.

There is a rationale for pharmacological treatment of obesity in adults as well as in children and adolescents. If permanent weight loss and/or the optimal body weight for optimal health could be achieved exclusively with behavioural reductions in food intake and increase in energy expenditure, medications for obesity would not be needed. However, for most patients weight management is difficult to achieve satisfactorily since restricting food intake and increasing physical activity are counteracted by adaptive biological responses [69,70]. The decrease in energy expenditure (out of proportion to reduction in body mass) and the increase in appetite that follow weight loss are associated with changes in a range of hormones, which alter physiology to promote weight regain.

With the exception of orlistat, drugs with an indication for obesity target appetite mechanisms. Such currently available drugs act primarily in the arcuate nucleus to stimulate POMC neurons that promote satiety. Some of these medications are serotoninergic, dopaminergic or norepinephrine-releasing agents/reuptake inhibitors.

Phentermine is a noradrenergic and probably also a dopaminergic sympathomimetic amine. Lorcaserin is a serotonin agent stimulating the serotonin type 2c receptor. The combination of phentermine and topiramate (a neurostabiliser and antiseizure medication) seems to be additive. Bupropion is a dopamine and norepinephrine reuptake inhibitor that stimulates POMC neurons. Its combination with naltrexone enhances efficacy due to the release of feedback inhibition of POMC neurons that naltrexone potentiates. GLP-1 agonists also affect POMC neurons to increase satiety. Orlistat is not absorbed systematically but blocks absorption of up to 30% of fat calories in the gut.

The following table summarises advantages and disadvantages associated with weight loss medications (according to table 2 in Apovian et al).

Several patients will profit from pharmacological treatment of obesity when safety issues are concerned since weight loss medications reinforce behavioural strategies to create a negative energy balance. As most weight loss medications affect appetite, they can promote the adherence to a diet. However, to get maximal efficacy, such drugs should always be used as adjuncts to lifestyle change therapy. Many of these medications are not approved in children and adolescents and should only be prescribed for adults. Children and adolescents who need pharmacological treatment should only receive drugs that are approved in this age group or should only be treated within registered clinical trials.

Advantages and disadvantages associated with weight loss medications

Drug	Advantages	Disadvantages
Phentermine	Inexpensive, greater weight loss[a]	Side effect profile, no long-term data[b]
Topiramate/ phentermine	Robust weight loss, long-term data[b]	Expensive, teratogen
Lorcaserin	Side effect profile, long-term data[b]	Expensive
Orlistat, prescription	Nonsystemic, long-term data[b]	Less weight loss[a], side effect profile
Orlistat, over-the-counter	Inexpensive	Less weight loss[a], side effect profile
Natrexone/ bupropion	Greater weight loss[a], food addiction, long-term data[b]	Side effect profile, mid-level price range
Liraglutide	Side effect profile, long-term data[b]	Expensive, injectable

[a] Less weight loss: 2–3%; greater weight loss: >3–5%; robust weight loss: >5%
[b] Long term: 1–2 years

Ontogeny of taste preferences: basic biology and implications for health

Mennella JA
Monell Chemical Senses Centre, Philadelphia, PA, USA
mennella@monell.org
Am J Clin Nutr 2014;99:704S–711S

Background: Recommendations to encourage healthy nutrition and exercise aim at reducing the prevalence of obesity in children and adults. A major challenge for these health initiatives is that neither adults nor children are complying with these recommendations. The question is whether this is due to a lack of self-control or to biological reasons which can or cannot be modified.
Methods: This is a review by Dr Julie Mennella who is a biopsychologist specialised in the development of food and flavour preferences in humans. The review is based on a summary of clinical and experimental studies, and the experiences of the author.
Results: This review highlights the biological drives of food acceptance during infancy and childhood, and how early-life experiences may be able to interact with inherent plasticity of chemical senses to mould preferences for foods. Scientific evidence suggests that early feeding experiences can influence the foods preferred later in life. The tastes sweet, salty and bitter which have been most extensively studied are directly involved in choices of specific foods of concern, and exhibit age-related changes in function.
Conclusion: Although food choices are widely viewed as a cultural trade not directly related to our biology, recent research suggests that children's biology makes them especially vulnerable to the current food environment of processed foods high in salt and refined sugars. Although it is not easy to change children's innate liking of sweets and salts and disliking of bitterness, the current scientific knowledge supports that beginning very early in life, sensory experience can shape and modify flavour and food preferences.

Flavour (taste, smell, texture, chemical irritation) and taste perception (quality, intensity, hedonics) interact in the brain and activate strong drive when choosing and eating foods. Neonates and infants like the sweet taste and later on also the salty taste, and dislike the bitter taste. The food industry is aware of these early taste preferences, which are much stronger in infancy and early childhood than in adulthood, and has found that adding sugar and salt to food products developed for children increases their consumption. The taste preferences of children reflect mainly their basic biology. Experimental research studies indicate that the rewarding properties of sweet and salt are more pronounced during childhood.

However, it has also been shown that early life experiences can modify later food preferences. Evidence suggests positive consequences of healthy dietary trajectories from infancy to adulthood, and how learning to like 'healthy' foods is modifiable and begins early in life. Infants weaned to complementary foods learn through both repeated exposure (8–10 exposures) to a particular food and exposure to foods that vary in both flavour and texture. Current research results suggest that arrays of dietary flavours are transmitted from the maternal diet to both amniotic fluid and mother's milk. Therefore mothers can get their infants off to a good start by eating a diet rich in healthy foods, both while they are pregnant and while they breastfeed. Investigating whether there are optimal periods, when experience promotes greater liking, will go a long way toward promoting healthy eating by clinical studies with measurable outcome parameters. The review here is a basis for further readings and explorations of this field of research.

References

1. Cummings G, Hervey J. The effects of lesions in the hypothalamus in parabiotic rats. Physiology 1959;145:336–352.
2. Coleman DL. Effects of parabiosis of obese with diabetes and normal mice. Diabetologia 1973;9(4):294–298.
3. Tartaglia LA, Dembski M, Weng X, Deng N, Culpepper J, Devos R, et al. Identification and expression cloning of a leptin receptor, OB-R. Cell 1995;83(7):1263–1271.
4. Chen H, Charlat O, Tartaglia LA, Woolf EA, Weng X, Ellis SJ, et al. Evidence that the diabetes gene encodes the leptin receptor: identification of a mutation in the leptin receptor gene in db/db mice. Cell 1996;84(3):491–495.
5. Chua SC, Jr., Chung WK, Wu-Peng XS, Zhang Y, Liu SM, Tartaglia L, et al. Phenotypes of mouse diabetes and rat fatty due to mutations in the OB (leptin) receptor. Science 1996;271(5251):994–996.
6. Peelman F, Zabeau L, Moharana K, Savvides SN, Tavernier J. 20 years of leptin: insights into signaling assemblies of the leptin receptor. J Endocrinol 2014;223(1):T9–23.
7. Allison MB, Myers MG, Jr. 20 years of leptin: connecting leptin signaling to biological function. J Endocrinol 2014;223(1):T25–T35.
8. Chehab FF. 20 years of leptin: leptin and reproduction: past milestones, present undertakings, and future endeavors. J Endocrinol 2014;223(1):T37–T48.

9. Chou SH, Mantzoros C. 20 years of leptin: role of leptin in human reproductive disorders. J Endocrinol 2014;223(1):T49–T62.
10. Farooqi IS, O'Rahilly S. 20 years of leptin: human disorders of leptin action. J Endocrinol 2014;223(1):T63–T70.
11. DePaoli AM. 20 years of leptin: leptin in common obesity and associated disorders of metabolism. J Endocrinol 2014;223(1):T71–T81.
12. Rosenbaum M, Leibel RL. 20 years of leptin: role of leptin in energy homeostasis in humans. J Endocrinol 2014;223(1):T83–T96.
13. Patton GC, Coffey C, Carlin JB, Sawyer SM, Williams J, Olsson CA, et al. Overweight and obesity between adolescence and young adulthood: a 10-year prospective cohort study. J Adolesc Health 2011;48(3):275–280.
14. Gordon-Larsen P, Adair LS, Nelson MC, Popkin BM. Five-year obesity incidence in the transition period between adolescence and adulthood: the National Longitudinal Study of Adolescent Health. Am J Clin Nutr 2004;80(3):569–575.
15. Blum RW, Garell D, Hodgman CH, Jorissen TW, Okinow NA, Orr DP, et al. Transition from child-centered to adult health-care systems for adolescents with chronic conditions. A position paper of the Society for Adolescent Medicine. J Adolesc Health 1993;14(7):570–576.
16. Reinehr T, Wiegand S, Siegfried W, Keller KM, Widhalm K, l'Allemand D, et al. Comorbidities in overweight children and adolescents: do we treat them effectively? Int J Obesity 2013;37(4):493–499.
17. Xu Q, Song Y, Hollenbeck A, Blair A, Schatzkin A, Chen H. Day napping and short night sleeping are associated with higher risk of diabetes in older adults. Diabetes Care 2010;33(1):78–83.
18. Karlsson B, Knutsson A, Lindahl B. Is there an association between shift work and having a metabolic syndrome? Results from a population based study of 27,485 people. Occup Environ Med 2001;58(11):747–752.
19. Roenneberg T, Allebrandt KV, Merrow M, Vetter C. Social jetlag and obesity. Curr Biol 2012;22(10):939–943.
20. Reutrakul S, Hood MM, Crowley SJ, Morgan MK, Teodori M, Knutson KL, et al. Chronotype is independently associated with glycemic control in type 2 diabetes. Diabetes Care 2013;36(9):2523–2529.
21. Guidolin M, Gradisar M. Is shortened sleep duration a risk factor for overweight and obesity during adolescence? A review of the empirical literature. Sleep Med 2012;13(7):779–786.
22. Roenneberg T, Kuehnle T, Pramstaller PP, Ricken J, Havel M, Guth A, et al. A marker for the end of adolescence. Curr Biol 2004;14(24):R1038–R1039.
23. Fleig D, Randler C. Association between chronotype and diet in adolescents based on food logs. Eat Behav 2009;10(2):115–118.
24. Mountjoy KG, Mortrud MT, Low MJ, Simerly RB, Cone RD. Localization of the melanocortin-4 receptor (MC4-R) in neuroendocrine and autonomic control circuits in the brain. Mol Endocrinol 1994;8(10):1298–1308.
25. Kishi T, Aschkenasi CJ, Lee CE, Mountjoy KG, Saper CB, Elmquist JK. Expression of melanocortin 4 receptor mRNA in the central nervous system of the rat. J Comp Neurol 2003;457(3):213–235.
26. Coll AP, Farooqi IS, O'Rahilly S. The hormonal control of food intake. Cell 2007;129(2):251–262.
27. van den Berg L, van Beekum O, Heutink P, Felius BA, van de Heijning MP, Strijbis S, et al. Melanocortin-4 receptor gene mutations in a Dutch cohort of obese children. Obesity 2011;19(3):604–611.
28. Lubrano-Berthelier C, Cavazos M, Le Stunff C, Haas K, Shapiro A, Zhang S, et al. The human MC4R promoter: characterization and role in obesity. Diabetes 2003;52(12):2996–3000.
29. Wankhade UD, Good DJ. Melanocortin 4 receptor is a transcriptional target of nescient helix-loop-helix-2. Mol Cell Endocrinol 2011;341(1–2):39–47.
30. Blondet A, Gout J, Durand P, Begeot M, Naville D. Expression of the human melanocortin-4 receptor gene is controlled by several members of the Sp transcription factor family. J Mol Endocrinol 2005;34(2):317–329.
31. Stutzmann F, Tan K, Vatin V, Dina C, Jouret B, Tichet J, et al. Prevalence of melanocortin-4 receptor deficiency in Europeans and their age-dependent penetrance in multigenerational pedigrees. Diabetes 2008;57(9):2511–2518.
32. Wabitsch M, Tews D, Denzer C, Moss A, Brandt S, Lennerz B, et al. Obesity and weight regulation. In: Ong K, Hochberg Z, editors. Yearbook of Pediatric Endocrinology 2014. Basel, Karger: Endorsed by the European Society for Paediatric Endocrinology (ESPE); 2014. p. 149–169.
33. Michaud JL, Rosenquist T, May NR, Fan CM. Development of neuroendocrine lineages requires the bHLH-PAS transcription factor SIM1. Genes Dev 1998;12(20):3264–3275.
34. Kublaoui BM, Holder JL, Jr., Gemelli T, Zinn AR. Sim1 haploinsufficiency impairs melanocortin-mediated anorexia and activation of paraventricular nucleus neurons. Mol Endocrinol 2006;20(10):2483–2492.
35. Traurig M, Mack J, Hanson RL, Ghoussaini M, Meyre D, Knowler WC, et al. Common variation in SIM1 is reproducibly associated with BMI in Pima Indians. Diabetes 2009;58(7):1682–1689.
36. Swarbrick MM, Evans DS, Valle MI, Favre H, Wu SH, Njajou OT, et al. Replication and extension of association between common genetic variants in SIM1 and human adiposity. Obesity 2011;19(12):2394–2403.
37. Ghoussaini M, Stutzmann F, Couturier C, Vatin V, Durand E, Lecoeur C, et al. Analysis of the SIM1 contribution to polygenic obesity in the French population. Obesity 2010;18(8):1670–1675.
38. Ramachandrappa S, Raimondo A, Cali AM, Keogh JM, Henning E, Saeed S, et al. Rare variants in single-minded 1 (SIM1) are associated with severe obesity. J Clin Investig 2013;123(7):3042–3050.
39. Holder JL, Jr, Butte NF, Zinn AR. Profound obesity associated with a balanced translocation that disrupts the SIM1 gene. Hum Molecular Genet 2000;9(1):101–108.
40. Faivre L, Cormier-Daire V, Lapierre JM, Colleaux L, Jacquemont S, Genevieve D, et al. Deletion of the SIM1 gene (6q16.2) in a patient with a Prader-Willi-like phenotype. J Med Genet 2002;39(8):594–596.

41. Bonnefond A, Raimondo A, Stutzmann F, Ghoussaini M, Ramachandrappa S, Bersten DC, et al. Loss-of-function mutations in SIM1 contribute to obesity and Prader-Willi-like features. J Clinical Investig 2013;123(7):3037–3041.
42. Schwartz MF, Kaffe S, Wallace S, Desnick RJ. Interstitial deletion of the long arm of chromosome 6 [del(6) (q16q22)]: case report and review of the literature. Clin Genet 1984;26(6):574–578.
43. Rosenfeld JA, Amrom D, Andermann E, Andermann F, Veilleux M, Curry C, et al. Genotype-phenotype correlation in interstitial 6q deletions: a report of 12 new cases. Neurogenetics 2012;13(1):31–47.
44. McIntosh BE, Hogenesch JB, Bradfield CA. Mammalian Per-Arnt-Sim proteins in environmental adaptation. Ann Rev Physiol 2010;72:625–645.
45. Goldfield GS, Lorello C, Doucet E. Methylphenidate reduces energy intake and dietary fat intake in adults: a mechanism of reduced reinforcing value of food? Am J Clin Nutr 2007;86(2):308–315.
46. Leddy JJ, Epstein LH, Jaroni JL, Roemmich JN, Paluch RA, Goldfield GS, et al. Influence of methylphenidate on eating in obese men. Obes Res 2004;12(2):224–232.
47. Leonard MB, Shults J, Wilson BA, Tershakovec AM, Zemel BS. Obesity during childhood and adolescence augments bone mass and bone dimensions. Am J Clin Nutr 2004;80(2):514–523.
48. Wu J, Bostrom P, Sparks LM, Ye L, Choi JH, Giang AH, et al. Beige adipocytes are a distinct type of thermogenic fat cell in mouse and human. Cell 2012;150(2):366–376.
49. Cypess AM, White AP, Vernochet C, Schulz TJ, Xue R, Sass CA, et al. Anatomical localization, gene expression profiling and functional characterization of adult human neck brown fat. Nat Med 2013;19(5):635–639.
50. Lidell ME, Betz MJ, Dahlqvist Leinhard O, Heglind M, Elander L, Slawik M, et al. Evidence for two types of brown adipose tissue in humans. Nat Med 2013;19(5):631–634.
51. Jespersen NZ, Larsen TJ, Peijs L, Daugaard S, Homoe P, Loft A, et al. A classical brown adipose tissue mRNA signature partly overlaps with brite in the supraclavicular region of adult humans. Cell Metab 2013;17(5):798–805.
52. Tews D, Schwar V, Scheithauer M, Weber T, Fromme T, Klingenspor M, et al. Comparative gene array analysis of progenitor cells from human paired deep neck and subcutaneous adipose tissue. Mol Cell Endocrinol 2014;395(1–2):41–50.
53. Heaton JM. The distribution of brown adipose tissue in the human. J Anat 1972;112(Pt 1):35–39.
54. Sharp LZ, Shinoda K, Ohno H, Scheel DW, Tomoda E, Ruiz L, et al. Human BAT possesses molecular signatures that resemble beige/brite cells. PloS One 2012;7(11):e49452.
55. Gilsanz V, Smith ML, Goodarzian F, Kim M, Wren TA, Hu HH. Changes in brown adipose tissue in boys and girls during childhood and puberty. J Pediatr 2012;160(4):604.e1–609.e1.
56. Feldmann HM, Golozoubova V, Cannon B, Nedergaard J. UCP1 ablation induces obesity and abolishes diet-induced thermogenesis in mice exempt from thermal stress by living at thermoneutrality. Cell Metabolism 2009;9(2):203–9.
57. Liu X, Wang S, You Y, Meng M, Zheng Z, Dong M, et al. Brown adipose tissue transplantation reverses obesity in Ob/Ob mice. Endocrinology 2015;156(7):2461–2469.
58. Yoneshiro T, Aita S, Matsushita M, Kayahara T, Kameya T, Kawai Y, et al. Recruited brown adipose tissue as an antiobesity agent in humans. J Clin Investig 2013;123(8):3404–3408.
59. Vosselman MJ, van der Lans AA, Brans B, Wierts R, van Baak MA, Schrauwen P, et al. Systemic beta-adrenergic stimulation of thermogenesis is not accompanied by brown adipose tissue activity in humans. Diabetes 2012;61(12):3106–3113.
60. Arch JR. Challenges in beta(3)-adrenoceptor agonist drug development. Ther Adv Endocrinol Metab 2011;2(2):59–64.
61. Pers TH, Karjalainen JM, Chan Y, Westra HJ, Wood AR, Yang J, et al. Biological interpretation of genome-wide association studies using predicted gene functions. Nat Commun 2015;6:5890.
62. Oude Luttikhuis H, Baur L, Jansen H, Shrewsbury VA, O'Malley C, Stolk RP, et al. Interventions for treating obesity in children. Cochrane Database Syst Rev 2009(1):CD001872.
63. Ho M, Garnett SP, Baur LA, Burrows T, Stewart L, Neve M, et al. Impact of dietary and exercise interventions on weight change and metabolic outcomes in obese children and adolescents: a systematic review and meta-analysis of randomized trials. JAMA Pediatr 2013;167(8):759–768.
64. Kaitosaari T, Ronnemaa T, Viikari J, Raitakari O, Arffman M, Marniemi J, et al. Low-saturated fat dietary counseling starting in infancy improves insulin sensitivity in 9-year-old healthy children: the Special Turku Coronary Risk Factor Intervention Project for Children (STRIP) study. Diabetes Care 2006;29(4):781–5.
65. Hebebrand J, Herpertz-Dahlmann B. Psychological and psychiatric aspects of pediatric obesity. Child Adolesc Psychiatr Clin N Am 2009;18(1):49–65.
66. Bjorkhem-Bergman L, Asplund AB, Lindh JD. Metformin for weight reduction in non-diabetic patients on antipsychotic drugs: a systematic review and meta-analysis. J Psychopharmacol 2011;25(3):299–305.
67. Das C, Mendez G, Jagasia S, Labbate LA. Second-generation antipsychotic use in schizophrenia and associated weight gain: a critical review and meta-analysis of behavioral and pharmacologic treatments. Ann Clin Psychiatry 2012;24(3):225–239.
68. Fiedorowicz JG, Miller DD, Bishop JR, Calarge CA, Ellingrod VL, Haynes WG. Systematic review and meta-analysis of pharmacological interventions for weight gain from antipsychotics and mood stabilizers. Curr Psychiatry Rev 2012;8(1):25–36.
69. Rosenbaum M, Hirsch J, Gallagher DA, Leibel RL. Long-term persistence of adaptive thermogenesis in subjects who have maintained a reduced body weight. Am J Clin Nutr 2008;88(4):906–912.
70. Sumithran P, Prendergast LA, Delbridge E, Purcell K, Shulkes A, Kriketos A, et al. Long-term persistence of hormonal adaptations to weight loss. New Engl J Med 2011;365(17):1597–1604.

Type 2 Diabetes, Metabolic Syndrome and Lipid Metabolism

Orit Pinhas-Hamiel

Pediatric Endocrine and Diabetes Unit, Edmond and Lily Safra Children's Hospital, Sheba Medical Center, Ramat-Gan, and Juvenile Diabetes Center, Maccabi Health Care Services, Tel-Aviv University Sackler School of Medicine, Israel

The overall prevalence of type 2 diabetes (T2DM) for US youth aged 10 to 19 years increased by 30% between 2001–2009, accounting for one in three new cases of diabetes in patients <18 years old. These numbers are concerning, considering reports of a linear dose-response relation between pancreatic adenocarcinoma and fasting blood glucose concentration across prediabetes and diabetes. It is thus important to identify those adolescents who are at risk of developing T2DM. Three separate studies analysed pathophysiologic changes that lead to the onset of T2DM in adolescents. A study from Australia reported that elevated fasting insulin concentrations in early childhood among three to six year olds, but not in adolescence, are independently associated with an elevated risk of T2DM in adulthood. In a study from Cincinnati, Ohio a rapid deterioration in beta-cell function was determined among obese adolescents followed longitudinally and a study from Pittsburgh demonstrated that an incretin defect may precede glucose dysregulation and be an early, inherent component of T2DM pathogenesis.

Exciting data from animal studies shed light on the impact of non-caloric artificial sweeteners on modulation of microbiota composition and function, and the resultant effects on host glucose metabolism. Further data on risk factors for the development of the metabolic syndrome reveal that small for gestational (SGA) children with compensatory catch-up growth in the first year of life show mild disturbances of glucose tolerance already at four years of age, suggesting impairment of beta-cell function. In animal models, exposure to antibiotics during a critical developmental window had lasting metabolic consequences through changes in intestinal microbiota. When antibiotics were combined with a high-fat diet the effect was potentiated.

A landmark review on cholesterol metabolism, by the Nobel Laureates Brown and Goldstein, was published. 10-year follow-up of statin therapy in children with familial hypercholesterolaemia showed benefits on atherosclerosis. Yet, there is poor adherence to the current guidelines for lipid lowering among children with elevated LDL. Finally, new hope was reported for the new drug evolocumab to treat patients with severe familial hypercholesterolaemia, with only partial response to statins or requiring apheresis.

Type 2 diabetes

New concerns

Prevalence of type 1 and type 2 diabetes among children and adolescents from 2001 to 2009

Dabelea D, Mayer-Davis EJ, Saydah S, Imperatore G, Linder B, Divers J, Bell R, Badaru A, Talton JW, Crume T, Liese AD, Merchant AT, Lawrence JM, Reynolds K, Dolan L, Liu LL, Hamman RF

Department of Epidemiology, Colorado School of Public Health, Aurora, CO, USA

JAMA 2014;311:1778–1786

Objective: To estimate changes in the prevalence of T1DM in US youth aged 0 through 19 years and T2DM in youth aged 10 through 19 years by sex, age and race/ethnicity between 2001 and 2009.
Methods: Case patients were ascertained in four geographic areas and one managed health care plan.
Results: The prevalence of T1DM increased from 1.48/1,000 in 2001 to 1.93/1,000 in 2009. Over eight years T1DM increased in all sex, age and race/ethnic subgroups (except for those aged 0–4 years and

American Indians) a 21.1% (95% CI, 15.6%–27.0%) increase. In 2001, 588 of 1.7 million youth were diagnosed with T2DM; prevalence was 0.34/1,000 (95% CI, 0.31–0.37). In 2009, 819 of 1.8 million were diagnosed with T2DM; prevalence was 0.46/1,000 (95% CI, 0.43–0.49). In 2009, the prevalence of T2DM was 1.20/1,000 among American Indian youth (95% CI, 0.96–1.51), 1.06/1,000 among black youth (95% CI, 0.93–1.22), 0.79/1,000 among Hispanic youth (95% CI, 0.70–0.88) and 0.17/1,000 among white youth (95% CI, 0.15–0.20). Significant increases occurred between 2001 and 2009 in both sexes, all age groups and in white, Hispanic and black youth, with no changes for Asian Pacific Islanders and American Indians. Adjusted for completeness of ascertainment, there was a 30.5% (95% CI, 17.3%-45.1%) overall increase in T2DM.
Conclusions: Between 2001 and 2009, the prevalence of both T1DM and T2DM diabetes among children and adolescents increased.

This is the largest ever study of childhood diabetes in diverse populations in the USA. It includes children residing in five states - California, Colorado, Ohio, South Carolina and Washington - as well as from selected American Indian reservations. The overall prevalence of T2DM for youth ages 10-19 years increased by an estimated 30.5% between 2001-2009 (among a population of 1.7 million and 1.8 million youth, respectively). Increases occurred in white, Hispanic and black youth, whereas no changes were found in Asian/Pacific Islander and American Indian youth. Increases were seen in both sexes and all age-groups. One in three new cases of diabetes mellitus diagnosed in patients younger than 18 years of age was T2DM. The authors speculate that the increase in T2DM may result from minority population growth, obesity, exposure to diabetes in utero and perhaps endocrine-disrupting chemicals.

This increase has important public health consequences. T2DM is harder to treat in children than in adults and more children will enter adulthood at increased risk of early complications. Younger patients also have their reproductive years ahead of them. Diabetes in pregnancy is a risk factor for diabetes in the next generation. This study is ongoing, to examine trends over time, as well as to study serious complications of diabetes.

Important for clinical practice

Blood glucose concentration and risk of pancreatic cancer: systematic review and dose-response meta-analysis

Liao WC, Tu YK, Wu MS, Lin JT, Wang HP, Chien KL
Department of Internal Medicine, National Taiwan University Hospital, National Taiwan University College of Medicine, Taipei, Taiwan
BMJ 2015;349:g7371

Objective: To evaluate potential linear and non-linear dose-response relations between blood glucose and risk of pancreatic cancer.
Methods: Systematic review and dose-response meta-analysis of prospective observational studies evaluating the association between blood glucose concentration and pancreatic cancer.
Results: Nine studies were included for analysis, with a total of 2,408 patients with pancreatic cancer. There was a strong linear dose-response association between fasting blood glucose concentration and the rate of pancreatic cancer across the range of prediabetes and diabetes. No non-linear association was detected. The pooled rate ratio of pancreatic cancer per 0.56mmol/L (10mg/dL) increase in fasting blood glucose was 1.14 (95% confidence interval 1.06–1.22; P<0.001) without significant heterogeneity. Sensitivity analysis excluding blood glucose categories in the range of diabetes showed similar results (pooled rate ratio per 0.56mmol/L increase in fasting blood glucose was 1.15, 95% confidence interval 1.05–1.27; P=0.003), strengthening the association between prediabetes and pancreatic cancer.
Conclusions: Every 0.56mmol/L increase in fasting blood glucose is associated with a 14% increase in the rate of pancreatic cancer. As prediabetes can be improved or even reversed through lifestyle changes, early detection of prediabetes coupled with lifestyle changes could represent a viable strategy to curb the increasing incidence of pancreatic cancer.

The incidence and mortality of pancreatic adenocarcinoma are increasing; it is the fifth leading cause of cancer mortality in the USA and the fourth in the UK. As about 85% of tumours are non-resectable at diagnosis, it is the most lethal cancer, with a five year survival rate <5%. Identifying and modifying risk factors is therefore crucial.

Epidemiological studies show that T2DM is a risk factor for pancreatic cancer. Chronic hyperinsulinaemia and hyperglycaemia are proposed underlying mechanisms. Insulin promotes proliferation and reduces apoptosis in pancreatic cancer cells, and hyperglycaemia enhances proliferation and invasion ability of pancreatic cancer cells. As hyperinsulinaemia and hyperglycaemia are already present in prediabetes, it is possible that prediabetes also increases the risk of pancreatic cancer, but previous studies were inconsistent.

The authors performed a dose-response meta-analysis to evaluate both linear and non-linear relations, and pooled multiple studies to optimise statistical power. They found a linear relation between fasting blood glucose concentration and pancreatic cancer across prediabetes and diabetes. Every 0.56mmol/L (10.08mg/dL) increment in fasting blood glucose was associated with a 14% increase in the risk of pancreatic cancer. Sensitivity analysis that excluded blood glucose categories in the range of diabetes showed similar results. The authors concluded that early detection of prediabetes and lifestyle changes are an important strategy to avoid pancreatic cancer. The prevalence of impaired fasting glucose (IFG) according to the ADA criteria, among adolescents in the USA is 13%, in a German cohort 5.7% and in Sweden, 17.1%. Considering these high rates in young children, the above findings are particularly important.

New paradigms

Insulin sensitivity is an important determinant of renal health in adolescents with type 2 diabetes

Bjornstad P, Maahs DM, Cherney DZ, Cree-Green M, West A, Pyle L, Nadeau KJ
Department of Pediatrics, University of Colorado School of Medicine, Aurora, CO, USA
petter.bjornstad@childrenscolorado.org
Diabetes Care 2014;37:3033–3039

Objective: Diabetic nephropathy (DN) remains the most common cause of end-stage renal disease and is a major cause of mortality in T2DM. Insulin sensitivity is an important determinant of renal health in adults with T2DM, but limited data exist in adolescents. It was hypothesised that measured insulin sensitivity (glucose infusion rate [GIR]) would be associated with early markers of DN reflected by estimated glomerular filtration rate (eGFR) and albumin-creatinine ratio (ACR) in adolescents with T2DM.
Methods: T2DM (n=46), obese (n=29) and lean (n=19) adolescents (15.1 ± 2.2 years) had GIR measured by hyperinsulinaemic-euglycaemic clamps.
Results: Adolescents with T2DM had lower GIR and higher eGFR and ACR than obese or lean adolescents. Moreover, 34% of T2DM adolescents had albuminuria (ACR ≥30mg/g) and 24% had hyperfiltration (≥135mL/min/1.73m^2). Stratifying ACR and eGFR into tertiles, adolescents with T2DM in the highest tertiles of ACR and eGFR had respectively lower GIR than those in the mid and low tertiles, after adjusting for age, sex, Tanner stage, BMI and HbA_{1c} (P=0.02 and P=0.04). GIR, but not HbA_{1c}, LDL or systolic blood pressure, was also associated with eGFR after adjusting for sex and Tanner stage (beta ± SE: -2.23 ± 0.87; P=0.02).
Conclusions: A significant proportion of adolescents with T2DM show evidence of early DN. Insulin sensitivity, rather than HbA_{1c}, blood pressure or lipid control, was the strongest determinant of renal health.

Microalbuminuria is often present already at diagnosis of T2DM in adolescents. Furthermore, adolescents with T2DM have a two-fold higher risk of microalbuminuria compared with youth with T1DM, despite shorter duration of diabetes [1]. Diabetic nephropathy (DN) is a major cause of morbidity and mortality in T2DM. Its natural history is characterised by a long silent period without overt clinical signs or symptoms. However, during that time, renal parenchyma damage progresses. Thus, a major challenge in preventing DN in T2DM is to accurately identify high-risk patients. There s paramount importance to identify adolescents at risk of lifetime morbidity during their most productive years.

The authors examined associations between DN and insulin sensitivity. Despite a short duration of T2DM (2.0 ± 1.8 years), a higher proportion of adolescents with T2DM had renal hyperfiltration and microalbuminuria than did obese or lean patients. One third of T2DM adolescents had microalbuminuria and one quarter had hyperfiltration, both parameters are early preclinical markers of DN and are also associated with early cardiovascular abnormalities. Importantly, among T2DM adolescents, insulin sensitivity measured by hyperinsulinaemic-euglycaemic clamp studies, was associated with lower risk of albuminuria and hyperfiltration. Furthermore, insulin sensitivity appeared to be a stronger determinant of renal health than conventional risk factors including blood pressure, HbA_{1c} and lipids. These observations show the importance of optimising insulin sensitivity in adolescents with T2DM to improve renal outcomes.

Important for clinical practice

Insulin and BMI as predictors of adult type 2 diabetes mellitus

Sabin MA, Magnussen CG, Juonala M, Shield JP, Kahonen M, Lehtimäki T, Ronnemaa T, Koskinen J, Loo BM, Knip M, Hutri-Kahonen N, Viikari JS, Dwyer T, Raitakari OT
Murdoch Childrens Research Institute, Royal Children's Hospital and University of Melbourne, Melbourne, VIC, Australia
matthew.sabin@mcri.edu.au
Pediatrics 2015;135:e144–e151

Background: Fasting insulin concentrations are increasingly being used as a surrogate for insulin resistance and risk for T2DM. The authors aimed to determine whether fasting insulin concentrations in childhood associate with later T2DM.
Methods: Fasting insulin values were available from 2,478 participants in the longitudinal Cardiovascular Risk in Young Finns Study at baseline age three to 18 years, along with data on adult T2DM (n=84, mean age 39.6 years).
Results: Among three- to six-year-olds, a 1-SD increase in fasting insulin was associated with a relative risk (RR) of 2.04 (95% CI, 1.54–2.70) for later T2DM, which remained significant after adjusting for BMI and parental history of T2DM. For those aged nine to 18 years, a 1-SD increase in insulin was associated with an RR of 1.32 (95% CI, 1.06–1.65) for T2DM, however after adjusting for BMI and parental history of T2DM it became non-significant. In nine- to 18-year-olds, a 1-SD increase in BMI was associated with an RR of 1.45 (95% CI, 1.21–1.73) for T2DM; adjustment for insulin and parental history of T2DM did not improve this association. BMI in younger children was not associated with later T2DM. In life course analyses, those with T2DM had higher fasting insulin levels in early childhood and later adulthood but not in peripubertal years.
Conclusions: Elevated fasting insulin concentrations in early childhood, but not adolescence, are independently associated with an elevated risk of T2DM in adulthood.

The association between childhood obesity and later T2DM is well known. However, data are limited on childhood insulin levels and later T2DM. The authors tested the association between childhood fasting insulin and the development of T2DM in early and mid-adult life by following 2,478 children for a mean of 29.1 ± 3.3 years. Analyses were stratified into two age groups (three to six years and nine to 18 years). In the three to six year age group (n=795) there was a clear positive association between fasting insulin levels and later T2DM, which was independent of BMI, but no association between childhood BMI and later T2DM. The opposite was seen in the nine to 18 year age group (n=1,683): baseline BMI, but not fasting insulin, was associated with later T2DM. Furthermore, of the 84 participants who developed T2DM as adults, 61 had normal BMI and insulin levels in childhood. The authors conclude that caution is warranted in interpreting elevated fasting insulin levels in older children and adolescents as an indicator of the risk of developing later T2DM.

Rapid deterioration of insulin secretion in obese adolescents preceding the onset of type 2 diabetes

Elder DA, Hornung LN, Herbers PM, Prigeon R, Woo JG, D'Alessio DA
Division of Endocrinology, Department of Pediatrics, Cincinnati Children's Hospital Medical Center, Cincinnati, OH, USA
deborah.elder@cchmc.org
J Pediatrics 2015;166:672–678

Objective: To identify pathophysiologic changes that lead to the onset of T2DM in adolescents.
Methods: Forty-one obese adolescents with normal glucose tolerance were studied longitudinally over the course of four years with serial measure of the acute insulin response to glucose (AIRg) as well as proinsulin (PI) concentrations. Insulin resistance was estimated with the homeostatic model assessment of insulin resistance (HOMA-IR), the disposition index (DI) computed as AIRg x 1/HOMA-IR and intravenous glucose tolerance estimated as the glucose disappearance constant.
Results: Four of 41 adolescents developed T2DM during the study. Baseline PI exceeded the IQR of the nondiabetic group in three of four subjects with T2DM and all had >85% reduction from baseline AIRg and DI within six months of diagnosis. All the subjects with T2DM gained weight over the course of the study, but these changes paralleled those for the nondiabetic group. HOMA-IR increased substantially in one of the subjects with T2DM at the time of diagnosis but was comparable with baseline in the other three. The DI and glucose disappearance constant of the subjects with T2DM was less than the 10th percentile of the nondiabetic group before and after diagnosis.
Conclusion: Conversion from normal glucose tolerance to T2DM in adolescents can occur rapidly, and the onset of T2DM is heralded by a substantial decrease in AIRg and DI, as well as increased release of PI. These results support loss of beta-cell function as the proximate step in the development of T2DM in this age group.

There are limited data on the pace of progression from prediabetes to T2DM in adolescents. The current study aimed to identify the key changes involved in the transition from normal glucose tolerance to adolescent T2DM; 41 obese adolescents were followed for four years (mean age: 14.4 years; mean BMI: 35kg/m^2). All had acanthosis nigricans and a family history of T2DM. All had normal baseline oral glucose tolerance tests (OGTT). Those who converted from nondiabetes to T2DM had higher baseline BMI and higher fasting glucose, insulin and proinsulin levels than those who did not develop diabetes. All four adolescents who developed T2DM had a unique deviation of some parameters of beta-cell function. However, deviations in these parameters were also observed among those who did not develop T2DM.

Importantly, in the year before diagnosis of T2DM, the four adolescents shared a low disposition index (DI; the product of insulin secretion and insulin sensitivity). Insulin secretion is the amount of insulin secreted during the first 10 minutes following an intravenous bolus of glucose. Insulin sensitivity is determined by examining the disappearance of glucose following an intravenous bolus of insulin. Here, DI was the most consistent abnormality among the DM group, always below the normative range. The authors conclude that a normal OGTT may be misleading in adolescents with impending T2DM, whereas a low DI and high proinsulin levels may be better predictors.

Another key finding was the abrupt reduction in acute insulin response to intravenous glucose, a parameter of beta-cell function, preceding the onset of adolescent T2DM. This contrasts with the widely held view that adults progress gradually to T2DM. This rapid deterioration in adolescents was not obviously related to changes in BMI, and indeed BMI trajectories were similar between those who did and did not convert to T2DM.

New mechanism

Beta-cell function, incretin effect, and incretin hormones in obese youth along the span of glucose tolerance from normal to prediabetes to type 2 diabetes

Michaliszyn SF, Mari A, Lee S, Bacha F, Tfayli H, Farchoukh L, Ferrannini E, Arslanian S
Division of Weight Management, Children's Hospital of Pittsburgh, University of Pittsburgh Medical Center, Pittsburgh, PA, USA
silva.arslanian@chp.edu
Diabetes 2014;63:3846-3855

Background: Impaired beta-cell function in obese youth with increasing dysglycaemia was demonstrated using the hyperglycaemic and euglycaemic clamp.
Objective: To describe oral glucose tolerance test (OGTT)-modelled beta-cell function and incretin effect in obese adolescents spanning the range of glucose tolerance.
Methods: Beta-cell function parameters were derived from established mathematical models yielding beta-cell glucose sensitivity (betaCGS), rate sensitivity and insulin sensitivity in 255 obese adolescents (173 with normal glucose tolerance [NGT], 48 with impaired glucose tolerance [IGT] and 34 with T2DM. The incretin effect was calculated as the ratio of the OGTT-betaCGS to the 2-h hyperglycaemic clamp-betaCGS. Incretin and glucagon concentrations were measured during the OGTT.
Results: Compared with NGT, betaCGS was 30 and 65% lower in youth with IGT and T2DM, respectively; rate sensitivity was 40% lower in T2DM. Youth with IGT or T2DM had 32 and 38% reduced incretin effect compared with NGT in the face of similar changes in GLP-1 and glucose-dependent insulinotropic polypeptide (GIP) in response to oral glucose.
Conclusions: Glucose sensitivity deteriorates progressively in obese youth across the spectrum of glucose tolerance in association with impairment in incretin effect without reduction in GLP-1 or GIP, similar to that seen in adult dysglycaemia.

The incretin hormones, glucagon-like peptide-1 (GLP-1) and glucose-dependent insulinotropic polypeptide (GIP), are gut hormones that are secreted from enteroendocrine cells into the blood within minutes after eating and act to augment insulin secretion. The incretin effect is the higher insulin response to oral glucose than to intravenous glucose at similar prevailing glucose concentrations.

The authors investigated the interplay of incretin hormones and beta-cell function in the evolution of prediabetes and T2DM in obese youth. The novel finding is that youth with IGT or T2DM have a reduced incretin effect, by 32% and 38% respectively. But this reduction was not associated with reductions in GLP-1 and GIP concentrations, which may suggest beta-cell resistance to GLP-1 actions. These findings support the postulate that a defective incretin effect may precede glucose dysregulation and may be an early, inherent part of T2DM pathogenesis, rather than a consequence of chronic hyperglycaemia.

Metabolic syndrome

Concepts revised

Artificial sweeteners induce glucose intolerance by altering the gut microbiota

Suez J, Korem T, Zeevi D, Zilberman-Schapira G, Thaiss CA, Maza O, Israeli D, Zmora N, Gilad S, Weinberger A, Kuperman Y, Harmelin A, Kolodkin-Gal I, Shapiro H, Halpern Z, Segal E, Elinav E
Department of Immunology, Weizmann Institute of Science, Rehovot 76100, Israel
Nature 2014;514:181-186

Background: Non-caloric artificial sweeteners (NAS) are among the most widely used food additives worldwide, regularly consumed by lean and obese individuals alike. NAS consumption is considered

safe and beneficial owing to their low caloric content, yet supporting scientific data remain sparse and controversial.
Objective: To assess NAS-mediated modulation of microbiota composition and function, and the resultant effects on host glucose metabolism.
Results: The authors demonstrate that consumption of commonly used NAS formulations drives the development of glucose intolerance through induction of compositional and functional alterations to the intestinal microbiota. These NAS-mediated deleterious metabolic effects are abrogated by antibiotic treatment and are fully transferrable to germ-free mice upon fecal transplantation of microbiota configurations from NAS-consuming mice, or of microbiota anaerobically incubated in the presence of NAS. NAS-altered microbial metabolic pathways that are linked to host susceptibility to metabolic disease were identified. A similar NAS-induced dysbiosis and glucose intolerance in healthy human subjects was demonstrated.
Conclusions: These data link NAS consumption, dysbiosis and metabolic abnormalities, thereby calling for a reassessment of massive NAS usage.

Obese people who wish to reduce their food energy intake, and also people with diabetes who need to regulate blood glucose levels, often use noncaloric artificial sweeteners (NAS), such as saccharine, sucralose and aspartame. In the current study, mice that consumed NAS developed marked glucose intolerance, compared with mice that consumed sucrose or glucose or water. The effect of NAS was amplified by a high-fat diet. The effect of NAS on glucose intolerance was abolished by treatment with a Gram-negative targeting broad-spectrum antibiotic regimen. This suggests that glucose intolerance was mediated through alterations to the commensal microbiota, with contributions from diverse bacterial taxa. To show that the microbiota role was causal, feces from mice given NAS were transferred into germ-free mice, which then exhibited impaired glucose tolerance.

Examination of the fecal microbiota composition revealed that saccharin-consuming mice displayed considerable dysbiosis, with more than 40 operational taxonomic units significantly altered. The effect of long-term sweeteners in humans was examined among 381 non-diabetic individuals. Significant differences in the gut bacteria were demonstrated between persons who habitually consumed NAS and those who did not, as well as positive correlations between NAS consumption and several metabolic-syndrome-related clinical parameters.

Thus, it appears that artificial sweeteners may promote rather than alleviate, obesity-related metabolic conditions, by altering the composition and function of bacterial populations in the gut.

Food for thought

SGA children with moderate catch-up growth are showing the impaired insulin secretion at the age of 4

Milovanovic I, Njuieyon F, Deghmoun S, Chevenne D, Levy-Marchal C, Beltrand J
INSERM Unite d'epidemiologie clinique, Hopital Robert Debre, Paris, France
PloS One 2014;9:e100337

Background: Being born small for gestational age (SGA) is a risk factor for later development of T2DM. The development of glucose tolerance disorders in adults involves insulin resistance and impaired insulin secretion.
Objective: To evaluate insulin secretion and insulin sensitivity in a four-year-old cohort of SGA children.
Methods: 85 children were prospectively followed from mid-gestation to four years of age. Fetal growth velocity (FGV) was measured using ultrasound measurements. Body composition and hormonal profile were measured at birth, one and four years.
Results: 23 SGA babies had lower birthweight compared with 62 appropriate for gestational age (AGA) babies (-1.9 ± 0.3 versus -0.6 ± 0.8 z-score; P<0.0001) and they were thinner at birth (ponderal index 24.8 ± 1.8 versus 26.3 ± 3.1kg/m^3; P=0.01 and fat mass 11 ± 2.6 versus 12.9 ± 3.1%; P=0.01). No differences in other measured metabolic and hormonal parameters were observed between the two groups at birth. SGA infants experienced an early catch-up growth in weight during the first year of life. At four

years, SGA children remain lighter than AGA, but with weight z-score in the normal range (–0.1 ± 1.3 versus 0.5 ± 0.3 z-score; P=0.05). No excess of fat mass was observed (19 ± 4.8 versus 19.7 ± 4.1%; P=0.45). 120-min plasma glucose was higher (6.2 ± 1.1 versus 5.6 ± 0.9mmol/L; P=0.006) and insulinogenic index was lower (0.28 ± 0.15 versus 0.40 ± 2.4; P=0.02) in the SGA group at four years of life contrasting with a preserved insulin sensitivity (QUICKI 0.47 ± 0.09 versus 0.43 ± 0.05; P=0.06).
Conclusion: SGA children with compensatory catch-up growth in first year of life show mild disturbances of glucose tolerance associated to a lower insulinogenic index at four years of age suggesting impairment of beta-cell function.

During the early 1900s death rates in newborns in Britain differed considerably between geographic areas, being highest in deprived areas. The common certified cause of death in newborn babies at that time was low birthweight. Several decades later, death rates from coronary heart disease were highest in the same geographical areas. Based on this observation, Professor David Barker suggested that growth restriction before birth is linked to the development of coronary heart disease in adult life (Barker's Hypothesis). This phenomenon is now termed the 'Developmental Origins of Health and Disease (DOHaD)' and applies to a panoply of adverse outcomes.

Individuals who displayed poor growth in utero are at higher risk for later life obesity, hypertension, dyslipidaemia, T2DM, insulin resistance and the metabolic syndrome and cardiovascular disease. Inherent in this concept is the idea of a critical period of plasticity and increased sensitivity to the environment, followed by a period of fixed functional capacity. Subsequent studies demonstrated that postnatal growth, specifically weight gain during the first three postnatal months is an important cofactor. The mechanisms are largely unknown. In adults, both insulin resistance and impaired insulin secretion are reported. Among children, the questions remain: 'How early can we detect hormonal changes and what is the mechanism?'

Here, the authors assessed hormonal profiles as early as four years of age. They found no difference in insulin sensitivity compared with AGA children, but the insulinogenic index (increment in plasma insulin/increment in plasma glucose during the first 30 min of OGTT) was impaired. This suggests a defect in beta-cell function, possibly due to pancreatic beta-cell maldevelopment during fetal life.

Mechanism of the year

Altering the intestinal microbiota during a critical developmental window has lasting metabolic consequences

Cox LM, Yamanishi S, Sohn J, Alekseyenko AV, Leung JM, Cho I, Kim SG, Li H, Gao Z, Mahana D, Zarate Rodriguez JG, Rogers AB, Robine N, Loke P, Blaser MJ
Harbor Department of Veterans Affairs Medical Center, New York, NY, USA
martin.blaser@nyumc.org
Cell 2014;158:705-721

Background: Acquisition of the intestinal microbiota begins at birth and a stable microbial community develops from a succession of key organisms.
Objective: To assess whether disruption of the microbiota during maturation by low-dose antibiotic exposure can alter host metabolism and adiposity.
Results: Low-dose penicillin (LDP) delivered from birth induced metabolic alterations and affected ileal expression of genes involved in immunity. LDP limited to early life transiently perturbed the microbiota, which was sufficient to induce sustained effects on body composition, indicating that microbiota interactions in infancy may be critical determinants of long-term host metabolic effects. In addition, LDP enhanced the effect of high-fat diet induced obesity. The growth promotion phenotype was transferrable to germ-free hosts by LDP-selected microbiota, showing that the altered microbiota, not antibiotics per se, play a causal role.
Conclusions: These studies characterise important variables in early-life microbe-host metabolic interaction and identify several taxa consistently linked with metabolic alterations.

For decades, farmers have exposed livestock to low doses of antibiotics to promote growth; the earlier in life that exposure begins the more profound the effects. The findings of the current study suggest that antibiotic exposure during a critical window of early development disrupts the gut's bacterial milieu and permanently reprogrammes the body's metabolism, setting up a predisposition to obesity.

Mice given long-term, low-dose penicillin (LDP) starting in the last week of pregnancy were more susceptible to obesity and metabolic abnormalities than mice exposed to LDP at four weeks after weaning or unexposed controls. When LDP was combined with a high-fat diet the effect was potentiated. LDP suppressed early-life *Lactobacillus, Allobaculum, Rikenellaceae* and *Candidatus Arthromitus*. This finding may suggest a protective role for these organisms in the modulation of host metabolism.

Furthermore, LDP induced substantial histopathologic effects in ileal tissues, notably shortened villi. Transcriptional profiling analysis of intestinal tissue revealed that the ileal atrophy was associated with a general decreased expression of genes involved in intestinal immune responses. Most intriguing, by transferring bacterial populations from penicillin-exposed mice, inoculated mice were fatter than controls inoculated with bacteria from unexposed donors. This shows that altered gut bacteria, rather than antibiotics, was responsible for promoting obesity and metabolic effects.

Another recent paper reported an association between infancy treatment with broad-spectrum antibiotics and early childhood obesity, particularly repeated exposure to antibiotics at ages 0 to 23 months [2]. While that observational study cannot prove causation, the link is plausible and highlights a need for judicious clinical use of antibiotics in early life.

Important for clinical practice

Sleep duration predicts cardiometabolic risk in obese adolescents

Iglayreger HB, Peterson MD, Liu D, Parker CA, Woolford SJ, Sallinen Gafka BJ, Hassan F, Gordon PM
The Laboratory for Physical Activity and Exercise Intervention Research, Department of Physical Medicine and Rehabilitation, University of Michigan, Ann Arbor, MI, USA
Paul_M_Gordon@baylor.edu
J Pediatr 2014;164:1085.e1–1090.e1

Objective: To examine the independent contributions of objectively measured sleep duration and fragmentation on cardiometabolic risk factors in obese adolescents.
Methods: Characteristics of the metabolic syndrome (MetS) were measured in obese adolescents and standardised residuals (z-scores) were summed (inverse high-density lipoprotein cholesterol) to create a continuous cardiometabolic risk score (cMetScore), adjusted for age, sex and race. Sleep and physical activity were measured in habitual conditions for seven days; n=37; 54% female, ages 11–17 years.
Results: BMI, total sleep time and sleep session length were each correlated with cMetScore (P<0.05 all). Total sleep time was inversely and independently associated with cMetScore (r=-0.535, P=0.001) and was the best independent predictor of metabolic risk.
Conclusions: Sleep duration inversely predicts cardiometabolic risk in obese adolescents, even when controlled for various measures of physical activity, anthropometry and adiposity. Further research should investigate the biological mechanism of this relationship and the potential treatment effect of sleep intervention in decreasing cardiometabolic risk in this population.

Among adults, short sleep duration has been associated with higher cardiometabolic risk and T2DM. In children, short sleep duration has been associated with overweight and obesity [3]. However, among adolescents, sleep duration was not previously associated with metabolic outcomes [4].

Here, the authors measured sleep duration objectively using a SenseWear armband in obese adolescents. This sensor also permits measurement of physical activity duration and intensity. Unlike previous studies, the authors analysed a continuous MetS score, rather than just its individual components. Total sleep time was inversely related to MetS score. The authors suggest that cardiometabolic risk might potentially be reduced in this population by targeting sleep enhancement interventions!

Of note, a review of historical trends in recommendations for sleep durations for children and adolescents acknowledged the lack of empirical evidence [5]. Sleep recommendations have generally been considered 'largely a matter of opinion'. Interestingly, all of the recommendations dating from 1897 to 2009 assumed that children need longer than their actual sleeping hours!

Lipid metabolism

Review of the year

A century of cholesterol and coronaries: from plaques to genes to statins

Goldstein JL, Brown MS
Department of Molecular Genetics, University of Texas Southwestern Medical Centre, Dallas, TX, USA
joe.goldstein@utsouthwestern.edu
Cell 2015;161:161–172

One-quarter of all deaths in industrialised countries result from coronary heart disease. A century of research has revealed the essential causative agent: cholesterol-carrying low-density lipoprotein (LDL). LDL is controlled by specific receptors (LDLRs) in liver that remove it from blood. Mutations that eliminate LDLRs raise circulating LDL and cause heart attacks in childhood, whereas mutations that raise LDLRs reduce LDL and diminish heart attacks. If we are to eliminate coronary disease, lowering LDL should be the primary goal. Effective means to achieve this goal are currently available. The key questions are: who to treat, when to treat and how long to treat.

The 1985 Nobel Prize in Physiology or Medicine was awarded jointly to Michael Brown and Joseph Goldstein for their discoveries concerning the regulation of cholesterol metabolism. They identified a cell surface receptor for the plasma cholesterol transport protein 'low density lipoprotein' (LDL) and elucidated the mechanism by which this receptor mediates feedback control of cholesterol synthesis. Their studies led to the development of lipid-lowering statin drugs.

This review highlights key discoveries from the early 19th century onwards, considered to be milestones in the research of cholesterol and coronaries: from the initial understanding about atherosclerotic plaques and their association to heart attacks, to the understanding of the importance of LDL and the discovery of the LDL receptor. In addition, the discoveries of molecular mechanisms and of cholesterol-lowering drugs are described. It is well worth reading!

Important for clinical practice

Patterns of lipid lowering therapy among children ages 8–20 years

Joyce N, Wellenius GA, Dore DD, Newburger JW, Zachariah JP
Department of Epidemiology, Brown University School of Public Health, Providence, RI, USA
nina_joyce@brown.edu
J Pediatr 2015;167(1):113.e1–119.e1

Background: Paediatric guidelines in 2008 and 2011 recommended lipid-lowering therapy in children $\geq$8 years of age with high-risk cardiovascular conditions, such as familial hypercholesterolaemia (FH).

Objective: To describe the patterns and predictors of lipid-lowering therapy initiation in commercially insured children between 2005 and 2010.
Methods: The rates of lipid-lowering therapy initiation were estimated using commercial health plan data on children ages 8–20 years from 2004–2010.
Results: Among >13 million children, 665 initiated lipid-lowering therapy; the overall incidence rate was 2.6/100,000 person-years (PY). Incidence rates were highest in 2005 (4.1/100,000 PY) and 2008 (3.9/100,000 PY), with no discernable secular trend. Rates of lipid-lowering therapy initiation were higher in children ≥15 years of age (OR 2.9 [95% CI 5.2–13.0]), males (2.1 [1.7–2.4]) and in those with a diagnosis of FH (165.2 [129.0–211.6]), other dyslipidaemia (175.5 [143.2–215.3]), T1DM (7.7 [4.7–12.4]), T2DM (13.6 [8.5–21.7]), hypertension (8.1 [4.9–13.3]), obesity (7.8 [4.7–12.7]) and number of outpatient visits ≥5 (1.5 [1.2–1.7]), and were lower in children with ≥2 non-lipid-lowering therapy prescriptions (0.2 [0.2–0.3]).
Conclusions: Despite new guidelines, lipid-lowering therapy initiation in children is low and has not increased since 2005. Although the diagnosis of FH and other dyslipidaemias was associated with higher probability of lipid-lowering therapy initiation, our findings suggest lipid-lowering therapy is underutilised in this population given the prevalence of these disorders.

This study has several important implications. Firstly, it shows that despite AAP/NHLBI recommendations for lipid-lowering therapy in children, initiation rates are extremely low. An estimated 0.85% of American children aged 12-17 years are eligible for lipid-lowering therapy. But the incidence of lipid-lowering therapy is only 2.6 per 100,000 patient years. Secondly, despite the AAP/NHLBI recommendation for statins as the first line therapy in children, 25-50% of initiated lipid-lowering therapies were non-statins! Finally, children who were prescribed ≥2 non-lipid lowering medications were less likely to be initiated lipid-lowering therapy. Of note, bile acid sequestrants taste unpleasant and are usually poorly tolerated and poorly adhered to.

The authors conclude that physicians remain hesitant to start children with genetic dyslipidaemia on lifelong medical treatment. Potential barriers include our lack of knowledge about the guidelines, our lack of agreement with the recommendations and our inability to overcome the inertia of previous practice and self-efficacy [6]. These conclusions are in agreement with a recent survey of paediatric providers, in which 83% felt uncomfortable with managing lipid disorders and 57% were opposed to lipid-lowering therapy in children [7]. Clearly, wider promulgation of the recommendations as well as more evidence is needed on treatment outcomes to persuade paediatricians of the benefits. A recent Cochrane review [8] included randomised controlled clinical trials in participants up to 18 years old, with average follow-up time of six months (maximum two years). Statins reduced the mean LDL cholesterol concentration by 23-40%. Highly elevated liver and muscle enzymes presented only rarely and rates were similar in the statin and control groups. There was no clinically important difference in the risk of myopathy or other clinical adverse events.

These findings are even more concerning, considering the next article.

Ten-year follow-up after initiation of statin therapy in children with familial hypercholesterolemia

Kusters DM, Avis HJ, de Groot E, Wijburg FA, Kastelein JJ, Wiegman A, Hutten BA
Department of Vascular Medicine, Academic Medical Center, Amsterdam, The Netherlands
JAMA 2014;312:1055-1057

Background: Familial hypercholesterolaemia (FH) is a prevalent (1:500 individuals) inherited disorder that strongly predisposes to premature atherosclerosis and cardiovascular disease. Consequently, guidelines for FH treatment advocate initiation of statins in children as young as eight years. In the current study the authors aimed to study the long-term efficacy and safety of statin therapy initiated during childhood.
Methods: A cohort study of 214 children heterozygous for FH, aged eight to 18 years, treated with (20–40mg/d) pravastatin. After 10 years, all participants underwent a physical examination, fasted blood sample, occurrence of adverse events and measurement of carotid intima-media thickness (IMT).
Results: After 10 years, mean carotid IMT was still higher in patients with FH compared with siblings (0.480mm [95% CI, 0.472–0.489mm] versus 0.469mm [95% CI, 0.459–0.480mm], respectively; P=0.02).

However, progression of carotid IMT from baseline was similar in both groups (FH, 0.039mm [95% CI, 0.032–0.046mm] versus siblings, 0.037 mm [95% CI, 0.032–0.042 mm]; P=0.52). In patients with FH, age at statin initiation was positively associated with carotid IMT at follow-up (regression coefficient, 0.003mm [SE, 0.001mm]; P=0.009).
Conclusions: Long-term statin treatment initiated during childhood in patients with FH was associated with normalisation of carotid IMT progression. Moreover, earlier statin initiation was associated with thinner carotid IMT at follow-up. No serious adverse events were reported during follow-up.

In 2011, the National Heart, Lung and Blood Institute expert panel issued guidelines for paediatric care providers to reduce cardiovascular disease risks in children. These guidelines suggest the consideration of pharmacologic intervention for patients eight years and older with an LDL concentration of ≥190mg/dL; or ≥160mg/dL with a family history of early heart disease or with two additional risk factors [9]. The recommendations were met with controversy; critics argued that the guidelines promoted medicating children without sufficient evidence on the long-term safety. The current study followed 214 children aged eight to 18 years, with FH, who received statin therapy until adulthood along with 95 unaffected siblings. After 10 years, all participants underwent a thorough evaluation. Statin treatment initiated during childhood in patients with FH was associated with normalisation of carotid IMT progression. Moreover, earlier statin initiation was associated with thinner carotid IMT at follow-up. Rhabdomyolysis or other serious major adverse events were not reported, nor were differences in growth and maturation. Nevertheless, LDL levels of patients with FH at follow-up did not meet current treatment standards and carotid IMT was thicker than in unaffected siblings.

The authors conclude that earlier initiation of statins and more robust lipid-lowering therapy may be required to completely restore arterial wall morphology and avert cardiovascular events later in life in this high-risk population.

Clinical trials, new treatments

PCSK9 inhibition with evolocumab (AMG 145) in heterozygous familial hypercholesterolaemia (RUTHERFORD-2): a randomised, double-blind, placebo-controlled trial

Raal FJ, Stein EA, Dufour R, Turner T, Civeira F, Burgess L, Langslet G, Scott R, Olsson AG, Sullivan D, Hovingh GK, Cariou B, Gouni-Berthold I, Somaratne R, Bridges I, Wasserman SM, Gaudet D
Carbohydrate and Lipid Metabolism Research Unit, Faculty of Health Sciences, University of Witwatersrand. Johannesburg, South Africa
frederick.raal@wits.ac.za
Lancet 2015;385:331-340

Background: Heterozygous familial hypercholesterolaemia (FH) is characterised by low cellular uptake of LDL-C, increased plasma LDL-C concentrations and premature cardiovascular disease. Despite intensive statin therapy, with or without ezetimibe, many patients are unable to achieve recommended target levels of LDL-C. The effect of PCSK9 inhibition with evolocumab (AMG 145) on LDL-C in patients with this disorder was studied.
Methods: In a multicentre, randomised, double-blind, placebo-controlled trial, 331 eligible patients (18–80 years), who met clinical criteria for heterozygous FH and were on stable lipid-lowering therapy for at least four weeks, with a fasting LDL-C concentration ≥2.6mmol/L (100mg/dL) were randomly allocated in a 2:2:1:1 ratio to receive subcutaneous evolocumab 140mg every two weeks (n=111), evolocumab 420mg monthly (n=110) or subcutaneous placebo every two weeks (n=55) or monthly for 12 weeks (n=55). The co-primary endpoints were percentage change from baseline in LDL-C at week 12 and at the mean of weeks 10 and 12, analysed by intention-to-treat.
Results: Compared with placebo, evolocumab at both dosing schedules reduced mean LDL-C at week 12 (every-two-weeks dose: 59.2% reduction [95% CI 53.4–65.1], monthly dose: 61.3% reduction

[53.6–69.0]; both P<0.0001) and at the mean of weeks 10 and 12 (60.2% reduction [95% CI 54.5–65.8] and 65.6% reduction [59.8–71.3], respectively; both P<0.0001). Evolocumab was well tolerated, with rates of adverse events similar to placebo. The most common adverse events seen more frequently in the evolocumab-treated patients were nasopharyngitis (in 19 patients [9%] versus five [5%] in the placebo group) and muscle-related adverse events (10 patients [5%] versus 1 [1%]).
Conclusions: In patients with heterozygous FH, evolocumab administered either 140mg every two weeks or 420mg monthly was well tolerated and yielded similar and rapid reductions in LDL-C, of about 60% compared with placebo.

Inhibition of PCSK9 with evolocumab in homozygous familial hypercholesterolaemia (TESLA Part B): a randomised, double-blind, placebo-controlled trial

Raal FJ, Honarpour N, Blom DJ, Hovingh GK, Xu F, Scott R, Wasserman SM, Stein EA
Carbohydrate and Lipid Metabolism Research Unit, Faculty of Health Sciences, University of Witwatersrand, Johannesburg, South Africa
Lancet 2015;385:341–350

Background: Homozygous FH is a rare, serious disorder caused by very low or absent plasma clearance of LDL, substantially raised LDL-C and accelerated development of cardiovascular disease. Conventional lipid-lowering treatments are modestly effective. Evolocumab, a monoclonal antibody to PCSK9, reduced LDL cholesterol by 16% in a pilot study.
Methods: In a randomised, double-blind, placebo-controlled phase 3 trial, 50 eligible patients (aged ≥12 years) with homozygous FH, on stable lipid-regulating therapy for at least four weeks and not receiving lipoprotein apheresis, were randomly allocated in a 2:1 ratio to receive subcutaneous evolocumab 420mg or placebo every four weeks for 12 weeks. The primary endpoint was percentage change in ultracentrifugation LDL-C from baseline at week 12 compared with placebo, analysed by intention-to-treat.
Results: Of the 50 eligible patients randomised, 49 received the study drug and completed the study (16 in the placebo group and 33 in the evolocumab group). Compared with placebo, evolocumab reduced ultracentrifugation LDL-C at 12 weeks by 30.9% (95% CI -43.9% to -18.0%; P<0.0001). Treatment-emergent adverse events occurred in 10 (63%) of 16 patients in the placebo group and 12 (36%) of 33 in the evolocumab group. No serious clinical or laboratory adverse events occurred and no development of anti-evolocumab antibodies was detected.
Conclusions: In patients with homozygous FH receiving stable background lipid-lowering treatment and not on apheresis, evolocumab 420mg administered every four weeks was well tolerated and reduced LDL cholesterol compared with placebo.

Proprotein convertase subtilisin/kexin type 9 (PCSK9) regulates levels of plasma LDL-C by interacting with the LDL receptor and directing it to lysosomal degradation. This process reduces the capacity of the liver to remove LDL-C from the circulation. Patients with PCSK9 gain-of function mutations have high LDL-C levels, whereas patients with PCSK9 loss-of function mutations have low LDL-C levels and low incidence of coronary heart disease. Monoclonal antibody therapy against PCSK9 substantially lowers LDL-C.

In the RUTHERFORD-2, the efficacy of evolocumab was assessed in 331 participants with heterozygous familial hypercholesterolaemia. All patients were on statins and 62% were also on ezetimibe. Evolocumab, whether given two-weekly or monthly, reduced plasma LDL-C by 60% relative to placebo (P<0.0001) from a baseline of 4 mmol/L (140mg/dL); more than 60% attained an LDL-C concentration <70mg/dL.

Homozygous FH affects only 1:160,000–300,000 people, however causes devastating early cardiovascular morbidity and mortality. More than 95% have mutations in both LDL receptor alleles; others have mutations in apolipoprotein B, PCSK9 or the LDL-receptor adapter protein. The residual level of LDL receptor activity is associated with disease severity. According to the mechanism of action of PCSK9 inhibitors, some functional LDL receptor activity is essential to reduce LDL-C [10]. In patients with heterozygous FH who usually have at least one normal LDL receptor allele, the benefit of PCSK9 inhibitors seems clear. However, in patients with homozygous FH, who have very little or no residual LDL receptor function, PCSK9 inhibitors might be less efficacious. This was the rationale for TESLA Part B. Evolocumab reduced LDL-C by 30% overall compared with placebo, and as expected the responses were related to the underlying genetic defect, ranging from a 40.8% reduction in patients with 2–25% residual receptor function to zero response in patients with less than 2% receptor function. Finally, a study to assess the long-term safety and efficacy of evolocumab in subjects with severe FH requiring apheresis is ongoing. If the results will be similar, this will truly be good news.

In mid-June 2015, the advisory panel to the FDA voted in favour of approval for evolocumab (Repatha) of Amgen, as well as for alirocumab (Praluent) of Sanofi and Regeneron. Although large clinical trials testing effectiveness in reducing heart attacks and deaths will be completed only in 2017, the FDA approved both of these drugs in July/August 2015.

Important for clinical practice

Ezetimibe reduces plant sterol accumulation and favourably increases platelet count in sitosterolemia

Othman RA, Myrie SB, Mymin D, Merkens LS, Roullet JB, Steiner RD, Jones PJ
Human Nutritional Sciences, University of Manitoba, Winnipeg, MB, Canada
peter_jones@umanitoba.ca
J Pediatr 2015;166:125-131

Objective: To assess if ezetimibe, a sterol-absorption inhibitor, improves platelet count and size relative to its effect on plasma plant sterol (PS) in patients with sitosterolaemia.
Methods: Patients with sitosterolaemia L (five males, three females, 16–56 years of age) receiving ezetimibe intervention as part of their routine care participated in this study. Ezetimibe was discontinued for 14 weeks (off) and then resumed for another 14 weeks (on). Haematology variables along with plasma and red blood cells plant sterol and total cholesterol (TC) levels were measured at the end of each phase.
Results: Ezetimibe increased platelet count (23 ± 9%) and decreased mean platelet volume (MPV; 10 ± 3%, all P<0.05). In patients off ezetimibe, platelet counts inversely correlated with plasma and RBC plant sterol to TC ratio and MPV positively correlated with plasma and RBC PS/TC. Ezetimibe reduced plasma and RBC sitosterol (-35 ± 4% and -28 ± 3%), total plant sterol (-37 ± 4% and -28 ± 3%, all P<0.0001) levels and plant sterol to TC ratio (-27 ± 4% and -28% ± 4%, P<0.01).
Conclusions: Ezetimibe reduces plasma and RBC plant sterol levels, while increasing platelet count and decreasing MPV, and thereby may reduce the risk for bleeding in sitosterolaemia. Plasma plant sterol levels and ABCG5/ABCG8 genes should be analysed in patients with unexplained haematologic abnormalities.

Sitosterolaemia (also known as phytosterolaemia) is a rare autosomal recessive sterol storage disease caused by mutations in either of the adenosine triphosphate (ATP) binding cassette transporter genes: *(ABC)G5* or *ABCG8*. The heterodimer transporter ABCG5/G8 is expressed in enterocytes, in the proximal small intestine and in hepatocytes, and function to rapidly excrete cholesterol, plant sterols and their saturated derivatives (stanols) from the body. Sitosterolaemia is characterised by significant elevation of serum plant sterols and stanols, as well as their accumulation in the arteries, skin (xanthomas) and tissues. Total cholesterol can be normal or reach extremely high levels. High plasma plant sterol levels reduce platelet counts, increase platelet size and cause severe bleeding episodes, as well as haemolytic anaemia. To date, only around 100 individuals with sitosterolaemia have been reported worldwide. However, since plant sterols are not usually measured in clinic, sitosterolaemia is likely to be underdiagnosed [11], and some population-based data suggest a much higher prevalence than currently known. These study findings show that ezetimibe effectively reduces plasma and RBC plant sterol levels and improves platelet indices, thereby potentially ameliorating bleeding tendency in patients with sitosterolaemia.

References

1. Pinhas-Hamiel O, Zeitler P. Acute and chronic complications of type 2 diabetes mellitus in children and adolescents. Lancet 2007;369(9575):1823–1831.
2. Bailey LC, Forrest CB, Zhang P, Richards TM, Livshits A, DeRusso PA. Association of antibiotics in infancy with early childhood obesity. JAMA Pediatr 2014;168(11):1063–1069.
3. Chen X, Beydoun MA, Wang Y. Is sleep duration associated with childhood obesity? A systematic review and meta-analysis. Obesity (Silver Spring) 2008;16(2):265–274.
4. Sung V, Beebe DW, Vandyke R, Fenchel MC, Crimmins NA, Kirk S, et al. Does sleep duration predict metabolic risk in obese adolescents attending tertiary services? A cross-sectional study. Sleep 2011;34(7):891–898.
5. Matricciani LA, Olds TS, Blunden S, Rigney G, Williams MT. Never enough sleep: a brief history of sleep recommendations for children. Pediatrics 2012;129(3):548–556.
6. Cabana MD, Rand CS, Powe NR, Wu AW, Wilson MH, Abboud PA, et al. Why don't physicians follow clinical practice guidelines? A framework for improvement. JAMA 1999;282(15):1458–1465.
7. Dixon DB, Kornblum AP, Steffen LM, Zhou X, Steinberger J. Implementation of lipid screening guidelines in children by primary pediatric providers. J Pediatr 2014;164(3):572–576.
8. Vuorio A, Kuoppala J, Kovanen PT, Humphries SE, Tonstad S, Wiegman A, et al. Statins for children with familial hypercholesterolemia. Cochrane Database Syst Rev 2014;7:CD006401.
9. Expert panel on integrated guidelines for cardiovascular health and risk reduction in children and adolescents: summary report. Pediatrics 2011;128 Suppl 5:S213–S256.
10. Santos RD, Watts GF. Familial hypercholesterolaemia: PCSK9 inhibitors are coming. Lancet 2015;385(9965):307–310.
11. Merkens LS, Myrie SB, Steiner RD, Mymin D. Sitosterolemia. In: Pagon RA, Adam MP, Ardinger HH, Wallace SE, Amemiya A, Bean LJH, et al, editors. GeneReviews®. Seattle (WA); 1993.

Evidence-based Paediatric Endocrinology

Roderick T Mitchell[a,b], Kathryn J Noyes[b], Tarini Chetty[b] and Christopher J H Kelnar[c]

[a] Centre for Reproductive Health, University of Edinburgh, Edinburgh, UK

[b] Department of Diabetes and Endocrinology, Royal Hospital for Sick Children, Edinburgh, UK

[c] Paediatric Endocrinology, University of Edinburgh, Edinburgh, UK

'An expert is a man who has made all the mistakes which can be made in a very narrow field.'
Niels Bohr
As quoted by Edward Teller (10 October 1972) and Alan L. Mackay: *A Dictionary of Scientific Quotations*, 1991, p. 35

Important for clinical practice

How are harms and risks best communicated to health care professionals, patients and the lay public? The 2014 Yearbook described a paper under the heading 'Public and professional prejudice' that demonstrated how misperception of data can lead to inappropriate health care policy and clinical practice (pp 225–6). That paper was in relation to the benefits and costs of mammography screening. However, misperception may continue to be abetted if treatment benefits and harms are expressed in suboptimal and potentially confusing ways.

Communicating relative risk changes with baseline risk: presentation format and numeracy matter

Bodemer N, Meder B, Gigerenzer G

Harding Center for Risk Literacy, and Center for Adaptive Behavior and Cognition (ABC), Max Planck Institute for Human Development, Berlin, Germany

Med Decis Making 2014;34(5):615–626

Background: Treatment benefits and harms are often communicated as relative risk reductions and increases, which are frequently misunderstood by doctors and patients. One suggestion for improving understanding of such risk information is to also communicate the baseline risk. The authors investigated 1) whether the presentation format of the baseline risk influences understanding of relative risk changes and 2) the mediating role of people's numeracy skills.

Methods: A hypothetical scenario about a treatment that decreased (experiments 1a, 2a) or increased (experiments 1b, 2b) the risk of heart disease was presented to members of the lay public (n=1,234). Baseline risk was expressed as a percentage or as a frequency. Participants' were asked to judge the risk in the treatment group given the relative risk reduction (or increase) and the baseline risk in a forced-choice paradigm. Numeracy was assessed using the Lipkus 11-item scale.

Results: The frequency format for communicating baseline risk facilitated correct understanding of the treatment benefits and harms across the numeracy spectrum. Participants with higher numeracy generally performed better but all participants benefitted from a frequency format. In contrast, a percentage format often impeded understanding. Many participants misinterpreted a relative risk reduction as referring to an absolute risk reduction.

Conclusions: Although numeracy skills are important for the correct interpretation of medical benefit and risk, presenting baseline risk in a frequency format improves understanding of relative risk information compared with a percentage. Overall, communicating treatment benefits and harms in the form of relative risk changes is still problematic, even when baseline risk is explicitly provided.

Treatment benefits and harms may be expressed in different ways. The transparent communication of health information is a major challenge in ensuring professional and lay comprehension, properly informed consent and shared and appropriate decision-making. Both healthcare professionals and patients are poor at understanding the magnitude of risk for potential treatment benefits and harms.

Participants chose between different estimates for the event rate in the treatment group after being given information on baseline risk (event rate in the control group) and the relative risk reduction (RRR) or the relative risk increase (RRI). The findings emphasise the importance of choosing the right presentation format to communicate baseline risk and the influence of numeracy skills on the perceived meaning of relative risk information.

The results may explain why people often overestimate treatment benefits when they are communicated as RRRs as interpreting a relative reduction as an absolute reduction results in an overestimation of treatment efficacy. Using information on baseline risk is beneficial only when there is an understanding that benefits and harms are evaluated based on a comparison between a control and a treatment group. If baseline risk is ignored, the incorrect assumption may be that the risk information refers directly to the event rate in the treatment group.

A 'fact box' (which presents information on event rates in the control and treatment groups in terms of frequencies, and dispenses with any measures of relative risk reduction) may provide patients, doctors and policy makers with a concise overview of the best evidence currently available (for example, based on the Cochrane Collaboration's systematic reviews - the example given again relates to breast cancer screening) in a transparent and intuitive manner.

Several Cochrane reviews have been published recently that are relevant for the paediatric endocrinologist and their collaboration with colleagues in other specialties such as respiratory medicine. These reviews often highlight therapeutic areas where prescribing habits have outstripped the evidence for efficacy and safety.

Bisphosphonate therapy for osteogenesis imperfecta

Dwan K, Phillipi CA, Steiner RD, Basel D
Department of Biostatistics, University of Liverpool, Liverpool, UK
Cochrane Database Syst Rev 2014 Jul 23;7:CD005088

Background: Osteogenesis imperfecta (OI) results from a genetic defect causing abnormal type I collagen bone matrix formation. Bisphosphonates are used in an attempt to increase bone mineral density and reduce the risk and frequency of the multiple fractures which otherwise typically occur following little or no trauma.
Objectives: To assess bisphosphonates safety and efficacy in increasing bone mineral density, reducing fractures and improving clinical function in people with OI.
Methods: The authors searched the Cochrane Cystic Fibrosis and Genetic Disorders Group Inborn Errors of Metabolism Trials Register. The authors also searched PubMed and major conference proceedings up to April 2014. The search criteria included randomised and quasi-randomised controlled trials comparing bisphosphonates to placebo, no treatment or comparator interventions in all types of OI. Extracted data and risk of bias in the included trials were independently assessed by two observers.
Results: Fourteen trials (n=819) were included. Trials were generally at a low risk of bias, although selective reporting was an issue in some.
Conclusions: Bisphophonates are widely prescribed to individuals with OI. Current evidence, albeit limited, demonstrates oral or intravenous bisphosphonates increase bone mineral density in children and adults with this condition. Most studies did not show a major reduction in fractures in affected individuals treated with bisphosphonates. Optimal treatment, long-term effectiveness and safety of bisphosphates, require further extended evaluation.

Lack of blinding, incomplete outcome data and selective reporting are problems in many of the studies reviewed. What is most important to measure is not always measured, often because this is more difficult to determine than other outcomes. Thus although the limited data that are available suggest that bisphosphonates increase bone mineral density in children with OI (and thus theoretically would reduce fracture *risk*), it remains unclear whether bisphosphonates consistently decrease fracture *numbers*. Both these outcomes should be 'easy' to measure. There is also no conclusive evidence as to whether other important clinical outcomes, which are more 'difficult' to measure but of particular relevance to patients and families (pain reduction, improved functional mobility and better growth) can be achieved. Quality of life indicators are generally more difficult to ascertain than biochemical or auxological measures. Dual-energy X-ray absorptiometry (DEXA) measurement may be difficult to standardise in the growing child and adolescent.

Randomised controlled trials are generally not designed to determine side-effects or harms. Amongst many additional and still unanswered questions: 1) What are the long-term effects of osteoclast inhibitors like bisphosphonates on the immature growing skeleton? 2) Will the efficacy of bisphosphonates in increasing BMD be confirmed in larger studies, and with more heterogeneous participants? 3) Does the efficacy of bisphosphonates differ by OI clinical type or mutation type? Biochemical markers of bone turnover should be carefully assessed to determine if they are an adequate proxy for dose efficacy and concordance with therapy. Quality of life outcomes should be properly assessed and broadened to include other factors such as hearing and dentition. The widespread current use of bisphosphonates in OI in children (and adults) is not as yet supported rigourously by evidence of functional improvement and fracture reduction.

Inhaled corticosteroids in children with persistent asthma: effects on growth

Zhang L, Prietsch SO, Ducharme FM
Faculty of Medicine, Federal University of Rio Grande, Rio Grande, Brazil; Department of Paediatrics, University of Montreal, Montreal, QC, Canada
Cochrane Database Syst Rev 2014;7:CD009471

Background: Treatment guidelines for asthma recommend inhaled corticosteroids (ICS) as first-line therapy for children with persistent asthma. Although ICS treatment is generally considered safe in children, potential systemic adverse effects (particularly on linear growth) related to regular ICS use continue to be a concern.
Methods: The authors searched the Cochrane Airways Group Specialised Register of trials (CAGR) and hand-searched respiratory journals and meeting abstracts. They sought potentially relevant unpublished studies by a search of ClinicalTrials.gov and manufacturers' clinical trial databases. Selection criteria were parallel-group randomised controlled trials comparing daily use of ICS, delivered by any type of inhalation device for at least three months, versus placebo or non-steroidal drugs in children up to 18 years of age with persistent asthma.
Results: 25 trials involving 8,471 (5,128 ICS-treated and 3,343 control) children with mild to moderate persistent asthma were included. Six molecules (beclomethasone dipropionate, budesonide, ciclesonide, flunisolide, fluticasone propionate and mometasone furoate) at low or medium daily doses were given during a period of three months to four to six years. Most trials were blinded. Over half had dropout rates of >20%. Compared with placebo or non-steroidal drugs, ICS resulted in a statistically significant reduction in linear growth velocity (14 trials with 5,717 participants, MD -0.48cm/year, 95% CI -0.65 to -0.30, moderate quality evidence) and in the change from baseline in height (15 trials with 3,275 participants; MD -0.61cm/year, 95% CI -0.83 to -0.38, moderate quality evidence) during a one-year treatment period. No statistically significant difference in linear growth velocity was found between participants treated with ICS and controls during the second year of treatment (five trials with 3,174 participants; MD -0.19cm/year, 95% CI -0.48 to 0.11, P=0.22). Among four trials reporting data on linear growth after treatment cessation, three did not describe statistically significant catch-up growth in the ICS group two to four months after treatment cessation. One trial showed accelerated linear growth velocity in the fluticasone group at 12 months after treatment cessation, but there remained a statistically significant difference of 0.7cm in height between the fluticasone and placebo groups at the end of the three-year trial. One trial with follow-up into adulthood showed participants of prepubertal age treated with budesonide 400 microgram/day for a mean duration of 4.3 years to have a mean reduction of 1.20cm (95% CI -1.90 to -0.50) in adult height compared with those treated with placebo.
Conclusions: In children with mild to moderate persistent asthma, regular use of ICS at low or medium daily doses is associated with a mean reduction of 0.48cm/year in linear growth velocity and a 0.61cm change from baseline in height over one year of treatment. Growth suppression appears maximal during the first year of therapy and less marked subsequently.

This meta-analysis suggests that children treated daily with ICS may grow ~0.5cm per year less during the first year of treatment than those not treated. However, the reduction in linear growth velocity did not persist into the second year of treatment. This publication coincided with a similar study by the same authors which demonstrated a modest difference in growth velocity (5.74 versus 5.94cm/year, 0.2cm over 12 months) favouring low (50 to 100 microgram) versus low to medium (200 microgram) doses of hydrofluoroalkane (HFA)-beclomethasone equivalent [1].

'Received wisdom' is that ICS are 'bad' for children's growth and this review confirmed that the regular use of ICS at low or medium daily doses is associated with statistically significant growth suppression during a one year treatment period in children with mild to moderate persistent asthma. However statistically significant differences do not always equate to clinically meaningful changes: whilst a reduction in growth velocity is maximal in the first year of therapy it equates only to just under and just over half a centimetre of growth and change from height baseline respectively. It is even less in subsequent years. Most clinicians and patients would agree that this is a small price to pay for adequate asthma control. The subgroup analysis indicated that the effect size of ICS on linear growth velocity appeared to be associated more strongly with the ICS molecule than with the device or dose. Participants in the trials included in the review included a wide age range, including toddlers/preschoolers and prepubertal and pubertal children. However we should be cautious when extrapolating the findings of this review to patients with more severe asthma who may need higher doses of ICS. In any case, ICS should be prescribed at the lowest effective dose and linear growth in children treated with ICS must be monitored as individual susceptibility to these drugs may vary considerably.

It is worrying that there was no or incomplete reporting of growth velocity in more than 86% (19/22) of eligible paediatric trials, including those using beclomethasone and budesonide. It is important that future paediatric trials comparing different doses of ICS with or without placebo should systematically document growth. Future trials involving ICS in children must 1) include growth assessment; 2) be pragmatic (that is, reflecting 'real-world' clinical practice); 3) be double-blind, parallel-group, adequately randomised, completely reported (including concordance, withdrawals and dropouts) and with intention-to-treat analysis; 4) measure and report change in standard deviation score (SDS) in height velocity, in absolute gain in height, in weight z-score, in BMI and in skeletal maturation between the beginning and end of treatment; 5) declare any concomitant use of non-steroidal anti-asthma drugs. It is important that paediatric endocrinologists work closely with their respiratory colleagues in the design of future studies.

Low-dose vs standard-dose insulin in paediatric diabetic ketoacidosis: A randomised clinical trial

Nallasamy K, Jayashree M, Singhi S, Bansal A
Department of Pediatrics, Postgraduate Institute of Medical Education and Research, Chandigarh, India
JAMA Pediatr 2014;168(11):999–1005

Background: The authors aimed to evaluate the safety and efficacy of low dose (0.05U/kg/hour) compared with standard dose (0.1U/kg/hour) insulin in the treatment of DKA in the paediatric population.
Methods: This prospective, open-label randomised clinical trial included 50 children aged 12 years or younger with a diagnosis of DKA. Participants were randomised to low-dose (n=25) and standard-dose (n=25) groups. They assessed the rate of decrease in blood glucose until a level of 250mg/dL or less was met. Time to resolution of acidosis, episodes of treatment failures and incidences of hypokalaemia and hypoglycaemia, were secondary outcomes.
Results: There was no difference in mean (SD) rate of blood glucose decrease (45.1 [17.6] versus 52.2 [23.4]mg/dL/hour), mean (SD) time taken to achieve this target (6.0 [3.3] versus 6.2 [2.2] hours) or mean (SD) length of time to achieve resolution of acidosis (16.5 [7.2] versus 17.2 [7.7] hours; P=0 .73) for low and standard dose groups respectively.
Conclusions: The authors conclude that low dose insulin is comparable to standard dose insulin regarding rate of blood glucose decrease and resolution of acidosis. They suggest that larger clinical trials are required prior to changing practice recommendations.

Current clinical practice consensus guidelines for paediatric DKA management recommend using a continuous infusion rate of insulin of 0.05–0.1U/kg/hour. Recently, uncontrolled retrospective observational studies have suggested that using 0.05U/kg/hour has comparable efficacy to standard dosing (0.1U/kg/hour). This paper represents the first prospective randomised controlled trial to compare an insulin infusion rate of 0.05U/kg/hour (low-dose) with a rate of 0.1U/kg/hour (standard dose) in children with DKA.

The authors found no difference in mean rate of BG decrease or time to resolution of acidosis, between the low dose and standard dose groups leading the authors to conclude that low dose insulin was non-inferior to standard dose insulin, adding to the evidence base supporting the use of low dose insulin in the management of DKA in the paediatric population. It differs from previous studies not only in regards to a prospective randomised design but also in length of follow up (until resolution of acidosis) and in the frequent and regular monitoring of parameters including blood glucose levels. However these findings must still be interpreted with caution. Reported rates of some secondary outcomes are low, including only one case of cerebral oedema, and most likely reflect the relatively small sample size of 50 subjects. Indeed, any reduction in a rare morbidity, such as severe cerebral oedema, would not be determined by such a study design (see also Glaser et al, discussed below). Additionally, the study was not blinded which may have inadvertently influenced treatment decisions. Finally we must also consider if this study population where malnutrition is reported to affect 28–32% of participants is generalisable to a developed word setting. As the authors state, further larger clinical trials are required to determine the optimal insulin dose for the treatment of DKA.

Diagnostic performance of random urine samples using albumin concentration vs ratio of albumin to creatinine for microalbuminuria screening in patients with diabetes mellitus: a systematic review and meta-analysis

Wu HY, Peng YS, Chiang CK, Huang JW, Hung KY, Wu KD, et al
Department of Internal Medicine, Far Eastern Memorial Hospital, New Taipei City, Taiwan
JAMA Intern Med 2014;174(7):1108–1115

Background: Measuring the albumin concentration (UAC) in a random urine sample is less expensive than measuring the ratio of albumin to creatinine (ACR); however, a meta-analysis comparing the diagnostic performance for microalbuminuria screening among patients with diabetes mellitus (DM) has not previously been undertaken.
Methods: Clinical studies assessing the use of ACR or UAC from random urine samples to detect the presence of microalbuminuria among diabetic patients were sought using electronic literature searches. A urinary albumin excretion rate of 30 to 300mg/day in 24-hour timed urine collections was used as the criterion standard. The primary end point was the diagnostic performance measures, and comparison between, the UAC and the ACR in random urine samples.
Results: 14 studies were identified, which included a combined total of 2,078 patients. Of these studies, nine studies reported on the UAC, whilst 12 studies reported on the ACR. The pooled sensitivities were 0.85 for UAC and 0.87 for ACR, whilst pooled specificities were 0.88 for UAC and 0.88 for ACR, There were no differences in sensitivity (P=0.70), specificity (P=0.63) or diagnostic odds ratios (P=0.59) between the two tests. The diagnostic performance of either test was not affected by the timing of urine collection.
Conclusions: Both tests (UAC and the ACR) were highly sensitive and specific for detecting microalbuminuria. These findings indicate that the UAC of random urine samples may become the screening tool of choice in patients with diabetes, considering the increasing incidence of diabetes and the constrained health care resources in many countries.

Financial constraints play an increasing role in modern healthcare, and they are particularly pertinent to the increasing number of mass screening programmes. Ensuring that screening strategies are cost-effective without sacrificing sensitivity and specificity is an important consideration. For patients with diabetes mellitus it is routine practice to screen for microalbuminuria as an independent risk factor for a decline in renal function and cardiovascular disease. The two most commonly used methods to detect microalbuminuria in a random urine sample are the urine albumin concentration (UAC) and the albumin to creatinine ratio (ACR). Previous studies evaluating the diagnostic performance of these tests have generally involved small numbers of participants. In this study the authors performed a systematic review and meta-analysis of studies that utilised the UAC and/or ACR in adults with T1DM. Including studies that looked at the performance of both tests in the same patients, there were no differences in sensitivity, specificity or diagnostic odds ratio between the two tests. Interestingly, the timing of the collection did not affect the performance of either test, albeit that the subgroup analyses had limited statistical power. The choice of test for patients may therefore be considered one of economics and available facilities rather than of diagnostic performance, although it should be noted that the analysis only included studies in adult patients and therefore cannot be directly applied to the paediatric population.

Clinical relevance of thyroid-stimulating autoantibodies in pediatric Graves' disease – a multicenter study

Diana T, Brown RS, Bossowski A, Segni M, Niedziela M, König J, et al
Thyroid Laboratory, Department of Medicine I, Johannes Gutenberg University Medical Center, Mainz, Germany
J Clin Endocrinol Metab 2014;99(5):1648–1655

Background: In paediatric Graves' disease (GD), controversy remains regarding the incidence of TSH receptor (TSHR) stimulating autoantibodies (TSAbs). This large, cross-sectional, multicentre study evaluated the clinical relevance of TSAbs in children with GD both with and without Graves' orbitopathy (GO).
Methods: Blood samples were collected across seven US and European academic referral centres, for measurement of TSAbs using a novel, chimeric TSHR bioassay and a cAMP response element-dependent luciferase. TSH binding-inhibitory Ig (TBII) and parameters of thyroid function were also determined. A total of 422 serum samples from 157 children with GD, 101 control individuals with other thyroid and non-thyroid autoimmune diseases and 50 healthy children were studied.
Results: In children with GD (n=82), TSAb and TBII were highly sensitive (100 and 92.68%; P=0.031) and specific (100 and 100%), with high positive (100 and 100%) and negative predictive values (100 and 96.15%). TSAbs and TBII were found in 147 (94%) and 138 (87.9%) of the 157 children with GD (P<0.039), respectively. TSAbs were noted in 100% and TBII in 96% (P<0.001) of children with GD and GO. There was a markedly higher TSAb level in hyperthyroid children with GD and GO compared with those with thyroidal GD only (P<0.0001), whilst no significant differences were noted for TBII between these two groups. After a three-year (median) medical treatment, TSAb levels had decreased by 69% in GD versus 20% in GD and GO (P<0.001). In euthyroid children with GO TSAb positive in all 31 cases, whilst only 24 were TBII positive (P=0.016). TSAb and TBII were negative in all children with Hashimoto's thyroiditis, non-autoimmune hyperthyroidism, type 1 diabetes and juvenile arthritis and in healthy controls.
Conclusions: For children with GD, serum TSAb level is a sensitive, specific and reproducible biomarker that correlates with disease severity and extrathyroidal manifestations.

The vast majority of adults with GD display TSAbs which may also predict the presence of GO; however, the relationship between these antibodies and GD/GO in children is less defined. The present study, the largest of TSAb in paediatric GD, utilised a novel TSAb assay and demonstrated a high specificity (100%) and sensitivity (100%) of TSAbs in patients with GD. Previous assays in commercial laboratories have reported detectable TSAbs in only 50% of children with GD, concluding that TSAbs are often negative in paediatric GD. This emphasises the importance of improved assays in ensuring adequate sensitivity and specificity. Importantly, using the reported assay, TSAbs were negative in patients with in non-GD thyroidal disorders as well as in the healthy controls, demonstrating that the higher true positive rate did not result in a higher false positive rate. Moreover, in patients with GD, the TSAb level was markedly higher in those who were hyperthyroid with GO than those without orbital manifestations. This study highlights the utility of TSAbs in the diagnosis of GD and monitoring of disease activity in the paediatric population.

Impact of hydrocortisone on adult height in congenital adrenal hyperplasia – the Minnesota cohort

Sarafoglou K, Addo OY, Turcotte L, Otten N, Wickremasinghe A, Pittock S, et al
Department of Pediatrics, University of Minnesota Amplatz Children's Hospital, Minneapolis, MN, USA
J Pediatr 2014;164(5):1141–1146.e1.

Background: The authors aimed to determine the impact of the average daily dose of hydrocortisone (HC) on predicted final adult height in children with congenital adrenal hyperplasia (CAH).
Methods: Triple logistic models estimating components of growth and maturation were applied to longitudinal data from 104 patients (including 3,664 clinical encounters) with classic CAH from three paediatric medical centres in Minnesota between 1955 and 2012. Logistical regression analysis was used to estimate the effect of HC therapy on linear growth.
Results: Predicted AH z-score (-0.7) was similar between the sexes and CAH subtypes. The mean growth period HC dose was 18.9 ± 5.6mg/m^2/day. HC dose was negatively associated with predicted AH, with each mg/m^2/day increase in average growth period HC dose predicting a 0.37cm decrease in AH (P<0.004).
Conclusion: Higher HC daily doses predicted fractional reductions in final AH. These findings should aid the decision making balance between HC replacement dose and adrenal androgen suppression in children with CAH.

Relationship between final height and health outcomes in adults with congenital adrenal hyperplasia: United Kingdom Congenital Adrenal Hyperplasia Adult Study Executive (CaHASE)

Han TS, Conway GS, Willis DS, Krone N, Rees DA, Stimson RH, et al; the UK Congenital Adrenal Hyperplasia Adult Study Executive (CaHASE)
Department of Endocrinology, St Peter's National Health Service Foundation Trust, Surrey, UK
J Clin Endocrinol Metab 2014;99(8):E1547–E1555.

Background: Growth and development is often the main clinical focus when treating children with congenital adrenal hyperplasia and final height (FH) represents treatment efficacy. The authors hypothesise that shorter adults will have more severe underlying disease and worse health outcomes.
Methods: Cross-sectional cohort study including 199 adults with CAH. They reported FH and quality of life z-scores adjusted for midparental target height or UK population height.
Results: FH was inversely associated with age (men, r=-0.38; women, r=-0.26, P<0.01). Z-scores adjusted for midparental target height were -2 and -1 for men and women respectively. The cohort had UK population height z-scores of -1 below the UK population (P<0.01). In females, FH was shorter in non-salt-wasting than salt-wasting classic CAH (P<0.05) and in moderately affected genotype group B females than either more severely affected groups null and A (P<0.01) or the mildest group C (P<0.001). Short stature was associated with a higher blood pressure in classic CAH patients diagnosed late (after one year) compared with those diagnosed early and in females treated solely with glucocorticoid compared with those treated with a combination of glucocorticoids and mineralocorticoids (P<0.05). FH did not correlate with insulin sensitivity, lipid profile, adiposity or quality of life.
Conclusions: Despite improvement in height prognosis over time, adult CAH patients remain short. The shortest adults are those diagnosed late with moderately severe CAH and who are at increased risk of hypertension in adulthood. The authors hypothesise that these patients are exposed in childhood to high androgens and/or excessive glucocorticoids with potential programming of hypertension. An alternative explanation is inadequate mineralocorticoid treatment early in life in the late-diagnosed patient group. Prospective studies are needed to examine these hypotheses.

When treating children with congenital adrenal hyperplasia (CAH) the clinician walks a fine line between over- and under-treatment, as both can adversely impact linear growth. It is well established that CAH is associated with shorter adult height compared with the normal population. Sarafoglou et al build on this evidence base by quantifying the impact of hydrocortisone (HC) on predicted adult height (PAH) in children with classic CAH. Mixed regression modelling found HC was not only negatively associated with PAH, but that each mg/m^2/day increase in HC dose predicted a 0.37cm decrease in adult height (P<0.004).

Whilst the treatment of children with CAH is often focused on achieving optimal growth and development, the impact of final height on adult health outcomes is not well described. The UK CaHASE study previously reported that adverse health outcomes in adults, including impaired quality of life, are associated with treatment rather than severity of enzyme deficiency. The group further hypothesised that short stature is a surrogate marker for disease severity and therefore shorter adults will have worse health outcomes. This insightful study found that adults with CAH had height Z-scores of -1 compared with the UK population (P<0.01). Perhaps contrary to expectation, final height did not associate with health outcomes such as insulin sensitivity, lipid profile, adiposity or quality of life. Interestingly, they reported that women with less severe classic CAH (non-salt wasting and genotype B) were shorter than those with a more severe clinical phenotype and genotype. In addition short stature was associated with hypertension, particularly in classic CAH patients diagnosed late (after one year). The authors postulate that a late presentation and subsequent prolonged androgen exposure in early life and/or excessive glucocorticoid treatment may play a role in programming hypertension. Further prospective studies are needed to investigate these hypotheses. Unfortunately Sarafoglou et al focused only on *predicted* adult height, which is an endpoint of doubtful clinical significance. Other outcomes such as bone health, the incidence of adrenal rest tumours, fertility, etc are of greater concern.

Evaluation of 451 Danish boys with delayed puberty: diagnostic use of a new puberty nomogram and effects of oral testosterone therapy

Lawaetz JG, Hagen CP, Mieritz MG, Blomberg Jensen M, Holm Petersen J, Juul A
Department of Growth and Reproduction, GR-5064, Copenhagen University Hospital (Rigshospitalet), Copenhagen, Denmark
J Clin Endocrinol Metab 2015;100(4):1376–1385

Background: There are few data on the diagnostic criteria for boys with constitutional delay in growth and puberty (CDGP) and on the effects of puberty induction in this group. The authors aimed to develop puberty nomograms based on normal Danish boys and to evaluate different diagnostic criteria and the effect of oral testosterone undecanoate (TU) in boys with CDGP.
Methods: A cross-sectional and longitudinal study of Danish boys with normal pubertal development (COPENHAGEN puberty study) and, in a tertiary referral centre for paediatric endocrinology, a retrospective observational study of boys evaluated for delayed puberty between 1990–2013 were carried out (n=451). A total of 287 (64%) of those evaluated for CDGP were eligible for analysis with 164 boys (36%) excluded due to missing data, reclassification or associated comorbidities. The main outcome measures were 1) the number of patients with CDGP classified by the puberty nomogram (genital stage <-2 SD for age) versus classical criteria for CDGP (genital stage 1 at ≥14 years) and 2) the effect of one year of oral TU treatment on pubertal progression, circulating hormones, height and predicted adult height (PAH).
Results: Seventy-eight (27%) of the 287 boys had delayed pubertal onset according to the classical criteria, whereas 173 (60%) of the 287 boys had impaired pubertal progression judged by the puberty nomogram. Ninety-six (56%) of these 173 boys were treated with oral TU for 0.8 years (0.5; 1.3) [median (25th; 75th percentiles)], resulting in beneficial effects on pubertal progression. Height increased from -1.9 SD (-2.5; -1.2) to -1.5 SD (-2.1; 0.7) (P<0.001) and PAH increased from 172.3cm (170.3; 182.8) to 178.1cm (171.4; 191.7) (P=0.001) after one year of treatment.
Conclusions: Use of the puberty nomogram allows detection of delayed pubertal onset and delayed pubertal progression. Oral TU treatment was followed by both pubertal induction and progression and short-term growth improved without compromising final height.

The correct classification of boys with pubertal delay can be difficult but is important for optimal management. At referral, boys and parents are often already impatient for 'something to be done', but very often explanation and reassurance after appropriate clinical and (not excessive) biochemical evaluation is most appropriate as puberty may be already imminent, starting or progressing. The administration of testosterone to adolescent boys with CDGP risks premature epiphyseal closure, resulting in reduced adult height and the widely used intramuscular depot injections of testosterone esters result in unphysiological peaks and troughs in testosterone exposure with gonadotrophin secretion completely suppressed. Theoretically, the daily administration of weak androgen would allow continuing gradual dose adjustment and endogenous gonadotrophin production without disproportionately rapid skeletal (bone age) maturation or final height compromise. TU was first studied in relation to pharmacokinetics and effects on growth and sexual maturation in this context nearly 25 years ago in a double blind, placebo-controlled study [2,3]. Despite the limitation of an observational study design (which potentially introduces bias), this is the largest evaluation TU treatment in CDGP boys.

Although bone age delay was not altered, 'predicted adult height' needs to be interpreted with caution. In the contexts of both precocious and delayed puberty, on repeated evaluations in the same individual bone age does not increase by one 'year' per year chronological age (CA), rather bone age accelerates/deviates from the cross-sectional reference in the same way as seen for height centile. Prediction equations are most accurate in children of 'average' height and normal puberty timing, but in CDGP will tend to overestimate adult height (in contrast to precocious puberty) [2].

The puberty nomogram was developed from the cross-sectional part of the COPENHAGEN Puberty Study (n=1,528 boys) and validated using data from the longitudinal part of the study (n=114). This defined delayed puberty as a genital stage <-2 SD for age. Because it evaluates both delayed pubertal onset and delayed pubertal progression, it allows the clinician to evaluate whether puberty is progressing appropriately. This should allow a more appropriate separation of normal from abnormal pubertal development than simply identifying prepubertal boys (in genital stage 1) aged 14 years or older. Although this large observational study does not show a dose- or time-response, it confirms the findings of the older smaller but double-blind, placebo-controlled prospective study that oral testosterone treatment of boys with CDGP is effective and safe in inducing puberty onset and progression and short-term growth considered safe, without (probably) compromising final height.

Food for thought

Recent advances in the technologies and regimens available for the management of type 1 diabetes have led to a focus on improvements in long-term outcomes. The following papers have investigated the change over time in life expectancy and the effect of intensive insulin therapy on the progression to retinopathy in patients with type 1 diabetes.

Estimated life expectancy in a Scottish cohort with type 1 diabetes, 2008-2010

Livingstone SJ, Levin D, Looker HC, Lindsay RS, Wild SH, Joss N, et al; Scottish Diabetes Research Network epidemiology group; Scottish Renal Registry
Diabetes Epidemiology Unit, University of Dundee, Dundee, Scotland, UK
JAMA 2015;313(1):37-44

Background: Type 1 diabetes (T1DM) is associated with significant reduction in life expectancy. However, given the advances in the treatment of diabetes over the last thirty years, contemporary estimates of life expectancy are required.
Methods: Prospective cohort study of 24,691 (67,712 person-years and 1,043 deaths) individuals aged 20 years or older with T1DM in Scotland using a nationwide register. The study investigated the differences in life expectancy between those with and those without T1DM and the contributions of specific causes (including kidney disease).
Results: Men with T1DM at age 20 years had an estimated loss in life expectancy of 11.1 years (95% CI, 10.1–12.1), and in women with T1DM it was 12.9 years (95% CI, 11.7–14.1), compared with those without T1DM. Life expectancy was even reduced in those with T1DM and an estimated glomerular filtration rate of 90mL/min/1.73m^2 or higher, in men by 8.3 years (95% CI, 6.5–10.1) and in women by

7.9 years (95% CI, 5.5–10.3). The largest contribution to loss in life expectancy overall was by ischaemic heart disease (36% in men, 31% in women), but in those under 50 years it was by diabetic coma or ketoacidosis (29.4% in men, 21.7% in women).
Conclusions: Estimated loss of life expectancy at age 20 for patients with T1DM in Scotland is approximately 11 years for men and 13 years for women compared with the general population without T1DM.

Whilst it is known that patients with T1DM have reduced life expectancies, the degree of reduction in life-years and the trends over time are largely unknown. With recent advances in the management of T1DM and the newer technologies available to patients it might be predicted that life expectancy will improve. This prospective cohort study took advantage of an extensive database that covers all patients with T1DM in >95% of Scottish GP practices. The accuracy and coverage of the database is extremely high, partly due to the financial incentive of the UK pay-for-performance programme. The study found that men aged 20 years with T1DM lived on average 11 years less than those from the general population without T1DM, whilst in women this was 12.9 years. Survival until age 70 years in both men and women with T1DM was reduced by around 30%. Interestingly, normal renal function (eGFR >90mL/min/1.73m^2) did not protect against the loss in life expectancy although the magnitude of loss from age 20 was slightly lower (8.3 years and 7.9 years in men and women, respectively). The paediatric dataset was less complete but showed slightly higher (0.6–0.7 years) loss in life expectancy compared with those at age 20 years. Overall, these predictions are more favourable than many previous estimates; however, given the lack of comparable datasets and analysis this cannot be easily extrapolated to demonstrate improvements in life expectancy over recent years.

Effect of intensive diabetes therapy on the progression of diabetic retinopathy in patients with type 1 diabetes: 18 years of follow-up in the DCCT/EDIC

Diabetes Control and Complications Trial (DCCT)/Epidemiology of Diabetes Interventions and Complications (EDIC) Research Group; Lachin JM, White NH, Hainsworth DP, Sun W, Cleary PA, Nathan DM
Diabetes 2015;64(2):631–642

Background: The Diabetes Control and Complications Trial (DCCT) showed a 76% reduction in the onset and progression of retinopathy after a mean of 6.5 years of intensive therapy compared with conventional treatment.
Methods: The Epidemiology of Diabetes Interventions and Complications (EDIC) study is the observational follow up study to DCCT. EDIC aimed to determine the risk of further progression of retinopathy after the end of the DCCT when both intensive and conventional groups switched to an intensive treatment regimen.
Results: The risk of progression of retinopathy at both four years and 10 years was markedly reduced in those who receiving intensive therapy compared with those receiving conventional treatment during the DCCT. This occurred despite that HbA_{1c} equalised between the groups.
Conclusions: The findings further support the concept of metabolic memory as the positive long-term result of early 'target' blood glucose control in type 1 diabetes.

The authors describe the outcome as a three-step progression of diabetic retinopathy (progression to proliferative retinopathy, clinically significant macular oedema and the need for intervention treatments) over the 18-year observational period. All participants in EDIC received intensive treatment, as the conventional treatment group switched to intensive treatment at the end of DCCT. The authors report remarkably high compliance with retinopathy data in the EDIC 'years 15–18': 88% of those enrolled in EDIC and impressively 84% of the original DCCT cohort.

Only 39% of the DCCT intensive treatment group showed progression of retinopathy compared with 56% of the original conventional treatment group. Of interest, at this stage the mean HbA_{1c} had equalised between the groups to 64mmol/mol (rising in the intensive group from 55mmol/mol at closeout, and falling in the conventional group from 76mmol/mol). This shows that the protective effect of target glycaemic control persists for up to 18 years although with smaller effects over time. This fall in effect is attributed to a decline in risk in the conventional group following their switch to intensive treatment at the end of DCCT. It is not seen as an increase in risk in the intensive treatment group, again highlighting the significance of metabolic memory. The incidence in the intensive group remains low and relatively stable for the three retinal outcomes. The key message is the importance of achieving a low target HbA_{1c} from diagnosis. Every effort must be made to maintain this for the paediatric and adolescent population, thereby reducing the likelihood of retinopathy and other complications.

New paradigms

Defining the role of common variation in the genomic and biological architecture of adult human height

Wood AR, Esko T, Yang J, Vedantam S, Pers TH, Gustafsson S, et al (298 authors and 359 collaborators!)
Genetics of Complex Traits, University of Exeter Medical School, University of Exeter, Exeter, UK
Nat Genet 2014;46(11):1173-1186

Background: Height is a classical polygenic trait that has provided general insights into the genetic architecture of common human traits and diseases and into the prospects and challenges of different methods used to identify genetic risk factors.
Methods, Results and Conclusions: Using genome-wide data from 253,288 individuals, the authors identified 697 variants at genome-wide significance that together explained one-fifth of the heritability for adult height. By testing different numbers of variants in independent studies, they demonstrate that the most strongly associated ~2,000, ~3,700 and ~9,500 SNPs explained ~21%, ~24% and ~29% of phenotypic variance. Furthermore, all common variants together captured 60% of heritability. The 697 variants clustered in 423 loci and were enriched for genes, pathways and tissue types known to be involved in growth and together also implicated genes and pathways not previously highlighted, including signalling by fibroblast growth factors, WNT/beta-catenin and chondroitin sulfate-related genes. Several genes and pathways not previously connected with human skeletal growth, including mTOR, osteoglycin and binding of hyaluronic acid were identified. These results indicate a genetic architecture for human height that is characterised by a very large number (thousands) of causal variants.

The additive genetic contribution to normal variation in adult height is thought to be around 80%. Increasing genome-wide association studies (GWAS) sample sizes to the order of 10^5 individuals (and the number of authors and collaborators to many hundreds!) now make possible the identification of associated variants and loci whilst improving knowledge of the biology of these traits. The authors identified variants that explain a substantial proportion of the heritability attributable to these common variants, suggesting that the genetic architecture for human height is characterised by a very large but finite number (thousands) of causal variants, located throughout the genome but clustered in both a biological and genomic manner.

The authors present strong evidence for multiple alleles at the same locus segregating in the population and for associated loci overlapping with Mendelian forms, suggesting a large but finite genomic mutational target for height and effect sizes ranging from minute (<1mm; ~0.01 s.d.) to gigantic (>300mm; >3 s.d.; in the case of monogenic mutations). The numerous associated gene sets and pathways were often overlapping and, therefore, represent multiple representations of a much smaller set of core biological mechanisms.

Individual genes at associated loci were often relevant to skeletal growth. Candidates that might contribute to syndromes of abnormal skeletal growth included *CHSY1*, recently identified as an underlying cause of a monogenic syndrome with short stature and brachydactyly.

The publicly available lists of genes and pathways provide a rich resource for future studies of skeletal growth. The authors speculate that increasing the number of associated loci for other traits and diseases could also yield similarly rich lists that would generate new biological hypotheses and motivate future research into other aspects of human biology and disease.

Brain cell swelling during hypocapnia increases with hyperglycaemia or ketosis

Glaser N, Bundros A, Anderson S, Tancredi D, Lo W, Orgain M, O'Donnell M
Department of Pediatrics, University of California Davis, School of Medicine, Sacraments, CA, USA
Pediatr Diabetes 2014;15(7):484–493

Background: Severe hypocapnia is a risk factor for cerebral oedema in paediatric diabetic ketoacidosis (DKA). This study, in ventilated rats with induced hypocapnia, aimed to identify specific metabolic conditions to inform the understanding of the cause of cerebral oedema and brain injury in paediatric DKA.
Methods: Cerebral blood flow (CBF) and apparent diffusion coefficient (ADC) were measured using magnetic resonance (MR) imaging in four experimental groups of rats (normal control, hypocapnia, hypocapnia plus hyperglycaemia and hypocapnia plus ketosis). pCO_2 levels were normalised in a subgroup of rats and the imaging studies were repeated.
Results: Low pCO_2 universally led to a decrease in CBF with no specific added effect of either hyperglycaemia or hyperketonaemia. There was also no difference in the effect of the increased CBF following normalisation of the pCO_2. However hyperglycaemia and hyperketonaemia led to a larger fall in ADC than in the hypocapnia group alone, which indicates increased brain swelling under these conditions.
Conclusions: Hyperglycaemia and ketonaemia, in addition to hypocapnia, may increase the susceptibility to brain injury.

Clinicians have clear guidelines for the management of paediatric DKA, yet the pathophysiology of the related cerebral oedema remains uncertain. Hypocapnia is a recognised risk factor in DKA and it is also known to significantly reduce CBF in other medical conditions. The authors previously reported that both hyperglycaemia and hyperketonaemia decrease CBF [4]. There is ongoing debate as to whether the metabolic derangements in DKA directly affect CBF or whether they increase susceptibility of the brain to injury over and above the reductions in CBF. The hypocapnia in DKA is a respiratory compensation to the metabolic acidosis and is often marked. However it is felt unlikely that hypocapnia is the sole cause of cerebral oedema and subsequent brain injury. This study suggests that both raised blood glucose and raised blood ketone levels have additional effects beyond that of hypocapnia-related reduced CBF, causing an increased likelihood of brain injury. Hypocapnia-related brain cell swelling is markedly increased, as identified by falling ADC values, in the presence of either a raised blood glucose value or ketonaemia. Caution must be taken in interpreting these animal study data and the duration of induced hypocapnia was shorter than that which occurs typically in a child in DKA.

Concepts revis(it)ed

Similar to the recognition of healthy and unhealthy fatness, so also not all thinness may be pathological and associated with broader health (including endocrine) consequences:

Constitutional thinness and anorexia nervosa: a possible misdiagnosis?

Estour B, Galusca B, Germain N
Service d'endocrinologie diabète et TCA, Centre Hospitalier Universitaire de Saint-Étienne, Saint Etienne, France
Front Endocrinol (Lausanne) 2014 20;5:175

Clinical and biological aspects of restrictive anorexia nervosa (R-AN) including genetic background, ineffectiveness of appetite regulating hormones on re-feeding, bone loss and the place of amenorrhoea in the definition, are widely studied and known: indeed more than 10,000 articles since 1911 and more than 600 in 2013 alone have addressed the psychiatric, somatic and biological aspects of R-AN. Constitutional thinness (CT), however, appears to be an almost unknown entity, with only 32 articles published on this topic since 1953. Whilst similar symptoms associating low body mass index (BMI), low fat and bone mass are reported in both CT and R-AN subjects, in CT menses are preserved and virtually the entire hormonal profile is normal, except for leptin and PYY. The confusing clinical presentation of these two situations is a potential source of misdiagnosis, especially since the revised definition of R-AN in the updated *Diagnostic and Statistical Manual of Mental Disorders* (DSM5; 2013).

For most clinicians finding a low BMI without obvious organic cause, the first likely diagnosis would be AN. However, the differential diagnosis should include the poorly-recognised entity 'constitutional thinness' (CT). One important distinguishing feature between R-AN and CT is the absence and presence (respectively) of menses, but this criterion cannot, of course, be applied to males, pre-menarcheal girls or women on the oral contraceptive pill. Characteristically, CT subjects want to gain weight (and this is the typical reason for seeking medical advice) but they fail to gain weight in a controlled overfeeding study [5].

What are the learning points? Firstly, a very thin girl who claims to eat a normal diet should be heard and not immediately considered to be deceiving herself and the clinician. This is particularly the case in the post-menarcheal adolescent or young woman whose menses are preserved and where other family members are constitutionally thin yet (by definition) reproductive function must be normal. CT is a well-defined condition of low BMI associated with a genuine desire to gain weight, normal nutritional markers except for a mildly low leptin (commensurate with the degree of thinness), a constitutive appetite-regulating hormone profile, the presence of menses in young women and low bone mass. Secondly, investigations including leptin, free-T3 and IGF-1 are valuable in order to prevent misdiagnosis. Thirdly, whilst the prevalence of CT is unknown, previous studies of 'AN' populations that have sometimes shown conflicting results may have, in fact, included heterogeneous groups of patients. More generally, classifications based on incomplete knowledge, whilst potentially useful, must be treated with caution so that the biology is not shoe-horned into the (sometimes arbitrary) classification – as knowledge increases a good classification should increasingly reflect (patho)physiology. Specifically, in this case, the revised definition of AN in DSM5 (based only on psychological and no organic symptoms) doubles the apparent risk of AN in (for example) dancers and in the general population.

In the above review, constitutional thinness is defined as a natural and physiologically low BMI (<18.5 kg/m^2), but how useful is BMI as a screening measure for identifying obesity in children and adolescents?

Diagnostic performance of body mass index to identify obesity as defined by body adiposity in children and adolescents: a systematic review and meta-analysis

Javed A, Jumean M, Murad MH, Okorodudu D, Kumar S, Somers VK, Sochor O, Lopez-Jimenez F
Department of Pediatric and Adolescent Medicine, Division of Pediatric Endocrinology, Mayo Clinic, Rochester, MN, USA
Pediatr Obes 2015 10(3):234–244

Background: The ideal measure for identifying obesity in children and adolescents has not been determined. Body mass index (BMI) has become a most widely used screening tool.
Methods: The authors carried out a systematic review and meta-analysis of studies assessing the diagnostic performance of BMI to detect adiposity in children aged up to 18 years using EMBASE, MEDLINE, the Cochrane Database of Systematic Reviews Cochrane CENTRAL, Web of Science and SCOPUS up to March 2013. Studies providing measures of diagnostic performance of BMI and employing a body composition technique for body fat percentage measurement were included.
Results: Thirty-seven eligible studies (n=53,521) with mean age between four and 18 years were included. Commonly used BMI cut-offs for obesity showed pooled sensitivity to detect high adiposity of 0.73 (confidence interval [CI] 0.67–0.79) and specificity of 0.93 (CI 0.88–0.96). The diagnostic odds ratio was 36.93 (CI 20.75–65.71). There was a lower sensitivity in males. Moderate heterogeneity between studies was observed (I2=48%). Meta-regression demonstrated that this was due to differences across studies in race, BMI cut-off, BMI reference criteria (Center for Disease Control versus International Obesity Task Force) and the method used to assess adiposity.

Conclusions: BMI has high specificity but low sensitivity to detect excess adiposity. As a result, BMI measurement fails to identify over a quarter of children with excess body fat percentage.

How is obesity in children and adolescents best determined? Although BMI is most widely used, its value has not properly evaluated. Indeed, whilst epidemiological data show a positive association between BMI and risk of cardiovascular events, there are *a priori* reasons why BMI may be inadequate for identifying those at risk: it inherently relies on body weight and fails to distinguish between lean and fat mass. Further limitations relate to difficulties with standardisation in the growing child and adolescent, the appropriateness of reference data (national versus racial/ethnic differences) and use of arbitrary cut-off centiles. Adiposity standards (for example, dual energy X-ray absorptiometry (DXA), hydrostatic weighing (HW), air-displacement plethysmography (ADP), isotope dilution, bioelectrical impedance analysis (BIA) and skinfold thickness measurement) lack reference data on 'normal' cut-offs for body fat percentage (BF%) values in children and are variably complex and cumbersome to perform.

This meta-analysis is the first to summarise the validity of BMI for detecting obesity as defined by excess adiposity in children and adolescents. They show that BMI has high specificity in identifying childhood obesity, but only moderate sensitivity – that is, over 25% of children considered non-obese by BMI have excess adiposity. Missed opportunities to institute lifestyle interventions to mitigate future health risks have important implications for policymakers, clinicians and affected families.

We can confidently state that a child deemed to be obese by their BMI is almost certainly obese. If BMI is 'normal', other tools may be helpful such as skinfold measurements (relatively easy to use and interpret despite high levels of inter-observer variability). Lowering the BMI cut-off to define 'obesity' is not the answer, as the decrease in specificity would result in many truly non-obese individuals being misclassified. At population level, BMI is a valuable tool to monitor obesity rates, but has limitations at the individual level and there is still a need to develop paediatric reference values for skinfold thickness, ADP, DXA and so on. and to assess their additive or independent ability to predict development of obesity-associated comorbidities. However, this is not the only area of paediatric endocrinology (or, indeed, medicine) where auxological or biochemical measures are used before their value is properly evaluated. Because something is 'easy' to measure does not mean it is informative for diagnosis, health-care policies, individual treatment interventions or long-term health outcomes.

References

1. Pruteanu AI, Chauhan BF, Zhang L, Prietsch SO, Ducharme FM. Inhaled corticosteroids in children with persistent asthma: is there a dose response impact on growth? An overview of Cochrane reviews. Paediatr Respir Rev 2015;16(1):51–52.
2. Brown DC, Butler GE, Kelnar CJ, Wu FC. A double blind, placebo controlled study of the effects of low dose testosterone undecanoate on the growth of small for age, prepubertal boys. Arch Dis Child 1995;73(2):131–135.
3. Butler GE, Sellar RE, Walker RF, Hendry M, Kelnar CJ, Wu FC. Oral testosterone undecanoate in the management of delayed puberty in boys: pharmacokinetics and effects on sexual maturation and growth. J Clin Endocrinol Metab 1992;75(1):37–44.
4. Glaser N, Ngo C, Anderson S, Yuen N, Trifu A, O'Donnell M. Effects of hyperglycemia and effects of ketosis on cerebral perfusion, cerebral water distribution, and cerebral metabolism. Diabetes 2012;61(7):1831–1837.
5. Germain N, Galusca B, Caron-Dorval D, Martin JF, Pujos-Guillot E, Boirie Y, et al. Specific appetite, energetic and metabolomics responses to fat overfeeding in resistant-to-bodyweight-gain constitutional thinness. Nutr Diabetes 2014;4:e126.

Science and Medicine

Ze'ev Hochberg[a] and Ken Ong[b]

[a] Technion-Israel Institute of Technology, Haifa, Israel

[b] Medical Research Council Epidemiology Unit, Wellcome Trust-MRC Institute of Metabolic Science, University of Cambridge, Cambridge, UK

An endocrine basis for 'man's best friend'

Social evolution. Oxytocin-gaze positive loop and the coevolution of human-dog bonds

Nagasawa M, Mitsui S, En S, Ohtani N, Ohta M, Sakuma Y, Onaka T, Mogi K, Kikusui T

Department of Animal Science and Biotechnology, Azabu University, Sagamihara, Kanagawa, Japan

kikusui@azabu-u.ac.jp

Science 2015;348(6232):333–336

Background: Human-like modes of communication, including mutual gaze, in dogs may have been acquired during domestication with humans.

Results: The authors show that gazing behaviour from dogs, but not wolves, increased urinary oxytocin concentrations in owners, which consequently facilitated owners' affiliation and increased oxytocin concentration in dogs. Further, nasally administered oxytocin increased gazing behaviour in dogs, which in turn increased urinary oxytocin concentrations in owners.

Conclusions: These findings support the existence of an interspecies oxytocin-mediated positive loop facilitated and modulated by gazing, which may have supported the coevolution of human-dog bonding by engaging common modes of communicating social attachment.

For 30,000 years, dogs have been rooted in human societies with mutual friendship and social attachments. This paper provides a biological mechanism for this interaction. Even as puppies, dogs respond to social signals, including gaze direction, use of communicative markers and even word learning. Thus, dogs show much of the same cognitive flexibilities and easygoing temperaments that characterise humans, but not their ancestral wolves. Direct comparisons show that unlike dogs, wolves do not expect humans to be cooperative social partners and do not look to humans for help when faced with an unsolvable problem. Dog psychology was shaped by domestication and includes a unique interspecies relationship that is surprisingly successful from an evolutionary perspective.

Oxytocin plays a role in this story. Oxytocin has long been known for its role in bonding among humans but now we learn that it can also facilitate social relationships between species. Both humans and dogs have increases in circulating oxytocin, as well as endorphins, dopamine and prolactin, when they interact with each other, and exogenous administration of oxytocin causes dogs to initiate more social contact with other dogs and humans, and allows dogs to more faithfully tune into human social cues. The authors measured changes in both the dogs' and owners' urinary oxytocin concentrations before and after the two interacted, and demonstrate that owners whose dogs gazed at them most had the largest change in urinary oxytocin, while their dogs, in return, experienced a similar oxytocin increase, the magnitude of which correlated with that of the owner. None of this was observed in wolves. Administration of oxytocin to dogs increased mutual gazing between owners and dogs, and increased oxytocin concentrations in the owners. Oxytocin administration to human parents can have parallel effects in their infants, as a result of increased bonded parental behaviour [1]. From an evolutionary perspective, dogs express behaviours that mimic the cues that elicit caregiving in humans towards our young. Once elicited, interspecies bonds are maintained through a positive hormone feedback loop, which originally evolved to promote bonding between parent and child.

Splicing for diversity

RNA splicing. The human splicing code reveals new insights into the genetic determinants of disease

Xiong HY, Alipanahi B, Lee LJ, Bretschneider H, Merico D, Yuen RK, Hua Y, Gueroussov S, Najafabadi HS, Hughes TR, Morris Q, Barash Y, Krainer AR, Jojic N, Scherer SW, Blencowe BJ, Frey BJ
Department of Electrical and Computer Engineering, University of Toronto, Toronto, ON, Canada
frey@psi.toronto.edu
Science 2015;347(6218):1254806

Background & Methods: To facilitate precision medicine and whole-genome annotation, the authors developed a machine-learning technique that scores how strongly genetic variants affect RNA splicing, whose alteration contributes to many diseases.
Results: Analysis of more than 650,000 intronic and exonic variants revealed widespread patterns of mutation-driven aberrant splicing. Intronic disease mutations that are more than 30 nucleotides from any splice site alter splicing nine times as often as common variants, and missense exonic disease mutations that have the least impact on protein function are five times as likely as others to alter splicing. Tens of thousands of disease-causing mutations were detected, including those involved in cancers and spinal muscular atrophy. Examination of intronic and exonic variants found using whole-genome sequencing of individuals with autism revealed misspliced genes with neurodevelopmental phenotypes.
Conclusion: This approach provides evidence for causal variants and should enable new discoveries in precision medicine.

The genomic code is activated by the transcription of a gene's DNA sequence into RNA, and the splicing of the primary RNA transcript to generate functional messenger RNAs, which are then translated into proteins. Alternative splicing is the mechanism by which the genome can generate multiple RNAs and proteins from a limited repertoire of genes. Alterations in the splicing process cause diseases such as spinal muscular atrophy. Using sophisticated machine-learning approaches, these authors built a mathematical model that predicts splicing in different tissues. The model predicts that intronic mutations associated with disease alter splicing nine times as often as common variants and argue that their approach is more sensitive than standard genome-wide association studies for capturing splicing-related disease single nucleotide variations (SNVs). The model explains disease penetrance of silent mutations in hereditary colorectal cancer and provides candidates for splicing alterations that may play a role in autism. Genetic variation in splicing-regulatory and particularly CpG sites might be related to disease predisposition. A recent paper identified 33 genes related to type 2 diabetes by investigating the impact of the corresponding coding sSNPs on splicing. SNPs, mostly epigenetic, in these genes were found to be prominent coding synonymous [2].

The human protein atlas

Proteomics. Tissue-based map of the human proteome

Uhlen M, Fagerberg L, Hallstrom BM, Lindskog C, Oksvold P, Mardinoglu A, Sivertsson A, Kampf C, Sjostedt E, Asplund A, Olsson I, Edlund K, Lundberg E, Navani S, Szigyarto CA, Odeberg J, Djureinovic D, Takanen JO, Hober S, Alm T, Edqvist PH, Berling H, Tegel H, Mulder J, Rockberg J, Nilsson P, Schwenk JM, Hamsten M, von Feilitzen K, Forsberg M, Persson L, Johansson F, Zwahlen M, von Heijne G, Nielsen J, Ponten F
Science for Life Laboratory, KTH-Royal Institute of Technology, SE-171 21 Stockholm, Sweden
Science 2015;347(6220):1260419

Background: Resolving the molecular details of proteome variation in the different tissues and organs of the human body will greatly increase our knowledge of human biology and disease.
Methods: The authors present a map of the human tissue proteome based on an integrated omics approach

that involves quantitative transcriptomics at the tissue and organ level, combined with tissue microarray-based immunohistochemistry, to achieve spatial localisation of proteins down to the single-cell level.
Results: This tissue-based analysis detected more than 90% of the putative protein-coding genes. The authors used this approach to explore the human secretome, the membrane proteome, the druggable proteome, the cancer proteome and the metabolic functions in 32 different tissues and organs. All the data are integrated in an interactive web-based database that allows exploration of individual proteins, as well as navigation of global expression patterns, in all major tissues and organs in the human body.

The human proteome (http://www.proteinatlas.org) has been developed using gene-centric and genome-wide antibody-based profiling on tissue microarrays. It therefore allows for tissue- and pathology-based annotation of protein expression, to be combined with deep-sequencing transcriptomics of the same tissue types. It has so far been performed for all 32 major tissues and organs in the human body, with a focus on the tissue-elevated proteins and all secreted and membrane proteins. It provides comprehensive metabolic maps for all 32 tissue types in order to identify differences in metabolism between tissues. The website is much worth a visit.

Evidence for a critical period in development

Effect of early institutionalization and foster care on long-term white matter development: a randomized clinical trial

Bick J, Zhu T, Stamoulis C, Fox NA, Zeanah C, Nelson CA
Division of Developmental Medicine, Department of Pediatrics, Boston Children's Hospital, Harvard Medical School, Boston, MA, USA
JAMA Pediatr 2015;169(3):211–219

Background: Severe neglect in early life is associated with compromises in brain development and associated behavioural functioning. Although early intervention has been shown to support more normative trajectories of brain development, specific improvements in the white matter pathways that underlie emotional and cognitive development are unknown.
Objective: To examine associations among neglect in early life, early intervention and the microstructural integrity of white matter pathways in middle childhood.
Methods: The Bucharest Early Intervention Project is a randomised clinical trial of high-quality foster care as an intervention for institutionally reared children in Bucharest, Romania, from 2000 through the present. During infancy, children were randomly selected to remain in an institution or to be placed in foster care. Those who remained in institutions experienced neglect, including social, emotional, linguistic and cognitive impoverishment. Developmental trajectories of these children were compared with a group of sociodemographically matched children reared in biological families at baseline and several points throughout development. At approximately eight years of age, 69 of the original 136 children underwent structural magnetic resonance imaging scans. Outcomes were four estimates of white matter integrity (fractional anisotropy [FA] and mean [MD], radial [RD] and axial [AD] diffusivity) for 48 white matter tracts throughout the brain were obtained through diffusion tensor imaging.
Results: Neglect in early life was associated with microstructural integrity of the body of the corpus callosum (FA, β=0.01 [P=0.01]; RD, β=-0.02 [P=0.005]; MD, β=-0.01 [P=0.02]) and tracts involved in limbic circuitry (fornix crus [AD, β=0.02 (P=0.046)] and cingulum [RD, β=-0.01 (P=0.02); MD, β=-0.01 (P=0.049)]), frontostriatal circuitry (anterior [AD, β=-0.01 (P=0.02)] and superior [AD, β=-0.02 (P=0.02); MD, β=-0.01 (P=0.03)] corona radiata and external capsule [right FA, β=0.01 (P=0.03); left FA, β=0.01 (P=0.03); RD, β=-0.01 (P=0.01); MD, β=-0.01 (P=0.03)]) and sensory processing (medial lemniscus [AD, β=-0.02 (P=0.045); MD, β=-0.01 (P=0.04)] and retrolenticular internal capsule [FA, β=-0.01 (P=0.002); RD, β=0.01 (P=0.003); MD, β=0.01 (P=0.04)]). Follow-up analyses revealed that early intervention promoted more normative white matter development among previously neglected children who entered foster care.
Conclusions: Removal from conditions of neglect in early life and entry into a high-quality family environment can support more normative trajectories of white matter growth. These findings have implications for public health and policy efforts designed to promote normative brain development among vulnerable children.

This was a controversial study at the time: to randomly select young children for high-quality foster care compared with those left in orphanages in Romania. As expected, children reared in institutions suffer setbacks, reflecting long-term changes in the brain. As we know from different contexts, the brain needs stimulation to develop and when these are prevented cognitive and emotional growths are stunted. The authors even claim that life without parenting can be more disastrous for brain development than living with an abusive caregiver. Child neglect is nearly three times as prevalent as physical and sexual abuse combined. The study reports that children in the institutional care group showed dramatic deficits on most measures when compared with the community group. Developmental quotient (DQ) score was 74 compared with 103 for the community group! In time, the children placed into foster care advanced toward the normal DQ, though they continued to lag behind the community group. The older the child when placed into foster care, the lower their cognitive score. Those who left the institution by age 18 months scored above 90, whereas those who left at 24 to 30 months scored just over 80. The first 24 months of life are essential for healthy attachment to a parent. Yet, as they reached eight years of age, the foster care children began to slow their climb into higher DQ and resemble the institutionalised group, with IQ scores hovering near 80, perhaps because their recovery from the effects of early neglect had reached a ceiling. Orphanages around the globe still house an estimated eight million children.

A trade-off between growth and metabolic demands

Neandertal growth: What are the costs?

Mateos A, Goikoetxea I, Leonard WR, Martín-González JÁ, Rodríguez-Gómez G, Rodríguez J
Centro Nacional de Investigación sobre la Evolución Humana (CENIEH), Paseo Sierra de Atapuerca 3, Burgos, Spain
ana.mateos@cenieh.es
J Hum Evol 2014;77:167–178

Background: Energetic approaches have been increasingly used to address key issues in Neanderthal palaeoecology and palaeobiology. Previous research has focused exclusively on the energy requirements of adults and highlights the high energy demands of these individuals compared with modern humans. Less attention has been paid to the energy requirements of sub-adult Neanderthals, even though this age group could provide clues for a better understanding of Neanderthal life history.
Methods: Accordingly, the authors here estimate the energy costs of maintenance and growth in Neanderthal infants and children from one to six years of age and compare these costs with values for modern humans. Statural growth models for two modern human populations (Beasain and Evenki) and an average Neanderthal model population are used to establish weight growth models. In turn, these models of body weight growth are used to estimate key components of energetic variables (basal metabolic rate, total energy expenditure, energy of growth and daily energy requirements).
Results: Between three and six years of age, Neanderthal children have slightly lower basal and growth energy costs than do modern humans of the same age, due primarily to their smaller body mass and slower growth rates. The reduction in energy allocated to growth is likely the result of metabolic adaptations to other somatic factors and thermal stress. Data from contemporary human infants and children suggest that even mild cold stress increases non-shivering thermogenesis, thus elevating metabolic needs by 50% or more.
Conclusions: These results suggest that thermal stress likely played a strong role in shaping the delayed developmental patterns and lower energy allocated to growth during early life in Neanderthals relative to *Homo sapiens*.

Linear growth rates of Neanderthal children aged two to six (which we now refer to as 'childhood' [3]) were much slower than those of modern human children. They obviously did not live in the type of energy-affluence that our children are exposed to, and accordingly their daily energy requirements were lower. The growth gap between their and our children was slight at age two to three and was markedly greater at age six, which is expected when 'childhood' gets shorter (five years for modern children and four years for Neanderthals) [4]. This is evidence of the modularity of development in body systems as recently proposed [5]. The slow linear growth of Neanderthals might be an adaptation to allow for faster growth of the brain. The positive correlation between basal metabolic rate and brain size in primates is well known, as is the potential trade-off between growth and the metabolic budget. Indeed, Neanderthal infants have cranial volumes at birth of 400cc (similar to those of modern human infants), but had greater brain capacity than ours at adulthood. The authors conclude that their European habitat and the associated thermal stress likely played a role in shaping the delayed developmental patterns and lower energy allocated to growth during childhood - a habitat that is still occupied by many contemporary children.

New methods: Genetic engineering

Enhanced homology-directed human genome engineering by controlled timing of CRISPR/Cas9 delivery

Lin S, Staahl BT, Alla RK, Doudna JA
Department of Molecular and Cell Biology, University of California, Berkeley, Berkeley, CA, USA
eLife 2015;3:e04766

Background: The CRISPR/Cas9 system is a robust genome editing technology that works in human cells, animals and plants based on the RNA-programmed DNA cleaving activity of the Cas9 enzyme.
Methods: Building on previous work (Jinek et al, 2013), the authors show that new genetic information can be introduced site-specifically and with high efficiency by homology-directed repair (HDR) of Cas9-induced site-specific double-strand DNA breaks using timed delivery of Cas9-guide RNA ribonucleoprotein (RNP) complexes.
Results: Cas9 RNP-mediated HDR in HEK293T, human primary neonatal fibroblast and human embryonic stem cells was increased dramatically relative to experiments in unsynchronised cells, with rates of HDR up to 38% observed in HEK293T cells. Sequencing of on- and potential off-target sites showed that editing occurred with high fidelity, while cell mortality was minimised.
Conclusions: This approach provides a simple and highly effective strategy for enhancing site-specific genome engineering in both transformed and primary human cells.

The molecular biology literature is now dominated by a single motto: 'CRISPR'. It is a genome-editing technique that emerged only a couple of years ago but is exploding. In these two years, scientists have CRISPRed dozens of cell types and organisms that traditionally have not been edited genetically. The technology allows scientists to quite easily edit mutations in and out of a genome.

The RNA-guided enzyme Cas9 originates from the CRISPR-Cas adaptive bacterial immune system, identified in *staphylococcus aureus*. When injected into adult mice with tyrosinaemia, it provided sufficient editing in the liver to alleviate the Fah mutation [6]. The problem was that Cas9 and RNA molecules that guide CRISPR to its target are too large to be efficiently transported into most human cells. This is almost resolved now by a Cas9 enzyme that is encoded by a much smaller gene. While technical in nature, this could open the door to new treatments for a host of genetic maladies (see Yin et al, below). The latest in CRISPR adventures is its role deciphering sex determination. Sex determination in the mosquito is governed by the dominant male-determining Nix gene in a Y chromosome-like region. Nix knockout with CRISPR/Cas9 resulted in largely feminised genetic males and the production of female isoforms of two key regulators of sexual differentiation: doublesex and fruitless. This is a control strategy to convert female mosquitoes into harmless males [7].

Genome editing with Cas9 in adult mice corrects a disease mutation and phenotype

Yin H, Xue W, Chen S, Bogorad RL, Benedetti E, Grompe M, Koteliansky V, Sharp PA, Jacks T, Anderson DG
David H. Koch Institute for Integrative Cancer Research, Massachusetts Institute of Technology, Cambridge, MA, USA
Nat Biotechnol 2014;32(6):551-553

Background: The authors demonstrate CRISPR-Cas9-mediated correction of a Fah mutation in hepatocytes in a mouse model of the human disease hereditary tyrosinaemia.

Methods: Delivery of components of the CRISPR-Cas9 system by hydrodynamic injection resulted in initial expression of the wild-type Fah protein in approximately 1/250 liver cells.
Results: Expansion of Fah-positive hepatocytes rescued the body weight loss phenotype.
Conclusions: This study indicates that CRISPR-Cas9-mediated genome editing is possible in adult animals and has potential for correction of human genetic diseases.

Hereditary tyrosinaemia type I (HTI) is a fatal disease caused by mutation of fumarylacetoacetate hydrolase (FAH), the last enzyme in the tyrosine catabolic pathway. FAH deficiency results in accumulation of toxic metabolites leading to liver damage. It can be caused by a mutation affecting a single critical nucleotide ('point mutation'), which causes skipping of a whole exon during splicing and leading to a truncated, unstable FAH protein. In such cases, only that one nucleotide needs to be repaired. Another key characteristic that makes this condition amenable to this novel genetic therapy is that repaired liver cells, with restored metabolic capacity, have a selective advantage over defective cells and can expand and repopulate the liver. Therefore, even the minor rate of successful cell repair (1/250 cells) proved sufficient to restore liver function in this mouse model. The hydrodynamic injection administration used here involves the rapid injection of a large volume of solution and is unlikely to be feasible in humans. They therefore consider these findings to show proof-of-principle for correction of genetic disease in vivo with CRISPR-Cas9 DNA technology. Despite such technical challenges, there is growing debate regarding the need for laws to restrict how widely we should edit the human genome [8].

New mechanisms: mTORC and FGF21 control whole-body physiology

Hepatic mTORC1 controls locomotor activity, body temperature, and lipid metabolism through FGF21

Cornu M, Oppliger W, Albert V, Robitaille AM, Trapani F, Quagliata L, Fuhrer T, Sauer U, Terracciano L, Hall MN
Biozentrum, University of Basel, Basel, Switzerland
M.Hall@unibas.ch
Proc Natl Acad Sci U S A 2014;111(32):11592–11599

Background: The liver is a key metabolic organ that controls whole-body physiology in response to nutrient availability. Mammalian target of rapamycin (mTOR) is a nutrient-activated kinase and central controller of growth and metabolism that is negatively regulated by the tumour suppressor tuberous sclerosis complex 1 (TSC1).
Methods: The authors generated liver-specific Tsc1 (L-Tsc1 KO) knockout mice to investigate the role of hepatic mTOR complex 1 (mTORC1) in whole-body physiology.
Results: L-Tsc1 KO mice displayed reduced locomotor activity, body temperature and hepatic triglyceride content in a rapamycin-sensitive manner. Ectopic activation of mTORC1 also caused depletion of hepatic and plasma glutamine, leading to peroxisome proliferator-activated receptor gamma coactivator-1-alpha (PGC-1-alpha)-dependent fibroblast growth factor 21 (FGF21) expression in the liver. Injection of glutamine or knockdown of PGC-1α or FGF21 in the liver suppressed the behavioural and metabolic defects due to mTORC1 activation.
Conclusions: mTORC1 in the liver controls whole-body physiology through PGC-1-alpha and FGF21. Finally, mTORC1 signalling correlated with FGF21 expression in human liver tumours, suggesting that treatment of glutamine-addicted cancers with mTOR inhibitors might have beneficial effects at both the tumour and whole-body level.

Since 2008, the fibroblast growth factor 21 (FGF21) has taken centre stage as a key metabolic hormone that helps the body to adapt to starvation (Yearbook 2008). FGF21 expression levels in the liver rise on fasting, stimulates the release of fatty acids from adipose tissue and promotes their conversion in the liver to ketone bodies, an energy source when carbohydrates are scarce, and mediates direct activation of brown fat thermogenesis during the fetal-to-neonatal transition. FGF21 treatment improves systemic insulin resistance and inhibits STAT5 signalling and the expression of IGF-1 through its PPAR effect, and thereby blunts GH action as part of its broader role in promoting energy conservation during starvation. As the FGF21 story has unfolded, Mechanism of Target of Rapamycin (mTOR) has become as important as a highly conserved protein kinase that is found in two structurally and functionally distinct protein complexes: TOR complex-1 (TORC1) and TORC2. TORC1 is a key regulator of cell growth and proliferation and mRNA translation, whereas TORC2 promotes actin cytoskeletal rearrangement, cell survival and cell cycle progression. These authors, who discovered its role in cell growth control, show now the mechanism of its action in whole-body physiology is through PGC-1-alpha and FGF21. Activation of mTORC1 caused depletion of hepatic and plasma glutamine, leading to PPAR gamma-dependent FGF21 expression in the liver. Injection of glutamine or knockdown of PGC-1-alpha or FGF21 in the liver suppressed the behavioural and metabolic defects due to mTORC1 activation. And, mTORC1 signalling correlated with FGF21 expression in human liver tumours, suggesting that treatment of glutamine-addicted cancers with mTOR inhibitors might have beneficial effects at both the tumour and whole-body level.

'Reading' about human history

Genome sequence of a 45,000-year-old modern human from western Siberia

Fu Q, Li H, Moorjani P, Jay F, Slepchenko SM, Bondarev AA, Johnson PL, Aximu-Petri A, Prufer K, de Filippo C, Meyer M, Zwyns N, Salazar-Garcia DC, Kuzmin YV, Keates SG, Kosintsev PA, Razhev DI, Richards MP, Peristov NV, Lachmann M, Douka K, Higham TF, Slatkin M, Hublin JJ, Reich D, Kelso J, Viola TB, Paabo S
Key Laboratory of Vertebrate Evolution and Human Origins of Chinese Academy of Sciences, IVPP, CAS, Beijing, China
Nature 2014;514(7523):445-449

Methods: The authors present the high-quality genome sequence of a ~45,000-year-old modern human male from Siberia.
Results: This individual derives from a population that lived before – or simultaneously with – the separation of the populations in western and eastern Eurasia and carries a similar amount of Neanderthal ancestry as present-day Eurasians. However, the genomic segments of Neanderthal ancestry are substantially longer than those observed in present-day individuals, indicating that Neanderthal gene flow into the ancestors of this individual occurred 7,000–13,000 years before he lived. The estimated autosomal mutation rate is 0.4 to $0.6x10^{-9}$ per site per year, Y chromosomal mutation rate 0.7 to $0.9x10^{-9}$ per site per year based on the additional substitutions that have occurred in present-day non-Africans compared with this genome and a mitochondrial mutation rate of $1.8x10^{-8}$ to $3.2x10^{-8}$ per site per year based on the age of the bone.

The genome sequence of this Siberian who lived some 45,000 years ago shows that our first episode of mixing with the Neanderthals occurred between 50,000 and 60,000 years ago, as soon as our species emerged from Africa, and before we ventured into Europe and Asia. The Siberian lived before we separated into different racial groups for Europe and Asia. Mostly, this paper provides the rates at which human DNA has changed or mutated over time. It is slower than previously suggested by fossil evidence and similar to that observed in contemporary families. If true, our evolutionary calendar may have to be redrawn: the very first species of hominids separated from apes might have happened 10 or 11 million years ago rather than five or six million years ago that we currently teach.

Food for thought: Equality and diversity

Special issue by *Nature* on diversity

In September 2014, *Nature* published a special issue with *Scientific American* that explored connections between diversity and the rigour of research, including how marginalisation affects study design that lead to misguided assumptions. Studies of social networks find that people tend to work and connect with their likes. Yet, greater ethnic diversity among authors is associated with a paper's publication in higher-impact journals and more citations. The conclusion is clear: inclusive science is better science.

Lack of reduction in racial disparities in cancer-specific mortality over a 20-year period

Aizer AA, Wilhite TJ, Chen MH, Graham PL, Choueiri TK, Hoffman KE, Martin NE, Trinh QD, Hu JC, Nguyen PL
Harvard Radiation Oncology Program, Harvard Medical School, Boston, MA, USA
Cancer 2014;120(10):1532–1539

Background: To the authors' knowledge, it remains unknown whether race-based differences in cancer outcomes have changed with time. The authors assessed whether racial disparities in cancer-specific mortality have improved over the last 20 years.
Methods: The Surveillance, Epidemiology and End Results program was used to identify 2,713,474 patients diagnosed between 1988 and 2007 with either lung, breast, prostate or colorectal cancer (the leading three causes of cancer-related mortality among each sex). After exclusions, 1,001,978 patients remained eligible for analysis. The impact of race on cancer-specific mortality was assessed using the regression model of Fine and Gray; an interaction model evaluated trends over time.
Results: African Americans presented with a more advanced stage of disease ($P<0.001$) and underwent definitive therapy less often ($P<0.001$) than whites. After adjustment for demographics and year of diagnosis, African Americans had higher cancer-specific mortality than whites for all cancers combined (hazards ratio, 1.28; 95% CI, 1.26–1.30 [$P<0.001$]) and within each individual cancer (each $P<0.05$). These differences did not change between 1988 through 1997 and 1998 through 2007, except among patients with breast cancer, in whom survival disparities increased. These findings remained after adjustment for stage of disease at presentation and receipt of definitive therapy (hazards ratio for breast cancer mortality in African Americans versus whites: 1.37 from 1988–1997 and 1.53 from 1998–2007; P for interaction, <0.001).
Conclusions: The survival gap for African Americans has not closed over time. Race-based differences in outcome persist independent of stage of disease and treatment, suggesting that additional strategies beyond screening and improving access to care, such as further research into tumour biologies disproportionately affecting African Americans, are needed to improve survival for African American patients with cancer.

Populations of non-European descent in the USA have higher rates of diseases such as asthma and cancer, and receive worse healthcare. Developed in biased samples of mostly Caucasian volunteers, many drugs work better in people of European origin than in others. Racial and ethnic minorities are harmed because they are not studied as often. Indeed, long-acting beta2-agonists are associated with higher mortality in African Americans. Study designers often see genetic diversity as a potential confounder. However, these differences can be leveraged to reveal new risk factors. This has been well known for a long time, but this study shows that nothing has changed; race-based differences in cancer outcomes persist. To close the gap we need research into the tumour biology of minority groups.

The impact of childhood experience on amygdala response to perceptually familiar black and white faces

Cloutier J, Li T, Correll J
University of Chicago, IL, USA
J Cogn Neurosci 2014;26(9):1992–2004

Background: Given the well-documented involvement of the amygdala in race perception, the authors aimed to investigate how interracial contact during childhood shapes amygdala response to racial outgroup members in adulthood.
Methods: Of particular interest was the impact of childhood experience on amygdala response to familiar, compared with novel, black faces. Results were controlled for a number of well-established individual difference measures related to interracial attitudes.

Results: Perceivers with greater childhood exposure to racial outgroup members displayed greater relative reduction in amygdala response to familiar black faces.
Conclusions: The implications of such findings are discussed in the context of previous investigations into the neural substrates of race perception and in consideration of potential mechanisms by which childhood experience may shape race perception.

If the human brain has evolved to support survival and prosperity in a complex social environment, then a research approach that considers this range of factors is needed to understand neural function. Research on the neural basis of prejudice has focused on the amygdala, the neural locus of emotion. It is essential for the processing of fear in facial expressions as well as other relevant social cues. Amygdala activation reflects an implied threat response to racial strangers. Thus, in white subjects viewing images of black faces, amygdala activation is greater in response to faces with darker rather than lighter complexion. By contrast, familiarity with racial outgroup members is associated with an attenuated difference in the amygdala response to strangers, both in children and adults. Social psychology theory regards prejudice as reflecting a form of threat processing as shaped by childhood experience. These findings have implications for social issues regarding inter-racial relations, and provide a context for understanding neural function as it relates to the real-world lives of human beings, social norms and social emotions as they relate to complex interpersonal behaviours.

Towards better research

How to make more published research true

Ioannidis JP
Meta-Research Innovation Center at Stanford (METRICS), Stanford University, Stanford, CA, USA
PLoS Med 2014;11(10):e1001747

Background: In a 2005 paper that has been accessed more than a million times, the author explained why most published research findings were false. Here he revisits the topic, this time to address how to improve matters.
Results: Currently, many published research findings are false or exaggerated. An estimated 85% of research resources are wasted. Possible practices to improve credibility and efficiency of research include: the adoption of large-scale collaborative research; reward a culture replication; registration, sharing and reproducibility of practices; standardisation of definitions and analyses; better statistical methods and (usually more stringent) statistical thresholds; and improvement in study design standards, peer review, reporting and dissemination of research and training of the scientific workforce.

It is very disheartening when the findings of our original experiments, or even publications, fail to be replicated by our own or others' larger-scale follow-up work. Yet our common goal should be to identify, validate and establish by replication 'true positive' findings, and to accept without recriminations subsequent repudiation of our 'false positive' findings. One of the biggest barriers to accepting this culture is that science funding and careers are rewarded for being the first to make new discoveries, and currently there is little kudos for publishing replication studies, let alone negative studies.

Genetic epidemiology is a discipline that managed to move on from two decades of reporting countless false positive association studies in underpowered (too small) studies. The last update of the Human Obesity Gene Map in 2005 catalogued 426 reported positive associations with 127 candidate genes; almost all of these have not been replicated in more recent very large-scale genome-wide association studies (GWAS). The game-changers included some of the measures described here by John Ioannidis. In addition to technological advances in genotyping, a consensus was universally adopted to use a highly stringent statistical threshold correcting for total common genomic variation ($P<5x10^{-8}$), and large-scale research collaborations were formed with sharing of data and analytical software. However, it remains a major challenge how to recognise and fund individual teams and early career scientists involved in such 'team science'.

Review on genomic imprinting

The role of genomic imprinting in biology and disease: an expanding view

Peters J
Medical Research Council Mammalian Genetics Unit, Harwell Science and Innovation Campus, Oxfordshire, UK
Nat Rev Genet 2014;15(8):517–530

Background: Genomic imprinting is an epigenetic phenomenon that results in monoallelic gene expression according to parental origin. It has long been established that imprinted genes have major effects on development and placental biology before birth. More recently, it has become evident that imprinted genes also have important roles after birth.
Results: In this review, the author brings together studies of the effects of imprinted genes from the prenatal period onwards. Recent work on postnatal stages shows that imprinted genes influence an extraordinarily wide-ranging array of biological processes, the effects of which extend into adulthood, and play important parts in common diseases that range from obesity to psychiatric disorders.

Paediatric endocrinologists are more familiar with the concepts of genomic imprinting than many other medical specialists because we look after children with imprinting disorders, such as Silver-Russell syndrome, Beckwith-Wiedemann syndrome, Angelman syndrome and pseudohypoparathyroidism types 1a and 1b. There are around 150 imprinted genes yet identified in the mouse and about half of those also have evidence of imprinting in humans – a key limitation to comprehensive assessment in humans is that imprinting may alter gene expression only in specific tissues. This genetic mechanism allows parental control of which genes are actively expressed or silenced after transmission to their in their offspring and it seems that fathers and mothers have different interests regarding the growth and development of their offspring. Genomic imprinting appears to have evolved at the same time as the placenta in mammals and concordantly the best characterised imprinted genes have key roles in fetal growth in mice and humans. However, there is growing evidence that imprinted genes also regulate postnatal and childhood traits, including infant feeding, growth, puberty timing, metabolism and neurological and behavioural processes. Furthermore, this review goes on to speculate on their possible influence on common diseases, such as obesity, diabetes mellitus, psychiatric disorders and cancer.

Placenta or egg?

The evolution of the placenta drives a shift in sexual selection in livebearing fish

Pollux BJ, Meredith RW, Springer MS, Garland T, Reznick DN
Department of Biology, University of California, Riverside, CA, USA
Nature 2014;513(7517):233–236

Background: The evolution of the placenta from a non-placental ancestor causes a shift of maternal investment from pre- to post-fertilisation. This creates a venue for parent-offspring conflicts during pregnancy. Theory predicts that the rise of these conflicts should drive a shift from a reliance on pre-copulatory female mate choice to polyandry in conjunction with post-zygotic mechanisms of sexual selection. This hypothesis has not yet been empirically tested.
Methods: The authors apply comparative methods to test a key prediction of this hypothesis, which is that the evolution of placentation is associated with reduced pre-copulatory female mate choice. They exploit a unique quality of the livebearing fish family *Poeciliidae*: placentas have repeatedly evolved or been lost, creating diversity among closely related lineages in the presence or absence of placentation.
Results: Post-zygotic maternal provisioning by means of a placenta is associated with the absence of bright coloration, courtship behaviour and exaggerated ornamental display traits in males. Furthermore, males

of placental species have smaller bodies and longer genitalia, which facilitate sneak or coercive mating and, hence, circumvents female choice. Moreover, post-zygotic maternal provisioning correlates with superfetation, a female reproductive adaptation that may result in polyandry through the formation of temporally overlapping, mixed-paternity litters.
Conclusions: These findings suggest that the emergence of prenatal conflict during the evolution of the placenta correlates with a suite of phenotypic and behavioural male traits that is associated with a reduced reliance on pre-copulatory female mate choice.

The main advantage of placentation versus egg-laying is the ability for the mother to closely nurture and nourish the fetus for longer before birth, compared with the egg's sealed system. The downside is the greater burden on the mother in terms of time, nutrient transfer and increased volume of embryonic waste. Placentation therefore allows for competition between mother and fetus over the transfer of resources, as well as ongoing competition between potential fathers even after mate choice, copulation and fertilisation. A remarkable range of phenotypic and behavioural changes in the parents following the 'emergence' of placentation is described here for the first time. 'Polyandry' is a form of polygamy whereby the mother mates with two or more potential fathers. Rather than rely on the father's physical appearance to choose her mate, in order to select the most viable offspring it is more reliable to allow direct competition between the embryos of different fathers. 'Superfetation' is the occurrence of a second conception during pregnancy, giving rise to the mother carrying embryos of different ages. This maternal reproductive behaviour is thought to avoid a single male monopolising an entire litter. It is reported only extremely rarely in humans, manifested as a small (range two to four weeks) discordance in gestational age between dizygotic twins.

Eating for our health and our planet

Global diets link environmental sustainability and human health

Tilman D, Clark M
Department of Ecology, Evolution and Behavior, University of Minnesota, St Paul, MN, USA
Nature 2014;515(7528):518–522

Background: Diets link environmental and human health. Rising incomes and urbanisation are driving a global dietary transition in which traditional diets are replaced by diets higher in refined sugars, refined fats, oils and meats.
Methods: The authors compiled and analysed global-level data to quantify relationships among diet, environmental sustainability and human health and to evaluate potential future environmental impacts of the global dietary transition.
Results: By 2050 these dietary trends, if unchecked, would be a major contributor to an estimated 80% increase in global agricultural greenhouse gas emissions from food production and to global land clearing. Moreover, these dietary shifts are greatly increasing the incidence of type 2 diabetes, coronary heart disease and other chronic non-communicable diseases that lower global life expectancies. Alternative diets that offer substantial health benefits could, if widely adopted, reduce global agricultural greenhouse gas emissions, reduce land clearing and resultant species extinctions and help prevent such diet-related chronic non-communicable diseases.
Conclusions: The implementation of dietary solutions to the tightly linked diet-environment-health 'trilemma' is a global challenge, and opportunity, of great environmental and public health importance.

The authors make a strong case that modern diets have adverse effects for both human health and for our planet. It is remarkable that despite our diverse international cultures and historical diets, rising incomes and urbanisation invariably lead to rising per capita demands for meat and 'empty calories' (from refined sugars, refined animal fats/oils and alcohol) as well as total calories. The authors project that from 2009 to 2050, the combined effects of ongoing global dietary shifts and the 36% rise in global population will cause an estimated 80% increase in global greenhouse gas emissions from food production. In contrast, there would be no net increase in emissions if we were to

adopt Mediterranean, pescetarian or vegetarian diets, and there would also be substantial reductions in rates of Type 2 diabetes, cardiovascular disease and other non-communicable diseases.

References

1. Weisman O, Zagoory-Sharon O, Feldman R. Oxytocin administration to parent enhances infant physiological and behavioral readiness for social engagement. Biol Psych 2012;72(12):982–989.
2. Karambataki M, MalousiA, Kouidou S. Risk-associated coding synonymous SNPs in type 2 diabetes and neurodegenerative diseases: genetic silence and the underrated association with splicing regulation and epigenetics. Mutat Res 2014;770:85–93.
3. Hochberg Z. Evo-devo of child growth II: human life history and transition between its phases. Eur J Endocrinol 2009;160(2):135–141.
4. Hochberg Z. Evo-Devo of child growth III: premature juvenility as an evolutionary trade-off. Horm Res Paediatr 2010;73(6)430–437.
5. Smith TM, Tafforeau P, Reid DJ, Pouech J, Lazzari V, Zemeno JP, et al. Dental evidence for ontogenetic differences between modern humans and Neanderthals. Proc Natl Acad Sci U S A 2010;107(49):20923–20928.
6. Yin H, Xue W, Chen S, Bogorad RL, Benedelti E, Grompe M, et al. Genome editing with Cas9 in adult mice corrects a disease mutation and phenotype. Nat Biotechnol 2014;32(6):550–553.
7. Cong L, Ran FA, Cox D, Lin S, Barretto R, Habib N, et al. Multiplex genome engineering using CRISPR/Cas systems. Science 2013;339(6121):819–823.
8. Lanphier E, Urnov F, Haecker SE, Werner M, Smolenski J. Don't edit the human germ line. Nature 2015;519(7544):410–411.

Editors' Choice

Ken Ong[a] and Ze'ev Hochberg[b]

[a] Medical Research Council Epidemiology Unit, Wellcome Trust-MRC Institute of Metabolic Science, University of Cambridge, Cambridge, UK

[b] Technion-Israel Institute of Technology, Haifa, Israel

Changing seasons

Widespread seasonal gene expression reveals annual differences in human immunity and physiology

Dopico XC, Evangelou M, Ferreira RC, Guo H, Pekalski ML, Smyth DJ, Cooper N, Burren OS, Fulford AJ, Hennig BJ, Prentice AM, Ziegler AG, Bonifacio E, Wallace C, Todd JA

JDRF/Wellcome Trust Diabetes and Inflammation Laboratory, Department of Medical Genetics, NIHR Cambridge Biomedical Research Centre, Cambridge Institute for Medical Research, University of Cambridge, Cambridge, UK

Nat Commun 2015;6:7000

Background: Seasonal variations are rarely considered a contributing component to human tissue function or health, although many diseases and physiological process display annual periodicities.
Results: The authors find more than 4,000 protein-coding mRNAs in white blood cells and adipose tissue to have seasonal expression profiles, with inverted patterns observed between Europe and Oceania. They also find the cellular composition of blood to vary by season, and these changes, which differ between the United Kingdom and The Gambia, could explain the gene expression periodicity. With regards to tissue function, the immune system has a profound pro-inflammatory transcriptomic profile during European winter, with increased levels of soluble IL-6 receptor and C-reactive protein, risk biomarkers for cardiovascular, psychiatric and autoimmune diseases that have peak incidences in winter.
Conclusions: Circannual rhythms require further exploration as contributors to various aspects of human physiology and disease.

We are familiar with seasonal differences in physiology (for example, growth) and behaviours across plant and animal species. In humans, many complex polygenic diseases, including cardiovascular, autoimmune and psychiatric illnesses, have established seasonal patterns of incidence and disease activity. These authors show how season might more broadly impact the underlying molecular details of human physiology. Initially, they hypothesised that anti-inflammatory circadian transcription factors, would also display seasonal gene expression differences, as daylight entrains circadian rhythms. But strikingly, they found ~23% of the genome (5,136 unique genes out of 22,822 genes tested) to show significant seasonal differences in expression. The findings include 2,311 genes that had increased expression in the summer while 2,826 genes were upregulated in the winter, demonstrating that different transcriptional landscapes are present. Given the remarkable seasonality of the peripheral immune system and their correlations with multiple health-associated phenotypes, they analysed gene expression data from a collection of subcutaneous adipose tissue samples. They report 4,027 genes to be seasonally expressed, including for example *PPARG*, targeted by thiazolidinediones as a current treatment of type 2 diabetes. We already know to treat differently data collected in morning or afternoon clinics; we now have to consider the seasons as well.

Does natural selection favour taller stature among the tallest people on earth?

Stulp G, Barrett L, Tropf FC, Mills M
Department of Population Health, London School of Hygiene and Tropical Medicine, London, UK
Proc Biol Sci 2015;282

Background: The Dutch are the tallest people on earth. Over the last 200 years, they have grown 20cm in height, a rapid rate of increase that points to environmental causes. This secular trend in height is echoed across all Western populations, but came to an end, or at least levelled off, much earlier than in The Netherlands. One possibility, then, is that natural selection acted congruently with these environmentally induced changes to further promote tall stature among the people of the lowlands.
Methods: Using data from the LifeLines study, which follows a large sample of the population of the north of The Netherlands (n=94,516), the authors examined how height was related to measures of reproductive success (as a proxy for fitness).
Results: Across three decades (1935–1967), height was consistently related to reproductive output (number of children born and number of surviving children), favouring taller men and average height women. This was despite a later age at first birth for taller individuals. Furthermore, even in this low-mortality population, taller women experienced higher child survival, which contributed positively to their increased reproductive success.
Conclusions: Natural selection in addition to good environmental conditions may help explain why the Dutch are so tall.

Firstly, this paper delivers the message that contemporary humans are still subject to natural selection. It also confirms our own perceptions when we visit the Netherlands - these youngsters are truly tall. In the 18th century, American men were five to eight centimeters taller than the Dutch. So, how did they become so tall? Genes and environment seem to influence stature about 50/50 and intuitively we thought that it would be the Dutch environment that would have augmented their height. But no, it is their genes. Tracking key life data for almost 100,000 people over 45 in the Netherlands, these researchers found that taller men had more children on average - extra 0.24 children for taller men, and taller men had a smaller chance of remaining childless and a higher chance of having a partner. The same effect wasn't seen in women, because the tallest women had a smaller chance of finding a mate. When this small change accumulates over six generations, it makes a difference. However, the authors don't show that genes that promote height are becoming more frequent. What is the mechanism for the fitness advantage of taller men? Is it a sexual selection? Dutch women may prefer taller men because they expect them to have more resources to invest in their children. But it could also be a natural selection, taller men may be more resistant to disease. Or a reproductive selection, they may be more likely to divorce and start a second family. Interestingly, natural selection in the USA has been suggested to pull in the opposite direction of environmental factors like diet, making people shorter instead of taller [1]. That may explain why the growth in average American height has levelled off. Humans often choose a partner who is not much shorter or taller than themselves. Because shorter women in the USA have more children, tall American men may be disadvantaged because they are less likely to partner with a short/fertile woman.

Exome sequencing for the diagnosis of 46,XY disorders of sex development

Baxter RM, Arboleda VA, Lee H, Barseghyan H, Adam MP, Fechner PY, Bargman R, Keegan C, Travers S, Schelley S, Hudgins L, Mathew RP, Stalker HJ, Zori R, Gordon OK, Ramos-Platt L, Pawlikowska-Haddal A, Eskin A, Nelson SF, Delot E, Vilain E
Departments of Human Genetics and Pathology and Laboratory Medicine, David Geffen School of Medicine, University of California-Los Angeles, Los Angeles, CA, USA.
J Clin Endocrinol Metab 2015;100:E333–E344

Background: Disorders of sex development (DSD) are clinical conditions where there is a discrepancy between the chromosomal sex and the phenotypic (gonadal or genital) sex of an individual. Such conditions can be stressful for patients and their families and have historically been difficult to diagnose, especially at the genetic level. In particular, for cases of 46,XY gonadal dysgenesis, once variants in SRY and NR5A1 have been ruled out, there are few other single gene tests available.
Methods: The authors used exome sequencing followed by analysis with a list of all known human DSD-associated genes to investigate the underlying genetic aetiology of 46,XY DSD patients who had not previously received a genetic diagnosis. Samples were either submitted to the research laboratory or submitted as clinical samples to the UCLA Clinical Genomic Center. Sequencing data were filtered using a list of genes known to be involved in DSD.
Results: A likely genetic diagnosis was identified in more than a third of cases, including 22.5% with a pathogenic finding, an additional 12.5% with likely pathogenic findings and 15% with variants of unknown clinical significance.
Conclusions: Early identification of the genetic cause of a DSD will in many cases streamline and direct the clinical management of the patient, with more focused endocrine and imaging studies and better-informed surgical decisions. Exome sequencing proved an efficient method toward such a goal in 46,XY DSD patients.

'Exome sequencing' is a high-throughput DNA sequencing approach that covers the coding exons of ~95% of known genes. Such 'research' tools used to require confirmation of detected mutations using more robust targeted sequencing methods, however recent progress has brought this nearer to become a routine test for the underlying genetic cause of disorders that affect our clinic patients. Notably, the authors describe that as of May 2013, a UCLA Clinical Genomics Center analysis showed that Sanger sequencing confirmation was unnecessary for those single-nucleotide variants with a high-quality score on exome sequencing.

A huge amount of data are produced by exome sequencing. The efficient analysis approach used here considers only the DNA sequences of genes already known to be disrupted in disorders of sex determination, sex differentiation or central causes of hypogonadism. They could reach a genetic diagnosis in 35% (14 of 40 cases), based on identified deleterious mutations in *MAP3K1, WT1, STAR, LHCGR, AMHR2, NR5A1/SF1, HSD17B3, CHD7* and even in *AR* (finding a mutation that had been missed on earlier targeted deletion analysis). The authors argue that exome sequencing should become a first-tier diagnostic test, and that reaching an early genetic diagnosis can guide subsequent biochemical and imaging investigations and therefore limit potentially unnecessary testing.

Large-scale whole-genome sequencing of the Icelandic population

Gudbjartsson DF, Helgason H, Gudjonsson SA, Zink F, Oddson A, Gylfason A, Besenbacher S, Magnusson G, Halldorsson BV, Hjartarson E, Sigurdsson GT, Stacey SN, Frigge ML, Holm H, Saemundsdottir J, Helgadottir HT, Johannsdottir H, Sigfusson G, Thorgeirsson G, Sverrisson JT, Gretarsdottir S, Walters GB, Rafnar T, Thjodleifsson B, Bjornsson ES, Olafsson S, Thorarinsdottir H, Steingrimsdottir T, Gudmundsdottir TS, Theodors A, Jonasson JG, Sigurdsson A, Bjornsdottir G, Jonsson JJ, Thorarensen O, Ludvigsson P, Gudbjartsson H, Eyjolfsson GI, Sigurdardottir O, Olafsson I, Arnar DO, Magnusson OT, Kong A, Masson G, Thorsteinsdottir U, Helgason A, Sulem P, Stefansson K
deCODE Genetics/Amgen Inc., Reykjavik, Iceland
Nat Genet 2015;47:435–444

Background and Methods: The authors describe the insights gained from sequencing the whole genomes of 2,636 Icelanders to a median depth of 20x. The density and frequency spectra of sequence variants

are described in relation to their functional annotation, gene position, pathway and conservation score.
Results: The authors found 20 million SNPs and 1.5 million insertions-deletions (indels). There was an excess of homozygosity and rare protein-coding variants in Iceland. By statistically imputing variants with minor allele frequency of 0.1% of more into 104,220 individuals they found a recessive frameshift mutation in *MYL4* that causes early-onset atrial fibrillation, several mutations in *ABCB4* that increase risk of liver diseases and an intronic variant in *GNAS* associated with increased thyroid-stimulating hormone levels when maternally inherited.
Conclusions: These data provide a study resource that can be used to determine how variation in the sequence of the human genome gives rise to human diversity.

GNAS gene variants have been associated with parathyroid hormone receptor sensitivity and effector function [2], and consequently impact on child growth and development. Among many other findings, the authors here describe an intronic variant in *GNAS* associated with increased TSH levels when maternally inherited, whereas paternally inherited copies are associated with decreased TSH levels. This is a deep intronic variant that would be missed by exome-focused sequencing methods.

The authors found fewer very rare variants in a small isolated population such as Iceland than in larger outbred populations. However, the small size of the population and the founder effect also allow deleterious variants to reach higher frequencies. Rare sequence variants tend to have a more recent origin than common ones and thus can help determine how variation in the sequence of the human genome gives rise to human diversity.

Ethnic differences – race, culture or nutrition?

Ethnic and sex differences in skeletal maturation among the Birth to Twenty cohort in South Africa

Cole TJ, Rousham EK, Hawley NL, Cameron N, Norris SA, Pettifor JM
Population Policy and Practice Programme, UCL Institute of Child Health, London, UK
Arch Dis Child 2015;100:138–143

Background and Methods: To examine ethnic and sex differences in the pattern of skeletal maturity from adolescence to adulthood using a novel longitudinal analysis technique (SuperImposition by Translation And Rotation (SITAR)). 607 boys and girls of black as well as white ethnicity from the Birth to Twenty bone health study, Johannesburg, South Africa, were assessed annually from nine to 20 years of age. Bone maturity scores (Tanner-Whitehouse III radius, ulna and short bones (TW3 RUS)) assessed longitudinally from hand-wrist radiographs were used to produce individual and mean growth curves of bone maturity and analysed by the SITAR method.
Results: The longitudinal analysis showed that black boys matured later by 7.0 SE 1.6 months ($P<0.0001$) but at the same rate as white boys, whereas black girls matured at the same age but at a faster rate than white girls (by 8.7% SE 2.6%, $P=0.0007$). The mean curves for bone maturity score consistently showed a mid-pubertal double kink, contrasting with the quadratic shape of the commonly used reference centile curves for bone maturity (TW3).
Conclusions: Skeletal maturity was reached 1.9 years earlier in girls than boys, and the pattern of maturation differed between the sexes. Within girls, there were no ethnic differences in the pattern or timing of skeletal maturity. However, skeletal maturity was delayed by seven months in black boys compared with white boys. Skeletal maturation, therefore, varies differentially by sex and ethnicity. The delayed maturity of black boys, but not black girls, supports the hypothesis that boys have greater sensitivity to environmental constraints than girls.

We are often asked whether we need national/racial/ethnic-specific standards for the assessment of bone maturation. Humans come in many different sizes, shapes and colours, and different forms of their eyes, hair nose and lips. These differences are immediately apparent, and thus some people assume they must be genetic. Yet, race and ethnicity are but two descriptions of human subjects, and are mostly historical and not natural. These two descriptive terms are typically used in an automatic and uncritical manner as a proxy for unmeasured biological, socioeconomic and/or sociocultural factors. Physiological traits, the rates of morbidity and mortality from particular diseases, growth and maturation are not uniformly distributed among socially defined racial and ethnic groups. The genetic variation among humans, which is continuous, complexly structured, constantly changing and predominantly within races, cannot be fully explained by race and ethnicity. Trait variations, which are usually based on social, familial and environmental differences, are much greater within races than between races. Descriptive statistics based on self-identified racial definitions are often not biological nor appropriate for an individual's medical assessment [3]. Moreover, no standard definition of race exists in medical, epidemiological or health services research [4]. The use of the terms 'African, Chinese or Swedish-origin' to describe an individual do not capture the complexity of human history, migrations, artificial boundaries and genetic drift and is scientifically unsupported and naive. In an era of individually tailored treatment, race and ethnicity should not be used to medically define a patient.

Childhood growth influenced by history

Intergenerational influences on the growth of Maya children: the effect of living conditions experienced by mothers and maternal grandmothers during their childhood

Azcorra H, Dickinson F, Bogin B, Rodriguez L, Varela-Silva MI
Departamento de Ecologia Humana, Centro de Investigacion y de Estudios Avanzados del Instituto Politecnico Nacional (Cinvestav)-Unidad Merida, Merida, Yucatan, Mexico
Am J Hum Biol 2015;8;27(4):494-500

Background: The authors tested the hypothesis that living conditions experienced by maternal grandmothers (F1 generation) and mothers (F2 generation) during their childhood are related to height and leg length (LL: height - sitting height) of their six to eight year old children (F3 generation).
Methods: From September 2011 to June 2012 the authors obtained and calculated z-score values for height and LL for 109 triads (F1, F2, F3) who are Maya living in Merida, Yucatan, Mexico. Multiple regression models were adjusted to examine the relation of anthropometric and intergenerational socioeconomic parameters of F1 (house index and family size during childhood) and F2 (paternal job loss during childhood) with the z-score values of height and LL of F3.
Results: Children's height and LL were positively associated with maternal height and LL. This association was relatively stronger in LL. Better categories of grand-maternal house index were associated with higher values of height and LL in grandchildren. Grand-maternal family size was positively related with LL, but not with height.
Conclusions: These findings partially support the hypothesis that living conditions experienced by recent maternal ancestors (F1 and F2) during their growth period influence the growth of descendants (F3). LL appear to be more sensitive to intergenerational influences than is total height and that the transition from a traditional rural lifestyle to urban conditions results in new exposures for risk in human physical growth.

Growth trajectories of children are influenced among others by factors that trace the nutritional history of maternal ancestors, including their nutrition during prenatal stage and first years of postnatal life [5]. Most of the accumulated evidence of intergenerational influences on growth is on the prenatal stage, but several studies suggest an association between parental and offspring height. This new study partially supports the hypothesis that living conditions experienced by recent maternal ancestors during their own childhoods contribute to the growth of children of the third (F3) generation. Height and leg length of children were more associated with mothers than with grandmothers. The results suggest that the grandmothers' house type is a good indicator of environmental quality during their growing years. Interestingly, the same group has previously shown that Maya children who immigrate to the USA show much better early childhood growth as compared with those remained in Guatemala [6]. This study did not mention mechanisms, but the trans-generation effects obviously raise the question of epigenetic mechanism.

Cold exposure: a treatment for obesity?

White-to-brown metabolic conversion of human adipocytes by JAK inhibition

Moisan A, Lee YK, Zhang JD, Hudak CS, Meyer CA, Prummer M, Zoffmann S, Truong HH, Ebeling M, Kiialainen A, Gerard R, Xia F, Schinzel RT, Amrein KE, Cowan CA
Roche Pharma Research and Early Development, Roche Innovation Center Basel, Basel, Switzerland
Nat Cell Biol 2015;17:57–67

Background: The rising incidence of obesity and related disorders such as diabetes and heart disease has focused considerable attention on the discovery of new therapeutics. One promising approach has been to increase the number or activity of brown-like adipocytes in white adipose depots, as this has been shown to prevent diet-induced obesity and reduce the incidence and severity of type 2 diabetes. Thus, the conversion of fat-storing cells into metabolically active thermogenic cells has become an appealing therapeutic strategy to combat obesity.
Methods: The authors designed a screening platform to identify small molecules capable of promoting a white-to-brown metabolic conversion in human adipocytes.
Results: The authors identified two inhibitors of Janus kinase (JAK) activity with no precedent in adipose tissue biology that stably confer brown-like metabolic activity to white adipocytes. Importantly, these metabolically converted adipocytes exhibit elevated UCP1 expression and increased mitochondrial activity. They further found that repression of interferon signalling and activation of hedgehog signalling in JAK-inactivated adipocytes contributes to the metabolic conversion observed in these cells.
Conclusions: These findings highlight a previously unknown role for the JAK-STAT pathway in the control of adipocyte function and establish a platform to identify compounds for the treatment of obesity.

Previous studies have reported the emergence of UCP1-expressing cells (indicative of brown fat) in white adipose tissue when stimulated by cold exposure, beta-adrenergic stimulation or PPARgamma activation, a phenomenon referred to as 'browning'. These 'brown-like' fat cells may arise from the recruitment of specific precursor cells or the conversion from white fat cells, or both. A clinical trial demonstrated that cold acclimatisation caused de novo generation of brown adipocytes, combined with increased non-shivering thermogenesis and decreased body fat mass [7]. Here, the authors confirm that repeated intermittent cold exposures in both men and women recruited brown adipocyte tissue and that this was accompanied by an increase in non-shivering thermogenesis. In addition, the subjective experience of cold shifted to a more comfortable experience. Thus, identifying inducers of browning in humans may ameliorate obesity-related diseases. Furthermore, the authors established a screening platform to discover small molecules capable of promoting white-to-brown metabolic conversion in human adipocytes and identified JAK inhibitors as molecules with browning potential. They also show that human pluripotent stem cell-derived adipocytes provide a scalable, robust and reliable cell model for adipocyte browning studies, compound screening and drug discovery. A variable indoor environment with frequent cold exposures might be an acceptable, economic and environmentally friendly way to increase energy expenditure and lose weight.

Or a pill?

Berberine activates thermogenesis in white and brown adipose tissue

Zhang Z, Zhang H, Li B, Meng X, Wang J, Zhang Y, Yao S, Ma Q, Jin L, Yang J, Wang W, Ning G
Shanghai Institute of Endocrine and Metabolic Diseases, Shanghai Clinical Center for Endocrine and Metabolic Diseases, State Key Laboratory of Medical Genomics, Ruijin Hospital, Shanghai Jiaotong University School of Medicine, Shanghai, China
Nat Commun 2014;5:5493

Background: Obesity develops when energy intake exceeds energy expenditure. Promoting brown adipose tissue formation and function increases energy expenditure and hence may counteract obesity.

Methods: The authors tested the effects of administration of berberine (BBR), a compound derived from the Chinese medicinal plant Coptis chinensis, in obese db/db mice.
Results: BBR increased energy expenditure, limited weight gain, improved cold tolerance and enhanced brown adipose tissue (BAT) activity. BBR markedly induced brown-like adipocytes in inguinal, but not epididymal adipose depots. BBR also increased expression of *UCP1* and other thermogenic genes in white and BAT and primary adipocytes via a mechanism involving AMPK and PGC-1alpha. BBR treatment also inhibited AMPK activity in the hypothalamus, but genetic activation of AMPK in the ventromedial nucleus of the hypothalamus did not prevent BBR-induced weight loss and activation of the thermogenic programme.
Conclusions: These findings establish a role for BBR in regulating organismal energy balance, which may have potential therapeutic implications for the treatment of obesity.

In addition to rodents and newborn humans, adult humans have functional brown adipose tissue (BAT), which is composed of single chambered lipid droplets and large numbers of mitochondria that contain uncoupling protein-1 (UPC1). This discovery has fuelled speculation that the pharmacologic enhancement of BAT development and activity could be a useful strategy for treating obesity. Berberine (BBR), a compound derived from Coptis chinesis, is a species of goldthread native to China. Will this Chinese herbal medicine that has traditionally been used as an anti-diarrhoea agent develop into a new therapy for obesity? Obese db/db mice that were given BBR exhibited increased energy expenditure, limited weight gain, improved tolerance to cold and enhanced brown adipose tissue activity in inguinal, but not epididymal, adipose deposits. When normalised to their lean mass, BBR mice showed higher oxygen consumption and carbon dioxide production rates through a 12-hour light/dark cycle compared with wild type animals. db/db mice treated with BBR showed significant increases in the whole-body energy expenditure. Other tests showed that BBR also ameliorated glucose tolerance. The combination of CT and PET images showed that the PET signal was more highly detected in the interscapular position of the BBR-treated mice and that BBR had a greater capacity to increase the activity of BAT in drug-treated mice. The number of mitochondria was increased as observed by means of transmission electronic microscopy after BBR treatment. The molecular target and mechanism of BBR is the transcription of UCP1 in brown and white adipocytes through AMPK activation and PGC-1-alpha recruitment. BBR may indeed be a new potential drug for treating patients with obesity.

It's in our bones

Bone marrow adipose tissue is an endocrine organ that contributes to increased circulating adiponectin during caloric restriction

Cawthorn WP, Scheller EL, Learman BS, Parlee SD, Simon BR, Mori H, Ning X, Bree AJ, Schell B, Broome DT, Soliman SS, DelProposto JL, Lumeng CN, Mitra A, Pandit SV, Gallagher KA, Miller JD, Krishnan V, Hui SK, Bredella MA, Fazeli PK, Klibanski A, Horowitz MC, Rosen CJ, MacDougald OA
Department of Molecular & Integrative Physiology, University of Michigan Medical School, Ann Arbor, MI, USA
macdouga@umich.edu
Cell Metab 2014;20:368–375

Background: The adipocyte-derived hormone adiponectin promotes metabolic and cardiovascular health. Circulating adiponectin increases in lean states such as caloric restriction (CR), but the reasons for this paradox remain unclear. Unlike white adipose tissue (WAT), bone marrow adipose tissue (MAT) increases during CR, and both MAT and serum adiponectin increase in many other clinical conditions.
Methods: The authors investigated whether MAT contributes to circulating adiponectin by using both mouse and human studies.
Results: We find that adiponectin secretion is greater from MAT than WAT. Notably, specific inhibition of MAT formation in mice results in decreased circulating adiponectin during CR despite unaltered adiponectin expression in WAT. Inhibiting MAT formation also alters skeletal muscle adaptation to CR, suggesting that MAT exerts systemic effects. Finally, we find that both MAT and serum adiponectin increase during cancer therapy in humans.

Conclusions: These observations identify MAT as an endocrine organ that contributes significantly to increased serum adiponectin during CR and perhaps in other adverse states.

We may know of bone marrow adipose tissue from its flavour when added to soup and as a delicacy for dogs, but now we learn that it is an endocrine organ making and secreting adiponectin and influence adaptive functions outside of the bone tissue, at least during calorie restriction. In fact, it seems to be a significant source of the 'good guy' adiponectin, which helps to maintain insulin sensitivity, break down fat and has been linked to lower risks of cardiovascular disease, diabetes and obesity-associated cancers. Previous work on bone marrow adipose tissue, which increases as body weight falls, has documented its relationship to reduced bone mass and increased risks of fractures and osteoporosis. Here, the authors show that both bone marrow adipose tissue and adiponectin were increased in anorexia and in patients undergoing chemotherapy or radiation treatment for cancer. Here is a new player in energy balance worth exploring - the bone marrow adipose tissue.

The importance of adrenarche

Childhood environment influences adrenarcheal timing among first-generation Bangladeshi migrant girls to the UK

Houghton LC, Cooper GD, Booth M, Chowdhury OA, Troisi R, Ziegler RG, Katki HA, Hoover RN, Bentley GR
Division of Cancer Epidemiology and Genetics, National Cancer Institute, National Institutes of Health, Bethesda, MA, USA
PLoS One 2014;9:e109200

Background: Adrenarche is a key early life event that marks middle childhood at around seven years of age. Earlier work with British-Bangladeshi migrant women suggested that environmental conditions experienced before adrenarche influence adult reproductive function. The authors therefore investigated whether Bangladeshi children who migrate to the UK reach adrenarche earlier than non-migrants in Bangladesh or the UK.
Methods: Healthy girls, aged five to 16 years, were recruited from schools in Sylhet, Bangladesh and London, England comprising four groups: Sylhetis (n=165), first-generation migrants to the United Kingdom (n=42), second-generation girls (n=162) and British girls of European origin (n=50). Anthropometric measurements were collected together with questionnaire data for migration and socioeconomic characteristics. Saliva samples were assayed for dehydroepiandrosterone (DHEAS) using enzyme-linked immunosorbent assays. Multiple linear regressions tested for group differences in anthropometric and socioeconomic variables and DHEAS levels. Median ages at adrenarche (DHEAS>400pg/ml) were estimated using Weibull regression models for parametric survival analysis. Hazard ratios for reaching adrenarche earlier and 95% confidence intervals (CI), both unadjusted and adjusted for anthropometric variables, were estimated from the survival analyses.
Results: First-generation migrants had a median age at adrenarche (5.3 years) that was earlier than Sylheti (7.2), second-generation (7.4) and European (7.1) girls. In univariate analyses, first-generation girls reached adrenarche earlier than Sylhetis [HR (CI): 2.8 (1.4–5.5)]. In multivariate models, first generation girls still reached adrenarche earlier than Sylhetis after adjusting for height [HR(CI): 1.9 (0.9–4.1)] and weight [HR(CI):1.7 (0.8–3.8)], but these results were attenuated.
Conclusions: The authors suggest that rapid catch-up growth experienced by first-generation girls during early childhood may explain their advanced adrenarche. The environmental conditions leading to an earlier adrenarche, as well as the health implications of this early transition, merit further exploration.

Plasticity in developmental programming has evolved in order to provide the best chances of survival and reproductive success under changing environments. Environmental conditions that are experienced in early life can profoundly influence human biology and long-term health. Developmental origins of health and disease and life-history transitions are purported to use placental, nutritional and endocrine cues for setting long-term biological, mental and behavioural strategies in response to local ecological and/or social conditions [8]. The window of developmental plasticity extends from preconception to early childhood and involves epigenetic responses to environmental changes, which exert their effects during life-history phase transitions. Houghton et al show here that environmental conditions experienced by British-Bangladeshi migrants before adrenarche influence adult reproductive function and that rapid catch-up growth experienced by first-generation girls during early childhood may explain their advanced adrenarche. The adrenarcheal transition is a key early life event that defines the transition from childhood to juvenility [9]. Such life-history transitions are the times when the child adaptively responds to environmental cues in order to enhance growth, body composition, lifespan, fecundity schedules and behavioural strategies that yield the highest fitness in a given environment [10]. Here, we learn that childhood environment prior to adrenarche might represent a key period influencing adult reproductive function that adrenarche itself might represent a critical childhood threshold for later life development and that rapid catch-up growth might provide the switch for this cascade of events.

Hormone changes in peripubertal girls

Biro FM, Pinney SM, Huang B, Baker ER, Walt Chandler D, Dorn LD
Cincinnati Children's Hospital Medical Center Cincinnati, OH, USA
J Clin Endocrinol Metab 2014;99:3829–3835

Background: Studies of circulating hormone concentrations in the peripubertal period report a temporal rise in adrenal hormones prior to the rise in sex steroid levels. The authors aimed to examine the relationships between changes in adrenal and sex hormones in 252 peripubertal girls.
Methods: A longitudinal observation study was conducted between 2004–2010 in school districts at the Cincinnati site of the Breast Cancer and the Environment Research Centers. Girls aged six to seven years old were recruited and assessed by female investigators every six months for height, weight and puberty status. At each visit a fasting blood sample was collected and analysed for concentrations of: androstenedione, estradiol, estrone and T by high-performance liquid chromatography (HPLC) with tandem mass spectrometry at Esoterix Laboratories (California, USA), and also for dehydroepiandrosterone-sulfate (DHEA-S) and SHBG. Changes in these concentrations were tested from 30 months prior to, and extending to six months after, breast development.
Results: A rise in DHEA-S concentrations was detectable between 30 to 18 months before breast development. Androstenedione and estrone increased between 12 to 18 months before breast development. Increases in estradiol and T, and declines in SHBG were detectable between six and 12 months before breast development. Girls with higher BMI had lower estradiol concentrations at start of breast development and also six months afterwards.
Conclusions: Sequential rises in serum DHEA-S, then estrone and then estradiol concentrations precede breast development. The lower estradiol levels observed in heavier peripubertal girls suggests breast development due to peripheral conversion of adrenal androgens to estrone.

These findings reveal interesting insights into the onset of puberty in girls. The authors used a novel hormone assay in a carefully designed study of girls with frequent clinical and biochemical evaluations during the pre- and peripubertal years. They propose the following messages.

Firstly, the findings support Ducharme's original suggestion that adrenal steroids trigger the re-initiation of the hypothalamic-pituitary-gonadal (HPG) axis [11]. This is inferred by remembering that, while T is aromatised to estradiol, androstenedione is converted to estrone (which accordingly is the most common estrogen in post-menopausal women). Pubertal onset, at least as indicated by breast development, followed around two years after the first detection of a rise in peripheral DHEA-S, followed first by a rise in estrone and only six months later by a rise in estradiol and a fall in SHBG.

Secondly, in contrast to this 'pubertal thelarche' pathway, girls with higher BMI reach thelarche with apparently less HPG axis activation. This is indicated by lower estradiol levels and the implied mechanism is greater local aromatisation of adrenal androgens at the target tissues. The authors suggest that this may explain why secular changes towards younger age at thelarche have been observed without similar secular changes in estradiol concentrations and with weaker trends in age at menarche [12].

The gradual rises in estrone and estradiol concentrations starting 18 to 12 months before breast development challenge our clinical paradigm of an abrupt onset of puberty coincident with the start of pulsatile GnRH secretion by the hypothalamus. Future clinical validation and use of such ultra-sensitive hormone assays may lead to greater appreciation of a continuum in pubertal onset and allow us to better understand the environmental factors that are promoting pubertal development at increasingly younger ages.

All-conquering metformin

Metformin as adjunct antituberculosis therapy

Singhal A, Jie L, Kumar P, Hong GS, Leow MK, Paleja B, Tsenova L, Kurepina N, Chen J, Zolezzi F, Kreiswirth B, Poidinger M, Chee C, Kaplan G, Wang YT, De Libero G
Singapore Immunology Network, Agency for Science, Technology and Research (A*STAR), Singapore
amit_singhal@immunol.a-star.edu.sg
Sci Transl Med 2014;6:263ra159

Background: The global burden of tuberculosis (TB) morbidity and mortality remains immense. A potential new approach to TB therapy is to augment protective host immune responses.
Methods: The authors tested the effects of the antidiabetic drug metformin (MET) to reduce the intracellular growth of *Mycobacterium tuberculosis* (Mtb) in an AMPK (adenosine monophosphate-activated protein kinase)-dependent manner.
Results: MET controlled the growth of drug-resistant Mtb strains, increased production of mitochondrial reactive oxygen species and facilitated phagosome-lysosome fusion. In Mtb-infected mice, use of MET ameliorated lung pathology, reduced chronic inflammation and enhanced the specific immune response and the efficacy of conventional TB drugs. Moreover, in two separate human cohorts, MET treatment was associated with improved control of Mtb infection and decreased disease severity.
Conclusions: Collectively, these data indicate that MET is a promising candidate host-adjunctive therapy for improving the effective treatment of TB.

Your Yearbook editors are unashamedly fans of metformin as current and potential future therapies in a handful of paediatric endocrine disorders, beyond its single licensed indication type 2 diabetes. Yet we are regularly surprised by its increasingly wide range of potential benefits. Here, the authors aimed to identify 'host-targeted' adjunct therapies that may augment the effects of antibiotics regimens. Autophagy is a mechanism used by the host to eliminate intracellular pathogens; it is activated by mammalian target of rapamycin (mTOR) complex 1, which is an adenosine monophosphate-activated protein kinase (AMPK). They therefore screened various known US FDA-approved AMPK modulators for their ability to control intracellular mycobacterial growth. Remarkably, they discovered that the AMPK-activating antidiabetic drug metformin inhibits the intracellular growth of *Mycobacterium tuberculosis* and enhances the efficacy of conventional anti-TB drugs.

Where next for metformin beyond diabetes, obesity, cardiovascular disease, reproductive disorders and cancer? In the US, the Targeting/Taming Ageing With Metformin (TAME) study aims to test the effectiveness of metformin in the elderly to delay the onset of multi-morbidities including cancer, CVD, T2DM, cognitive decline and mortality.

Human oocytes reprogram adult somatic nuclei of a type 1 diabetic to diploid pluripotent stem cells

Yamada M, Johannesson B, Sagi I, Burnett LC, Kort DH, Prosser RW, Paull D, Nestor MW, Freeby M, Greenberg E, Goland RS, Leibel RL, Solomon SL, Benvenisty N, Sauer MV, Egli D
The New York Stem Cell Foundation Research Institute, New York, NY, USA
Nature 2014;510:533–536

Background: The transfer of somatic cell nuclei into oocytes can give rise to pluripotent stem cells that are consistently equivalent to embryonic stem cells, holding promise for autologous cell replacement therapy. Although methods to induce pluripotent stem cells from somatic cells by transcription factors are widely used in basic research, numerous differences between induced pluripotent stem cells and embryonic stem cells have been reported, potentially affecting their clinical use.
Methods: Because of the therapeutic potential of diploid embryonic stem-cell lines derived from adult cells of diseased human subjects, the authors systematically investigated the parameters affecting efficiency of blastocyst development and stem-cell derivation.
Results: Improvements to the oocyte activation protocol, including the use of both kinase and translation inhibitors, and cell culture in the presence of histone deacetylase inhibitors, promoted development to the blastocyst stage. Developmental efficiency varied between oocyte donors, and was inversely related to the number of days of hormonal stimulation required for oocyte maturation, whereas the daily dose of gonadotropin or the total number of metaphase II oocytes retrieved did not affect developmental outcome. Because the use of concentrated Sendai virus for cell fusion induced an increase in intracellular calcium concentration, causing premature oocyte activation, diluted Sendai virus was used in calcium-free medium.
Conclusions: Use of this modified nuclear transfer protocol allowed diploid pluripotent stem-cell lines to be derived from somatic cells of a newborn and, for the first time, an adult, a female with type 1 diabetes.

Replacement of insulin-producing cells holds promise as a future 'cure' for type 1 diabetes. Organ donation has long been explored, however in 2013 only around 250 patients in USA received a pancreas transplant, largely due to limited availability of deceased organ donors. A number of sources are being explored to generate renewable insulin-producing cells. Human embryonic stem cells can be differentiated into insulin-expressing cells with ~25% conversion efficiency, however the resulting cells are not yet responsive to glucose stimulation. De-differentiation of adult cells to 'induced pluripotent stem cells' (iPSCs) represents an alternative approach, and using samples from patients with genetic disease also allows generation of disease-specific stem cells for detailed study of the molecular pathogenesis of those conditions; however, the transformation process can disrupt the genetic and epigenetic integrity of the iPSCs.

Here, the authors describe a third approach, to transfer the nuclear material from a differentiated somatic cell into an enucleated oocyte. In theory, this follows a more natural developmental pathway, and potentially even allows the generation of a whole organism from the nucleus of single differentiated somatic cell! The authors report successful production of cells that were able to secrete insulin upon potassium stimulation. While still far from the clinic, the hurdles are steadily being overcome.

Clinical implications of basic research

Cell-free fetal DNA – a trigger for parturition

Phillippe M
Vincent Center for Reproductive Biology, Department of Obstetrics and Gynecology, Massachusetts General Hospital, Boston, MA, USA
N Engl J Med 2014;370:2534–2536

Short fragments (~200 base-pairs long) of fetal DNA, derived from placental trophoblasts, can be detected in maternal plasma from very early gestation. This discovery is promising to revolutionise non-invasive prenatal testing, with particularly highly promising results for screening for Down syndrome and other fetal aneuploidy status, and also prediction of X-linked disorders and Rhesus or ABO incompatibility. Commercial providers even offer a paternity test from nine weeks of gestation.

Here, Mark Phillippe presents the hypothesis that cell-free DNA is not simply an accidental by-product of the close maternal-fetal interface, but rather the steady rise in the amount of circulating fetal DNA in the mother might have a functional role in triggering an inflammatory process that leads to the onset of labour. The potential implications for prediction and prevention of pre-term deliveries are enormous.

Coping without SHBG

Sex hormone binding globulin deficiency due to a homozygous missense mutation

Vos MJ, Mijnhout GS, Rondeel JM, Baron W, Groeneveld PH
Departments of Clinical Chemistry and Internal Medicine, Isala Hospital, 8025 AB Zwolle, The Netherlands
J Clin Endocrinol Metab 2014;99:E1798–E1802

Background: SHBG is known as the major sex steroid binding protein in plasma, and it regulates the bioavailability of both T and estradiol levels required for effects on target tissues. The authors identified a man with an undetectable SHBG concentration in combination with low total T. He presented with a seven-year history of muscle weakness, fatigue and a low libido.
Methods: To determine the cause of the SHBG deficiency, the authors used both genetic analysis of the SHBG gene and transgene SHBG expression.
Results: Genetic analysis identified a novel homozygous missense mutation that was predicted to be deleterious for protein function. Transgene expression showed that the mutation resulted in a block in SHBG secretion accompanied by increased expression of the endoplasmic reticulum molecular chaperone HSPA5. The mutation results in accumulation of the mutant SHBG within the cell and failure to secrete the mutant protein. Screening of family members identified one sister who was also deficient for SHBG.
Conclusions: This report describes a family with a missense mutation within the SHBG gene, which results in a complete deficiency of plasma SHBG in the homozygous state. Although total T level was low in the male patient, it did not interfere with normal gonadal development and spermatogenesis, suggesting a limited role of SHBG in sexual maturation and male physiology.

Sex hormone binding globulin (SHBG) functions as both a sex hormone transport protein and a regulator of sex hormone bioavailability. Numerous robust epidemiological associations have been described between circulating SHBG concentrations and various sex hormone sensitive conditions, but also with obesity, dyslipidaemia, cardiovascular disease and type 2 diabetes. The difficulty in establishing whether such associations are causal is that SHBG concentrations are strongly influenced by sex hormone and insulin concentrations, hence SHBG may simply be a passive marker of those other mechanisms. Genetic studies of common variants can be used to model the likely causal effects of targeted biological traits on common diseases and other outcomes, for example between SHBG and type 2 diabetes [13]. In the same way, detailed characterisation of rare cases with severe deleterious mutations is a powerful approach to shed light on the functional roles of SHBG.

Here, the authors describe the first report of a mutation resulting in the complete absence of plasma SHBG. The clinical features were surprisingly mild. The 27-year-old man had low total testosterone, but normal free testosterone concentrations. He had normal adult secondary sexual characteristics, but reported low libido, decreased spontaneous morning erections, fatigue, muscular weakness and decreased shaving frequency (once every four days). His affected sister reported a normal, although irregular, menstrual cycle and no signs of hirsutism or hyperandrogenism. The authors suggest that 'passive diffusion' of sex hormones into cells might make SHBG redundant, except when large amounts of sex hormone is needed, as in the adult male.

New treatment – for DIDMOAD

A calcium-dependent protease as a potential therapeutic target for Wolfram syndrome

Lu S, Kanekura K, Hara T, Mahadevan J, Spears LD, Oslowski CM, Martinez R, Yamazaki-Inoue M, Toyoda M, Neilson A, Blanner P, Brown CM, Semenkovich CF, Marshall BA, Hershey T, Umezawa A, Greer PA, Urano F
Department of Medicine, Division of Endocrinology, Metabolism, and Lipid Research, Washington University School of Medicine, St Louis, MO, USA
urano@dom.wustl.edu
Proc Natl Acad Sci U S A 2014;111:E5292–E5301

Background: Wolfram syndrome is a genetic disorder characterised by diabetes and neurodegeneration and considered as an endoplasmic reticulum (ER) disease. Despite the underlying importance of ER dysfunction in Wolfram syndrome and the identification of two causative genes, Wolfram syndrome 1 (*WFS1*) and Wolfram syndrome 2 (*WFS2*), a molecular mechanism linking the ER to death of neurons and beta-cells has not been elucidated.
Results: The authors implicate calpain 2 in the mechanism of cell death in Wolfram syndrome. Calpain 2 is negatively regulated by WFS2, and elevated activation of calpain 2 by WFS2-knockdown correlates with cell death. Calpain activation is also induced by high cytosolic calcium mediated by the loss of function of WFS1. Calpain hyperactivation is observed in the *Wfs1* knockout mouse as well as in neural progenitor cells derived from induced pluripotent stem (iPS) cells of Wolfram syndrome patients. A small-scale small-molecule screen targeting ER calcium homeostasis reveals that dantrolene can prevent cell death in neural progenitor cells derived from Wolfram syndrome iPS cells.
Conclusions: These findings demonstrate that calpain and the pathway leading to its activation provides potential therapeutic targets for Wolfram syndrome and other ER diseases.

Wolfram syndrome is a rare autosomal-recessive disease characterised by diabetes insipidus, juvenile-onset diabetes mellitus, optic atrophy and deafness (or DIDMOAD). Additional features include renal abnormalities, ataxia and mental retardation. Disruption of the underlying genes *WFS1* and *WFS2* leads to endoplasmic reticulum (ER) dysfunction and pancreatic beta-cell death. Furthermore, common variants in *WFS1* are robustly associated with susceptibility to type 2 diabetes. Therefore characterisation of the underlying molecular mechanisms may provide important information, not only for the treatment of this rare disorder, but also for the pathogenesis and future prevention and treatment of diabetes.

Calpains are calcium-dependent proteases, which regulate diverse biological functions including cell death. The authors chose to study calpain 2 because it was known to play a role in ER stress-induced apoptosis and beta-cell death. As well as clearly demonstrating its relevance to Wolfram syndrome, they searched for potential therapeutic targets by screening for chemical compounds that could prevent cell death by maintaining calcium homeostasis. In addition to GLP-1, pioglitazone and rapamycin, they found that dantrolene, a muscle relaxant drug, can prevent ER stress-mediated cell death in human and rodent cells, and in mouse models of Wolfram syndrome, and opens new potential treatment strategies in both type 1 and type 2 diabetes.

Prove untested 'established' treatments

A randomised, controlled trial of oral propranolol in infantile haemangioma

Leaute-Labreze C, Hoeger P, Mazereeuw-Hautier J, Guibaud L, Baselga E, Posiunas G, Phillips RJ. Caceres H, Lopez Gutierrez JC, Ballona R, Friedlander SF, Powell J, Perek D, Metz B, Barbarot S, Maruani A, Szalai ZZ, Krol A, Boccara O, Foelster-Holst R, Febrer Bosch MI, Su J, Buckova H, Torrelo A, Cambazard F, Grantzow R, Wargon O, Wyrzykowski D, Roessler J, Bernabeu-Wittel J, Valencia AM, Przewratil P, Glick S, Pope E, Birchall N, Benjamin L, Mancini AJ, Vabres P, Souteyrand P, Frieden IJ, Berul CI, Mehta CR, Prey S, Boralevi F, Morgan CC, Heritier S, Delarue A, Voisard JJ
Unité de Dermatologie Pédiatrique, Hópital Pellegrin-Enfants, Bordeaux, France
christine.labreze@chu-bordeaux.fr
N Engl J Med 2015;372:735–746

Background: Oral propranolol has been used to treat complicated infantile haemangiomas, although data from randomised, controlled trials to inform its use are limited.
Methods: The authors performed a multicentre, randomised, double-blind, adaptive, phase 2–3 trial assessing the efficacy and safety of a paediatric-specific oral propranolol solution in infants one to five months of age with proliferating infantile haemangioma requiring systemic therapy. Infants were randomly assigned to receive placebo or one of four propranolol regimens (1 or 3mg of propranolol base per kilogram of body weight per day for three or six months). A preplanned interim analysis was conducted to identify the regimen to study for the final efficacy analysis. The primary end point was success (complete or nearly complete resolution of the target haemangioma) or failure of trial treatment at week 24, as assessed by independent, centralised, blinded evaluations of standardised photographs.
Results: Of 460 infants who underwent randomisation, 456 received treatment. On the basis of an interim analysis of the first 188 patients who completed 24 weeks of trial treatment, the regimen of 3mg of propranolol per kilogram per day for six months was selected for the final efficacy analysis. The frequency of successful treatment was higher with this regimen than with placebo (60% versus 4%, $P<0.001$). A total of 88% of patients who received the selected propranolol regimen showed improvement by week five, versus 5% of patients who received placebo. A total of 10% of patients in whom treatment with propranolol was successful required systemic retreatment during follow-up. Known adverse events associated with propranolol (hypoglycaemia, hypotension, bradycardia and bronchospasm) occurred infrequently, with no significant difference in frequency between the placebo group and the groups receiving propranolol.
Conclusions: This trial showed that propranolol was effective at a dose of 3mg per kilogram per day for six months in the treatment of infantile haemangioma. (Funded by Pierre Fabre Dermatologie; ClinicalTrials.gov number, NCT01056341.)

We admit that the topic of this paper has little of relevance to the paediatric endocrinologist! However, we highlight it as an exemplar of good practice in clinical research. Propranolol was already widely considered to be first-line therapy for infantile haemangioma following numerous case reports, retrospective studies and two small, placebo-controlled trials. Yet there was a paucity of evidence on its efficacy, the optimal dose and duration of treatment. Another commendable feature of the trial was the two-stage adaptive design, with selection of the optimal propranolol dose and duration after an interim analysis at the end of stage 1. This selected the higher dose and longer treatment arm for continued testing in stage 2.

It is all too easy for us to use uncritically treatments (and also investigations) that are 'widely considered to be appropriate' based on case reports or historical clinical practice. Advantages of putting such 'established' treatments 'on trial' are to inform optimal dosing and duration, and also to provide quantifiable data on the risks of side effects. However, without 'equipoise' (defined as uncertainty regarding the balance of risks:benefits), there may be ethical considerations of allocating patients to not-receiving the 'established' treatment. To avoid such conflict, the authors excluded patients with life-threatening, function-threatening or severely ulcerated haemangiomas.

Undoubtedly harmful for health

Risks associated with obesity in pregnancy, for the mother and baby: a systematic review of reviews

Marchi J, Berg M, Dencker A, Olander EK, Begley C
School of Nursing and Midwifery, Trinity College Dublin, Dublin, Ireland
Obes Rev 2015;16:621–638

Background: Maternal obesity is linked with adverse outcomes for mothers and babies.
Methods: To get an overview of the risks related to obesity in pregnant women, the authors performed a systematic review of reviews. For inclusion, reviews had to compare pregnant women of healthy weight with women with obesity, and measure a health outcome for mother and/or baby. Authors conducted full-text screening, quality assurance using the AMSTAR tool and data extraction steps in pairs. A narrative analysis of the identified reviews was performed.
Results: 22 reviews were included. They show that gestational diabetes, pre-eclampsia, gestational hypertension, depression, instrumental and caesarean birth and surgical site infection are more likely to occur in pregnant women with obesity compared with women with a healthy weight. Maternal obesity is also linked to higher risks of preterm birth, large-for-gestational-age babies, fetal defects, congenital anomalies and perinatal death. Furthermore, breastfeeding initiation rates are lower and there is greater risk of early breastfeeding cessation in women with obesity compared with healthy weight women. These adverse outcomes may result in longer duration of hospital stay, with concomitant resource implications.
Conclusions: It is crucial to reduce the burden of adverse maternal and fetal/child outcomes caused by maternal obesity. Women with obesity need support to lose weight before they conceive, and to minimise their weight gain in pregnancy.

A systematic review was once considered as the authoritative answer on the clinical question in hand. However, as expertise has (appropriately) become disseminated, the numbers of such reviews has increased exponentially. There are over 100 systematic reviews on maternal obesity published on PubMed in the last five years! Hence, the 'review of reviews' (or 'umbrella review') is becoming a more efficient search strategy to comprehensively update ourselves with the evidence.

Here, the authors summarise the overwhelming evidence on the adverse effects of maternal obesity in pregnancy on both the mother and her baby. The 22 individual reviews covered 573 non-overlapping studies with wide representation across the world. There was strong evidence for five adverse maternal outcomes (gestational diabetes, pre-eclampsia, caesarean delivery, surgical site infection, mental health) as well as for several adverse outcomes in her offspring. In addition, there is even now a robust association between maternal obesity and higher infant mortality [14,15].

Two issues come to mind. Firstly, we do not need any more evidence to convince us of the harms of maternal obesity. Instead, efforts should focus on disseminating this evidence, including educating young people and also testing new interventions to support weight management before and during pregnancy. Secondly, while in utero developmental programming is a fascinating area of science, from the public health perspective, would the goal of avoiding offspring disease in 40–60 years time further motivate an obese mother beyond the obvious immediate benefits?

References

1. Stulp G, Mills M, Pollet TV, Barrett L. Non-linear associations between stature and mate choice characteristics for American men and their spouses. Am J Hum Biol 2014;26(4):530–537.
2. Freson K, Hoylaerts MF, Jaeken J, Eyssen M, Arnout J, Vermylen J, et al. Genetic variation of the extra-large stimulatory G protein alpha-subunit leads to Gs hyperfunction in platelets and is a risk factor for bleeding. Thromb Haemost 2001;86(3):733–738.
3. Braun L, Fausto-Sterling A, Fullwiley D, Hammonds EM, Nelson A, Quivers W, et al. Racial categories in medical practice: how useful are they? PLoS Med 2007;4(9):e271.
4. Krieger N, Rowley DL, Herman AA, Avery B, Phillips MT. Racism, sexism, and social class: implications for studies of health, disease, and well-being. Am J Prev Med 1993;9(6 Suppl):82–122.
5. Kuzawa CW. Fetal origins of developmental plasticity: are fetal cues reliable predictors of future nutritional environments? Am J Hum Biol 2005;17(1):5–21.
6. Bogin B, Smith P, Orden AB, Varela Silva MI, Loucky J. Rapid change in height and body proportions of Maya American children. Am J Hum Biol 2002;14(6):753–761.
7. van der Lans AA, Hoeks J, Brans B, Vijgen GH, Visser MG, Vosselman MJ, et al. Cold acclimation recruits human brown fat and increases nonshivering thermogenesis. J Clin Invest 2013;123(8):3395–3403.
8. Hochberg Z, Feil R, Constancia M, Fraga M, Junien C, Carel JC, et al. Child health, developmental plasticity, and epigenetic programming. Endocr Rev 2011;32(2):159–224.
9. Hochberg Z. Juvenility in the context of life history theory. Arch Dis Child 2008;93(6):534–539.
10. Hochberg Z. Evo-devo of child growth II: human life history and transition between its phases. Eur J Endocrinol 2009;160(2):135–141.
11. Ducharme JR, Forest MG, De Peretti E, Sempe M, Collu R, Bertrand J. Plasma adrenal and gonadal sex steroids in human pubertal development. J Clin Endocrinol Metab 1976;42(3):468–476.
12. Aksglaede L, Sorensen K, Petersen JH, Skakkebaek NE, Juul A. Recent decline in age at breast development: the Copenhagen Puberty Study. Pediatrics 2009;123(5):e932–e939.
13. Perry JR, Weedon MN, Langenberg C, Jackson AU, Lyssenko V, Sparso T, et al. Genetic evidence that raised sex hormone binding globulin (SHBG) levels reduce the risk of type 2 diabetes. Hum Mol Genet 2010;19(3):535–544.
14. Meehan S, Beck CR, Mair-Jenkins J, Leonardi-Bee J, Puleston R. Maternal obesity and infant mortality: a meta-analysis. Pediatrics 2014;133(5):863–871.
15. Johansson S, Villamor E, Altman M, Bonamy AK, Granath F, Cnattingius S. Maternal overweight and obesity in early pregnancy and risk of infant mortality: a population based cohort study in Sweden. BMJ 2014;349:g6572.

Author Index

C

D

E

F

G

H

I

J

K

L

M

N

O

P

Q

R

S

T

U

V

W

X

Y

Z

Subject Index

A

B

C

D

E

K

L

M

N

O

U

V

W

X